Tea in Health and Disease

Tea in Health and Disease

Special Issue Editor

Q. Ping Dou

MDPI • Basel • Beijing • Wuhan • Barcelona • Belgrade

MDPI

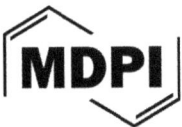

Special Issue Editor
Q. Ping Dou
Wayne State University School of Medicine
USA

Editorial Office
MDPI
St. Alban-Anlage 66
4052 Basel, Switzerland

This is a reprint of articles from the Special Issue published online in the open access journal *Nutrients* (ISSN 2072-6643) from 2018 to 2019 (available at: https://www.mdpi.com/journal/nutrients/special_issues/Tea_Health_Disease).

For citation purposes, cite each article independently as indicated on the article page online and as indicated below:

LastName, A.A.; LastName, B.B.; LastName, C.C. Article Title. *Journal Name* **Year**, *Article Number*, Page Range.

ISBN 978-3-03897-986-9 (Pbk)
ISBN 978-3-03897-987-6 (PDF)

Contents

About the Special Issue Editor

Q. Ping Dou is a professor of oncology, pharmacology, and pathology and a scientific member of the Molecular Therapeutics Program of the Barbara Ann Karmanos Cancer Institute, Wayne State University School of Medicine, Detroit, MI, USA. Dr. Dou obtained his B.S. degree in chemistry from Shandong University in 1981, his Ph.D. degree in chemistry from Rutgers University in 1988, and postdoctoral training at the Dana-Farber Cancer Institute and Harvard Medical School from 1988 to 1993. Dr. Dou has a broad background in chemistry and biochemistry, with specific training and expertise in molecular pharmacology and oncology. He has extensive experience in the fields of natural products, chemoprevention, drug discovery, proteasome inhibitors, and molecular targeting. Dr. Dou has published 245 peer-reviewed research and review articles, many of those in journals of the highest quality, and also holds numerous patents. Dr. Dou has mentored 12 Ph.D. students and many undergraduate/high school students, MD and MS students, postdoc fellows, junior faculty, physician scientists, and visiting scholars.

nutrients

MDPI

Editorial

Tea in Health and Disease

Q. Ping Dou

Barbara Ann Karmanos Cancer Institute and Departments of Oncology, Pharmacology and Pathology, School of Medicine, Wayne State University, Detroit, MI 48201-2013, USA; doup@karmanos.org; Tel.: +313-576-8301

Received: 19 April 2019; Accepted: 23 April 2019; Published: 25 April 2019

Tea, including green tea made from the leaves of the *Camellia senenisis* plant, is the second most consumed beverage worldwide after water, and is consumed by more than two-thirds of the world population [1–3]. Accumulating evidence from cellular, animal, clinical and epidemiological studies have linked tea consumption to various health benefits, such as chemoprevention of cancers, chronic inflammation, heart and liver diseases, diabetes, neurodegenerative diseases, ultraviolet B (UVB)-induced skin aging, bone fracture, etc., along with some other beneficial activities, e.g., chemo-sensitizing, antioxidizing stress-reducing, etc. [1–3]. Although some of these health benefits have not been consistently achieved by intervention trials, positive results from some clinical trials have provided direct evidence supporting the protective effect of tea against, at least, human cancer [1–5]. In addition, multiple mechanisms of action have been proposed to explain how tea exerts its disease-preventive effects.

This special issue of Nutrients, "*Tea in Health and Disease*", has collected nine (9) research articles and four (4) comprehensive review articles. All of these publications are timely, novel, and written by authors who are experts in the field of tea research.

Jang, Hwang and Choi found in their research article, that rosmarinic acid, a compound isolated from rosemary tea, modulates expression of histone deacetylase 2 and inhibits growth of prostate cancer cells via induction of the cell cycle arrest and apoptosis [6].

Heyza et al., reported, in their original study, that green tea polyphenol (–)-epigallocatechin-3-gallate (EGCG) acts as a potent inhibitor of the 5′-3′ structure-specific endonuclease ERCC1/XPF (Excision Repair Cross-Complementation Group 1/Xeroderma Pigmentosum Group F) in human cancer cells, serving as an ideal candidate for further pharmacological development with the goal of enhancing cisplatin response in human tumors [7].

Farabegoli et al., discovered that the combinational treatment of EGCG and a rexinoid, 6-OH-11-O-hydroxyphenanthrene [IIF] inhibits neuroblastoma cell growth and neurosphere formation in vitro [8]; the authors concluded that the association of EGCG to IIF might be able to overcome the incomplete success of retinoid treatments in neuroblastoma patient without toxic effects.

Zhao et al., reported that Fuzhuan brick-tea protects against UVB irradiation-induced photo-aging via MAPKs/Nrf2-mediated down-regulation of MMP-1, and suggested that this tea could be used as not only a functional food but also a good candidate in the development of cosmetic products and medicines for the remedy of UVB-induced skin photo-aging [9].

Annunziata et al., evaluated colon bioaccessibility and antioxidant activity of tea polyphenolic extract by using an in vitro simulated gastrointestinal digestion assay [10]. They found that after gastrointestinal digestion, the bioaccessibility and the antioxidant activity in the colon stage were significantly increased compared to the duodenal stage for both tea polyphenols and total phenol content. These results could be attributable in vivo to the activity of gut microbiota, which metabolize tea compounds and generate metabolites with a greater antioxidant activity [10].

Pan et al., report that polyphenols in Liubao tea prevent carbon tetrachloride-induced hepatic damage in mice through their antioxidant function [11]. Molecularly, Liubao tea modulates various enzymatic activities and reduces serum levels of several cytokines in mice with liver injury.

Shen et al., examined the association between tea consumption and risk of hospitalized fracture in 453,625 Chinese adults. Their study concluded that habitual tea consumption was associated with moderately decreased risk of any fracture hospitalizations, and the participants with decades of tea consumption and those who preferred green tea were also associated with lower risk of hip fracture [12].

Unno et al., determined the stress-reducing function of matcha green tea (that contain high levels of theanine, a major amino acid) in both animal experiments and clinical trials [13]. They found that high contents of theanine and arginine in matcha exhibited a high stress-reducing effect in mice, and that anxiety, a reaction to stress, was significantly lower in the matcha tea-consuming participants than in the placebo group.

Rode et al., determined, in a cross-sectional observational study among a population of 273 hypercalciuric stone-formers, whether daily green tea drinkers experienced increased stone risk factors (especially for oxalate) compared to non-drinkers, and found no evidence for increased stone risk factors or oxalate-dependent stones in daily green tea drinkers [14].

Furthermore, Khan and Mukhtar extensively reviewed the health-promoting effects of tea polyphenols [15], by summarizing recent studies on the role of tea polyphenols in the prevention of cancer, diabetes, cardiovascular and neurological diseases. Negri et al., presented another comprehensive updated summary on molecular targets of green tea polyphenol EGCG with a special focus on the involved signal transduction pathways in human cancer [16].

In another review article, Gan et al., summarized the distribution, composition, and health benefits of several caffeinated beverages from the genus *Ilex*, including the large-leaved Kudingcha (*Ilex latifolia* Thunb and *Ilex kudingcha* C.J. Tseng), Yerba Mate (*Ilex paraguariensis* A. St.-Hil), Yaupon Holly (*Ilex vomitoria*), and Guayusa (*Ilex guayusa* Loes), and suggested their potential applications in the pharmaceutical or nutraceutical industries [17].

Tea consumption is also considered a natural complementary therapy for neurodegenerative diseases such as Alzheimer's disease that affects an increasing patient population among the elderly. Polito et al., reviewed epidemiological studies on the association between tea consumption and the reduced risk of Alzheimer's disease, along with the anti-amyloid effects and the role of tea in preventing this neurodegenerative disease [18].

While beneficial effects by tea consumption have been documented in various human disease models as mentioned above, there are major challenges in developing some tea components (such as green tea polyphenols) as therapeutic agents, including how to improve their bioavailabilities, stability, efficacies, and specificity [5]. Further well-designed preclinical and clinical studies are warranted in the future.

I would like to thank all the authors for their exceptional contributions.

Conflicts of Interest: The author declares no conflict of interest.

References

1. Yang, C.S.; Wang, X.; Lu, G.; Picinich, S.C. Cancer prevention by tea: Animal studies, molecular mechanisms and human relevance. *Nat. Rev. Cancer* **2009**, *9*, 429–439. [CrossRef]
2. Mukhtar, H.; Ahmad, N. Tea polyphenols: Prevention of cancer and optimizing health. *Am. J. Clin. Nutr.* **2000**, *71*. [CrossRef]
3. Chen, D.; Dou, Q.P. Tea polyphenols and their roles in cancer prevention and chemotherapy. *Int. J. Mol. Sci.* **2008**, *9*, 1196–1206. [CrossRef] [PubMed]
4. Bettuzzi, S.; Brausi, M.; Rizzi, F.; Castagnetti, G.; Peracchia, G.; Corti, A. Chemoprevention of human prostate cancer by oral administration of green tea catechins in volunteers with high-grade prostate intraepithelial neoplasia: A preliminary report from a one-year proof-of-principle study. *Cancer Res.* **2006**, *66*, 1234–1240. [CrossRef] [PubMed]

5. Li, F.; Wang, Y.; Li, D.; Chen, Y.; Qiao, X.; Fardous, R.; Lewandowski, A.; Liu, J.; Chan, T.H.; Dou, Q.P. Perspectives on the recent developments with green tea polyphenols in drug discovery. *Expert Opin. Drug Discov.* **2018**, *13*, 643–660. [CrossRef] [PubMed]

6. Jang, Y.G.; Hwang, K.A.; Choi, K.C. Rosmarinic Acid, a Component of Rosemary Tea, Induced the Cell Cycle Arrest and Apoptosis through Modulation of HDAC2 Expression in Prostate Cancer Cell Lines. *Nutrients* **2018**, *10*, 1784. [CrossRef] [PubMed]

7. Heyza, J.R.; Arora, S.; Zhang, H.; Conner, K.L.; Lei, W.; Floyd, A.M.; Deshmukh, R.R.; Sarver, J.; Trabbic, C.J.; Erhardt, P. Targeting the DNA Repair Endonuclease ERCC1-XPF with Green Tea Polyphenol Epigallocatechin-3-Gallate (EGCG) and Its Prodrug to Enhance Cisplatin Efficacy in Human Cancer Cells. *Nutrients* **2018**, *10*, 1644. [CrossRef] [PubMed]

8. Farabegoli, F.; Govoni, M.; Spisni, E.; Papi, A. Epigallocatechin-3-gallate and 6-OH-11-O-Hydroxyphenanthrene Limit BE(2)-C Neuroblastoma Cell Growth and Neurosphere Formation In Vitro. *Nutrients* **2018**, *10*, 1141. [CrossRef] [PubMed]

9. Zhao, P.; Alam, M.B.; Lee, S.H. Protection of UVB-Induced Photoaging by Fuzhuan-Brick Tea Aqueous Extract via MAPKs/Nrf2-Mediated Down-Regulation of MMP-1. *Nutrients* **2018**, *11*, 60. [CrossRef] [PubMed]

10. Annunziata, G.; Maisto, M.; Schisano, C.; Ciampaglia, R.; Daliu, P.; Narciso, V.; Tenore, G.C.; Novellino, E. Colon Bioaccessibility and Antioxidant Activity of White, Green and Black Tea Polyphenols Extract after In Vitro Simulated Gastrointestinal Digestion. *Nutrients* **2018**, *10*, 1711. [CrossRef] [PubMed]

11. Pan, Y.; Long, X.; Yi, R.; Zhao, X. Polyphenols in Liubao Tea Can Prevent CCl4-Induced Hepatic Damage in Mice through Its Antioxidant Capacities. *Nutrients* **2018**, *10*, 1280. [CrossRef] [PubMed]

12. Shen, Q.; Yu, C.; Guo, Y.; Bian, Z.; Zhu, N.; Yang, L.; Chen, Y.; Luo, G.; Li, J.; Qin, Y. China Kadoorie Biobank Collaborative Group. Habitual Tea Consumption and Risk of Fracture in 0.5 Million Chinese Adults: A Prospective Cohort Study. *Nutrients* **2018**, *10*, 1633. [CrossRef] [PubMed]

13. Unno, K.; Furushima, D.; Hamamoto, S.; Iguchi, K.; Yamada, H.; Morita, A.; Horie, H.; Nakamura, Y. Stress-Reducing Function of Matcha Green Tea in Animal Experiments and Clinical Trials. *Nutrients* **2018**, *10*, 1468. [CrossRef] [PubMed]

14. Rode, J.; Bazin, D.; Dessombz, A.; Benzerara, Y.; Letavernier, E.; Tabibzadeh, N.; Hoznek, A.; Tligui, M.; Traxer, O.; Daudon, M. Daily Green Tea Infusions in Hypercalciuric Renal Stone Patients: No Evidence for Increased Stone Risk Factors or Oxalate-Dependent Stones. *Nutrients* **2019**, *11*, 256. [CrossRef] [PubMed]

15. Khan, N.; Mukhtar, H. Tea Polyphenols in Promotion of Human Health. *Nutrients* **2018**, *11*, 39. [CrossRef]

16. Negri, A.; Naponelli, V.; Rizzi, F.; Bettuzzi, S. Molecular Targets of Epigallocatechin—Gallate (EGCG): A Special Focus on Signal Transduction and Cancer. *Nutrients* **2018**, *10*, 1936. [CrossRef]

17. Gan, R.Y.; Zhang, D.; Wang, M.; Corke, H. Health Benefits of Bioactive Compounds from the Genus Ilex, a Source of Traditional Caffeinated Beverages. *Nutrients* **2018**, *10*, 1682. [CrossRef] [PubMed]

18. Polito, C.A.; Cai, Z.Y.; Shi, Y.L.; Li, X.M.; Yang, R.; Shi, M.; Li, Q.S.; Ma, S.C.; Xiang, L.P.; Wang, K.R. Association of Tea Consumption with Risk of Alzheimer's Disease and Anti-Beta-Amyloid Effects of Tea. *Nutrients* **2018**, *10*, 655. [CrossRef] [PubMed]

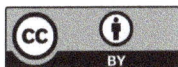

nutrients

MDPI

Review

Association of Tea Consumption with Risk of Alzheimer's Disease and Anti-Beta-Amyloid Effects of Tea

Curt Anthony Polito [1], Zhuo-Yu Cai [1], Yun-Long Shi [1], Xu-Min Li [1], Rui Yang [1], Meng Shi [1], Qing-Sheng Li [1], Shi-Cheng Ma [2], Li-Ping Xiang [3], Kai-Rong Wang [4], Jian-Hui Ye [1], Jian-Liang Lu [1], Xin-Qiang Zheng [1] and Yue-Rong Liang [1],*

[1]   Tea Research Institute, Zhejiang University, Hangzhou 310058, China; curtpolito@outlook.com (C.A.P.);
      21716160@zju.edu.cn (Z.-Y.C.); 11516051@zju.edu.cn (Y.-L.S.); 21616096@zju.edu.cn (X.-M.L.);
      21616106@zju.edu.cn (R.Y.); 11616052@zju.edu.cn (M.S.); qsli@zju.edu.cn (Q.-S.L.);
      jianhuiye@zju.edu.cn (J.-H.Y.); jllu@zju.edu.cn (J.-L.L.); xqzheng@zju.edu.cn (X.-Q.Z.)
[2]   Liupao Tea Academy, Wuzhou 543003, Guangxi, China; zjumasc@aliyun.com
[3]   National Tea and Tea product Quality Supervision and Inspection Center (Guizhou), Zunyi 563100, China;
      gzzyzj_2009@vip.sina.com
[4]   Ningbo Extension Station of Forestry & Specialty Technology, Ningbo 315012, China;
      wkrtea321hjytea@163.com
*   Correspondence: yrliang@zju.edu.cn; Tel.: +86-571-8898-2704

Received: 4 April 2018; Accepted: 21 May 2018; Published: 22 May 2018

Abstract: Neurodegenerative disease Alzheimer's disease (AD) is attracting growing concern because of an increasing patient population among the elderly. Tea consumption is considered a natural complementary therapy for neurodegenerative diseases. In this paper, epidemiological studies on the association between tea consumption and the reduced risk of AD are reviewed and the anti-amyloid effects of related bioactivities in tea are summarized. Future challenges regarding the role of tea in preventing AD are also discussed.

Keywords: *Camellia sinensis*; epigallocatechin gallate (EGCG); theanine; caffeine; Alzheimer's disease; Parkinson's disease

1. Introduction

Alzheimer's disease (AD) is progressive neurodegenerative disorder pathologically characterized by deposition of β-amyloid (Aβ) peptides as senile plaques in the brain and its prevalence is strongly correlated with aging [1]. AD is the second leading health concern among adults following cancer [2], being the sixth leading cause of death, and also the only disease among the top 10 that cannot be prevented, cured, or treated [3]. AD is characterized by a progressive cognitive decline, leading to dementia [4]. The increase in life expectancy due to modern society and the associated healthcare has been accompanied by an increase in the number of people with AD. It is estimated that 50% of people with aged 85 or older suffered from AD [5]. In the United States, someone develops AD every 67 seconds [3]. In China, 7.4 million elderly persons are estimated to have dementia, and this number is expected to grow to 18 million by 2030 if effective preventions are not identified and implemented [6]. Although many AD-related treatment hypotheses have been proposed, the exact causes and pathogenesis of AD are still unclear. Furthermore, along with other neurodegenerative dementias diseases, AD lacks any effective cure. For this reason, the prevention of AD and non-pharmacological treatments are important research [7].

Dietary interventions might play a role in the prevention of AD. Beverages containing plant polyphenolshave been recommended as a natural complementary therapy for alleviating the symptoms of AD [8]. Specifically, one study reported that language and verbal memory were positively associated with the intake of green tea catechins and black tea theaflavins [9]. Data from several cross-sectional studies consistently showed that tea drinking is associated with better performance on cognitive tests. Tea consumption is considered to be one simple lifestyle adjustment that may either prevent or treat the cognitive declines associated with neurodegenerative AD [10,11].

Many review articles focused on the subject of tea polyphenols and potential neuroprotective properties, in which the potential benefits of tea catechins for reducing the risk of AD by targeting the effects of oxidation, iron chelating, microglia activation, andmodulating intracellular neuronal signal transduction pathways [12–14]. The originality of the present review includes two aspects: (1) the neurodegenerative process in AD is characterized by the presence of cerebral extracellular deposition of Aβ and the published reviews rarely focused on the anti-Aβ effects of tea. The present review summarizes the advances in the anti-Aβ effects of tea with regards to its association with AD. (2) The latest review of the association of tea with AD updated the literature published until December 2016 [14]. Since then, more than 10 research papers have been published on this topic that involved epidemical surveys and mechanism studies. The most significant research advances regarding tea's potential role in the prevention and treatment of AD and other related neurodegenerative symptoms were included in the present review by searching the Web of Science database using keywords "tea" and "Alzheimer's disease" and the cited references were updated until February 2018.

2. Epidemiological Evidence

Considerable epidemiological evidence has associated tea consumption with a decreased risk of AD and other neurodegenerative diseases. The procedure for preparing a cup of tea was used to assess the action-based memory of people with AD dementia [15]. In Japan, a community-based comprehensive geriatric assessment involving 1003 Japanese residents aged 70 or older showed that a higher consumption of green tea was associated with a lower prevalence of cognitive impairment (CoI). At the cutoff cognitive function score of below 26 as evaluated by the Mini-Mental State Examination (MMSE), the odds ratios (OR) were 0.62 (95% confidence interval (95% CI): 0.33, 1.19) for four to six cups per week to one cup per day and 0.46 (95% CI: 0.30, 0.72) for two or more cups per day ($p = 0.0006$), compared to the OR = 1.00 for reference ($\leq$3 cups/week) [16]. A cohort study involving 13,988 Japanese people aged 65 or older showed that green tea consumption was significantly associated with a lower risk of incident functional disability, among which the three-year incidence of functional disability was 9.4% (1316 cases). The multiple-adjusted hazard ratio (HR) of the incidentfunctional disability was 0.90 (95% CI: 0.77, 1.06) among respondents who consumed one to two cups of green tea per day, 0.75 (95% CI: 0.64, 0.88) for those who consumed three to four, and 0.67 (95% CI: 0.57, 0.79) for those who consumed five or more cups per day, in comparison with those who consumed one or fewer cups/day ($p = 0.001$) [17]. A follow-up 4.9 $\pm$ 0.9 years' population-based prospective study with 490 Japanese residents aged 60 or older from Nakajima showed that the multiple-adjusted ORs for the incidence of overall cognitive decline (MCI) was 0.32 (95% CI: 0.16, 0.64) among individuals who consumed green tea every day and 0.47 (95% CI: 0.25, 0.86) among those who consumed green tea one to six days per week, compared with individuals who did not consume green tea at all. The multiple adjusted OR for the incidence of dementia was 0.26 (95% CI: 0.06, 1.06) among individuals who consumed green tea every day, compared with those who did not consume any green tea. No association was found between the consumption of coffee or black tea and the incidence of dementia or MCI [18]. A cross-sectional study including 1143 Japanese residents showed that low green tea consumption was independently associated with a higher prevalence of CoI ($p = 0.032$), with an OR for drinking tea daily of 0.65 (95% CI: 0.47, 0.89) [19]. However, a double-blind randomized controlled study involving 33 nursing home residents revealed that consumption of 2 grams per day of green tea powder for 12 months was not significantly associated with cognitive disfunction, compared with that of the placebo group (OR: −0.61 (95% CI: −2.97, 1.74, $p = 0.59$)) [20].

In Singapore, a cross-sectional study involving 2501 participants aged 55 or older showed that regular tea consumption was associated with a lower risk of CoI. Compared with the ORs for rare or no tea consumption, the ORs for low (<1 cup/day), medium (1–5 cups/day), and high levels (≥6 cups/day) of tea consumption were 0.56 (95% CI: 0.40, 0.78), 0.45 (95% CI: 0.27, 0.72), and 0.37 (95% CI: 0.14, 0.98), respectively ($p < 0.001$) [21]. Another cross-sectional study involving 716 adults aged 55 or older showed that the protective effect of tea consumption on cognitive function was not limited to a particular type of tea. Total tea consumption was independently associated with better performance on global cognition (regression coefficient (B) = 0.055, standard error (SE) = 0.026, $p = 0.03$), memory (B = 0.031, SE = 0.012, $p = 0.01$), executive function (B = 0.032, SE = 0.012, $p = 0.009$), and information processing speed (B = 0.04, SE = 0.014, $p = 0.001$) based on the MMSE total score. Both black and oolong tea and green tea consumption were associated with better cognitive performance. However, no association was found between coffee consumption and cognitive function [22]. A longitudinal aging study involving 1615 adults aged 55 to 93 examining the association between the amount of tea drinking and incident depressive symptoms from follow-up over an average period of 18 months showed that the proportion of participants with depression at the follow-up was 6.6% for participants with no tea consumption, 5.3% for low tea consumption participants (<1 cup/day), 3.2% for medium tea consumption participants (1–5 cups/day), and 1.8% for high tea consumption participants (≥6 cups/day). The ORs were 0.79 (95% CI: 0.42, 1.48) for low tea consumption participants, 0.47 (95% CI: 0.25, 0.88) for medium tea consumption participants, and 0.27 (95% CI: 0.11, 0.63) for high tea consumption participants ($p = 0.01$) [23]. A cohort study involving 614 adults aged 60 or older who were free of dementia and CoI showed that long-term tea consumption for at least 15 years was associated with reduced depressive and anxiety symptoms among community-living elderly persons [24].

In China, a cohort study revealed that among 681 unrelated Chinese aged 90 or older (67.25% women), men with CoI had significantly lower prevalence of tea drinking ($p = 0.041$ and 0.044, for former and current tea drinking, respectively); whereas in women, CoI was not associated with tea drinking [25]. A national population-based prospective nested case-control study involving 5691 elderly residents aged 65 or older showed an inverse association between tea drinking and cognitive decline (OR: 0.82; 95% CI: 0.69, 1.00, $p = 0.0468$) [26]. A town level population-based survey involving 4579 persons aged 60 or older from Weitang in Suzhou City showed that tea consumption was inversely associated with the prevalence of CoI (OR: 0.74, 95% CI: 0.57, 0.98, $p = 0.032$). The protective correlation of tea was more obvious in persons who never smoked (OR: 0.63) but vanished in current or former smokers (OR: 1.10) [27]. A rural population-based study involving 1368 rural community-dwelling individuals aged 60 or older (59.3% women) showed that daily tea consumption was associated with a lower likelihood of depressive symptoms in older people in rural communities. The association appeared to be independent of cerebrovascular disease and atherosclerosis. The ORs of having high depressive symptoms were 0.86 (95% CI: 0.56, 1.32) for weekly and 0.59 (95% CI: 0.43, 0.81) for daily tea consumption ($p = 0.001$) [28]. Another study involving 9375 persons aged 60–65 and 2015 persons aged 65 or older showed that tea consumption was inversely correlated with prevalence of CoI [29] and AD [30]. Data from the Chinese Longitudinal Healthy Longevity Surveys showed that drinking tea had a positive impact on cognitive function. A survey involving 32,606 individuals (13,429 men and 19,177 women) aged 65 or older showed that frequent tea consumption was significantly associated with reduced OR of CoI [31]. Another survey involving 7139 participants aged 80–115 years showed that regular tea drinking was associated with better cognitive function among the oldest of the living Chinese persons. In a linear mixed effects model that adjusted for age, gender, years of schooling, physical exercise, and activities, the regression coefficient was 0.72 ($p < 0.0001$) for daily drinking and 0.41 ($p = 0.01$) for occasional drinking. Tea drinkers had higher verbal fluency scores throughout the follow-up period but concurrently had a steeper slope of cognitive decline compared with non-drinkers [32]. A prevalence survey involving 1000 residents aged 60 or older in which the samples were collected by the multi-stage random cluster sampling method in

Huangshi City, China showed that drinking tea reduced the incidence of MCI ($p < 0.05$) [33]. However, a cross-sectional study including 870 residents aged 90 or older showed no significant correlation between tea consumption and the prevalence of MCI among this group [34].

In Norway, a cross-sectional study involving 2031 participants aged 70–74 (55% women) showed that participants who consumed chocolate, wine, or tea had significantly lower prevalence of poor cognitive performance than those who did not. Participants who consumed all three tested items had the best cognitive testing scores and the lowest risks for poor cognitive testing performance. The associations between intake of these foodstuffs and cognition were dose dependent, with an approximately linear relationship for tea consumption [35].

A large-scale population study involving participants from 23 developed countries given different genetic backgrounds found a significant inverse correlation between dietary consumption of flavonoids (also a group of polyphenols found in green tea) and disability-adjusted life year rates of AD and other related dementias [36]. A meta-analysis involving 52,503 participants from Asia, Europe, Australia, and North America showed that daily tea consumption was associated with a decreased risk of CoI, MCI, and cognitive decline in elderly persons. Tea consumption significantly reduced the risk of cognitive disorders (OR = 0.65, 95% CI: 0.58, 0.73). Tea consumption was inversely associated with the risk of CoI, MCI, cognitive decline, and other ungrouped cognitive disorders. However, another investigation also showed that the association between tea consumption and AD remained elusive [37] (Table 1).

Table 1. Epidemiological evidence for the association between tea intake and the risk of Alzheimer's disease (AD) and related cognitive decline.

Type of Study	Country	Number of Subjects	Main Results	Reference
Six-year follow up longitudinal study	U.K.	Nine community-dwelling men and women.	The action-based memory of people with dementia of AD can be judged by looking at the process of preparing a cup of tea.	Rusted et al., 2002 [12]
Cross-sectional study	Japan	1003 Japanese subjects aged 70 or older.	Consumption of ≥2 cups/day green tea was associated with a lower prevalence of CoI (OR: 0.46 (95% CI: 0.30, 0.72; p = 0.0006), compared to reference (≤3 cups/week)	Kuriyama et al., 2006 [13]
Prospective cohort study	Japan	13,988 Japanese subjects aged 65 or older.	Green tea consumption was significantly associated with a lower risk of incident functional disability, even after adjustment for possible confounding factors.	Tomata et al., 2012 [14]
Population-based prospective study	Japan	490 Japanese residents over 60 years old.	The multiple adjusted OR for the incidence of dementia was 0.26 (95% CI: 0.06, 1.06) among individuals who consumed green tea every day compared with those who did not consume green tea at all. No association was found between coffee or black tea consumption and the incidence of dementia or MCI.	Noguchi-Shinohara et al., 2014 [15]
Cross-sectional study	Japan	1143 subjects.	Low green tea consumption (p = 0.032) were independently associated with a higher prevalence of CoI. The OR for drinking tea every day was 0.65 (95% CI: 0.47, 0.89).	Kitamura et al., 2016 [16]
A double-blind, randomized controlled study	Japan	33 nursing home residents, consumed 2 g/day of green tea powder for 12 months.	Cognitive disfunction was not significantly different compared with that of the placebo group (OR: −0.61 (95% CI: −2.97, 1.74), p = 0.59).	Ide et al., 2016 [17]
Cross-sectional study	Singapore	2501 adults aged 55 or older.	Cognitive decline ORs were 0.74 (95% CI: 0.54, 1.00) for low level, 0.78 (95% CI: 0.55, 1.11) for medium level, and 0.57 (95% CI: 0.32, 1.03) for high level tea intake.	Ng et al., 2008 [18]
Cross-sectional study	Singapore	716 adults aged 55 or older.	Total tea consumption was independently associated with better performance on global cognition, memory, executive function, and information processing speed.	Feng et al., 2010 [19]

Table 1. Cont.

Type of Study	Country	Number of Subjects	Main Results	Reference
Longitudinal aging study	Singapore	1615 adults aged 55 to 93.	The ORs were 0.79 (95% CI: 0.42, 1.48) for low tea consumption participants, 0.47 (95% CI: 0.25, 0.88) for medium tea consumption participants and 0.27 (95% CI: 0.11, 0.63) for high tea consumption participants ($p = 0.01$).	Feng et al., 2012 [20]
Cohort study	Singapore	614 elderly aged 60 or older who were free of dementia and cognitive impairment.	Long-term tea consumption was associated with reduced depressive and anxiety symptoms among community-living elderly.	Chan et al., 2017 [21]
Cohort study	China	681 unrelated Chinese nonagenarians/centenarians (67.25% women).	Habits of tea drinking had a significantly positive impact on CoI in men, but no association of CoI with tea drinking in women.	Huang et al., 2009 [22]
Population-based, nest case-control study	China	5691 elderly residents aged 65 or older (1489 cognitive decline and 4822 normal cognitive function).	An inverse association between tea drinking and cognitive decline was found (OR: 0.82; 95% CI: 0.69, 1.00, $p = 0.0468$).	Chen et al., 2012 [23]
Population-based survey	China	4579 elders aged 60 or older from the town of Weitang in Suzhou, China.	An inverse association was found between tea consumption (of any type) and prevalence of CoI (OR: 0.74, 95%CI: 0.57–0.98, $p = 0.032$).	Gu et al., 2017 [24]
Population-based study	China	1368 rural community-dwelling individuals aged 60 or older (59.3% female).	Daily tea consumption was associated with a lower likelihood of depressive symptoms in older Chinese people living in a rural community. The association appears to be independent of cerebrovascular disease and atherosclerosis.	Feng et al., 2013 [25]
Cross-sectional Study	China	9375 adults aged 60 or older.	An inverse correlation was found between tea consumption and prevalence of CoI.	Shen et al., 2015 [26]
Cross-sectional study	China	2015 adults aged 65 or older (42.2% men).	Tea consumption was associated with low prevalence of AD.	Yang et al., 2016 [27]
Longitudinal Healthy Longevity Survey	China	32,606 subjects aged 65 or older (13,429 men and 19,177 women).	High frequency of tea consumption was significantly associated with reduced OR of CoI.	Qiu et al., 2012 [28]
Longitudinal Healthy Longevity Survey	China	7139 participants aged 80 to 115 years.	Regular tea drinking was associated with better cognitive function in oldest-old Chinese, with regression coefficient 0.72 ($p < 0.0001$) for daily drinking and 0.41 ($p = 0.01$) for occasional drinking.	Feng et al., 2012 [29]
Prevalence survey	China	1000 residents aged $\geq$60 years old.	Drinking tea reduced the incidence of MCI ($p < 0.05$)	Yang et al., 2017 [30]
Cross-sectional study	China	870 elders aged $\geq$90 years old.	Among the Chinese nonagenarians and centenarians, no significant correlation between tea consumption and the prevalence of MCI.	Wang et al., 2010 [31]
Cross-sectional study	Norway	2031 adults aged 70–74 years (55% women).	The associations between intake of tea and cognition were approximately linearly dose-dependent.	Nurk et al., 2009 [32]
Population-based study	23 developed countries	Adults from 23 developed countries and given different genetic backgrounds.	A significant inverse correlation was found between dietary consumption of flavonoids and rate of AD or related dementias.	Beking et al., 2010 [33]
Meta-analyses	Asia, Europe, Australia, and North America.	52,503 participants distributed in Asia, Europe, Australia, and America.	Daily tea drinking was associated with decreased risk of CoI, MCI and cognitive decline in the elderly. However, the association between tea intake and AD remained elusive.	Ma et al., 2016 [34]

3. Anti-Aβ Effects of Tea

The amyloid cascade hypothesis states that naturally occurring Aβ monomers aggregate via a nucleation-dependent pathway to form insoluble fibrils that are deposited as plaques in the brain. The self-assembly of Aβ into neurotoxic oligomers followed by fibrillar aggregates is a defining characteristic of AD. AD is characterized by misfolding, aggregation, and accumulation of amyloid fibrils in an insoluble form in the brain. Green tea polyphenols (GTPs) including (−)-epigallocatechin gallate (EGCG), (+)-catechin (C) and (−)-epicatechin (EC), myricetin, quercetin, and kaempferol can protect cells from Aβ-mediated neurotoxicity by dose-dependently inhibiting the formation of Aβ fibrils (fAβ) from fresh Aβ(1–40) and Aβ(1–42) through the destabilization of preformed fAβ. The effective concentrations (EC$_{50}$) of myricetin and quercetin for the formation, extension, and destabilization of fAβ are 0.1–1.0 μM. Although the mechanisms by which these polyphenols inhibit fAβ formation from Aβ and destabilize pre-formed fAβ in vitro are still unclear, polyphenols are considered to be valuable for the prevention and therapeutic treatment of AD [38].

GTPs are believed to combat neurodegenerative diseases by inhibiting amyloid fibril formation andprotectingneurons from toxicity induced by Aβ. Okadaicacid (OA) is a toxin that inducesneurotoxicity. GTPs considerablyreducedprimary hippocampal neurondamage induced by OA. In mice pretreated with OA, ethologic tests indicated that the staying time and swimming distance in the target quadrant significantly decreased, whereas mice pretreated with GTPs stayed longer in the target quadrant [39]. In "Swedish" mutant Aβ precursor protein (APP) over expressing mice (APPsw, Tg), intraperitoneal (i.p.) injection (20 mg/kg) of green tea EGCG decreased Aβ levels and plaques via promotion of the non-amyloidogenic α-secretase proteolytic pathway. Oral administration of 50 mg/kg EGCG in drinking water reduced Aβ deposition in the tested mice. A six-month EGCG treatment revealed that plaque burdens decreased in the cingulate cortex, hippocampus, and entorhinal cortex by 54, 43, and 51%, respectively. Congo red plaque burden were decreased in the cingulate cortex, hippocampus, and entorhinal cortex by 53, 53, and 58%, respectively, and were accompanied by a reduction in both Aβ(1–40) and Aβ(1–42). Radial Ann water maze (RAWM) testing for working memory indicated that EGCG provided a cognitive benefit to Tg mice with both i.p. and oral administration; however, i.p. treated benefited more [40]. The anti-Aβ mechanism of tea is summarized below.

3.1. Inhibiting APP Cleavage by Regulating Activity of Related Enzymes

EGCG reduced Aβ generation in both murine neuron-like cells (N2a) transfected with Swedish mutant APP mice and primary neurons derived from Swedish mutant APP-overexpressing mice (Tg APPsw line 2576). EGCG markedly promoted cleavage of the α-C-terminal fragment of APP and elevated the N-terminal APP cleavage product, soluble APP-α. These cleavage events are associated with elevated α-secretase activity and enhanced hydrolysis of tumor necrosis factor α-converting enzyme, a primary product of α-secretase. In vivo tests on Tg APPsw transgenic mice showed that EGCG administration decreased Aβ levels and plaques by promotingthe nonamyloidogenic α-secretase proteolytic pathway [41,42].

The β-site APP cleaving enzyme 1 (BACE1) is a rate-limiting enzyme in APP processing and Aβ generation. The nuclear receptor peroxisome proliferator-activated receptor γ (PPARγ) is a potential target for AD treatment because of its potent inhibitory effects on Aβ production by negatively regulating BACE1. EGCG reduced Aβ generation in N2a/APP695 cells similar to the PPARγ agonist pioglitazone by inhibiting the transcription and translation of BACE1. This effect was reduced by the PPARγ inhibitor GW9662. EGCG significantly reinforced the activity of PPARγ by promoting its mRNA and protein expressions. The therapeutic efficacy of EGCG in testing for AD is thought to be derived from the up-regulation of PPARγ mRNA and protein expressions [43]. EGCG modulated APP processing, which resulted in enhanced cleavage of the α-COOH-terminal fragment (α-CTF) of APP and the corresponding elevation of the NH2-terminal APP product [i.e., soluble APP-α (sAPP-α)]. These beneficial effects were associated with increased α-secretase cleavage activity. Furthermore, EGCG treatment markedly elevated active ADAM10 protein (a-disintegrin and metalloprotease) in N2a cells by increasing α-CTF cleavage and elevating sAPP-α.

ADAM10 is an important pharmacotherapeutic target for the treatment of cerebral amyloidosis in AD. ADAM10 activation is critical for EGCG promotion of non-amyloidogenic (α-secretase cleavage) APP processing [44]. Estrogen depletion following menopause has been correlated with an increased risk of developing AD. EGCG increased non-amyloidogenic processing of APP through ADAM10, which was mediated by the maturation of ADAM10 via an estrogen receptor-α/phosphatidylinositol 3-kinase/aserine/threonine-specific protein kinase (ERα/PI3K/Akt) signaling-dependent mechanism, independent of furin-mediated ADAM10 activation. Central selective ER modulation could be a

9

therapeutic target for AD, and EGCG could be used as a well-tolerated alternative to estrogen therapy in the prophylaxis and treatment of this disease [45]. Oral administration of EC, another type of tea catechin, showed the same effect on Aβ pathology by inhibiting BACE1 [46].

Prolyl endopeptidase (PEP) is a serine protease known to cleave peptide substrates on the C-terminal side of proline residues. PEP also plays an important role in the degradation of proline-containing neuropeptides such as oxytocin, vasopressin, substance P, neurotensin, and angiotensin, which have been suggested as participants in the learning and memory processes [47]. The PEP activity in persons with AD was significantly higher than that in those without AD [48]. PEP could be involved in the processing of the C-terminal portion of the APP in AD [49]. Specific PEP inhibitors could prevent memory loss and increase attention span in patients suffering from senile dementia. EGCG, (−)-epicatechin gallate (ECG), and (+)-gallocatechin gallate (GCG) extracted from tea leaves were PEP inhibitors, with IC_{50} values of 1.42×10^{-4} mM, 1.02×10^{-2} mM, and 1.09×10^{-4} mM, respectively. They were non-competitive with a substrate in Dixon plots and did not show any significant effects on any other serine proteases like elastase, trypsin, and chymotrypsin, suggesting that they were relatively specific inhibitors against PEP and may be useful for preventing AD [50].

The drug therapies for AD are based on the cholinergic hypothesis that AD begins as a deficiency in the production of the neurotransmitter acetylcholine. Cholinesterase inhibition might impact the processing of amyloid in AD [51] and cholinesterase inhibitors have been suggested as the standard drugs for the treatment of AD. The inhibitors of acetylcholinesterase (AChE) and butyrylcholinesterase (BChE) show potential in the treatment process of AD. A molecular docking study revealed that EGCG inhibited AChE and BChE, resulting in enhance cholinergic neurotransmission [52].

Caffeine, a major component in tea, induced an increase in specific cellular neutral endopeptidase (NEP) activity in neuroblastoma cell line SK-N-SH and its activity was stronger than theophylline, theobromine, or theanine. The combination of EC, EGC, and EGCG with caffeine, theobromine, or theophylline induced cellular neutral endopeptidase activity. The enhancement of cellular NEP activity by green tea extract and its natural products might be correlated with an elevated levelofintracellular cyclic adenosine monophosphate [53].

Lipopolysaccharide (LPS) impairsmemory through the accumulation of Aβ via the increase of β- and γ-secretase. Oral treatment with EGCG (1.5 and 3 mg/kg for three weeks) into drinking water ameliorated LPS (1 μg/mouse, i.c.v.)-induced memory deficiency in a dose dependent manner. EGCG also dose-dependently inhibited LPS-induced elevation of Aβ levels by reducing LPS-induced β- and γ-secretase activities and expression of its metabolic products such as C99 and Aβ. EGCG prevented LPS-induced neuronal cell death as well as the expression of inflammatory proteins through inducible nitric oxide synthetase and cyclooxygenase. EGCG prevented LPS-mediated apoptotic cell death through suppression of Aβ elevation by inhibiting β- and γ-secretase. As a result, EGCG might be a useful agent against the neuroinflammation-associated development or progression of AD [54].

The kinetics of inhibition tests using Dixon, Cornish-Bowden, and Lineweaver-Burk plots showed that green, oolong, and black tea extracts, EGCG, theaflavin-3,3'-digallate (TFDG), and tannic acid were competitive inhibitors of PPA, whereas ECG, theaflavin-3'-gallate (TFG), and theaflavin (TF) were mixed-type inhibitors with both competitive and uncompetitive inhibitory characteristics. Only catechins with a galloyl substituent at the three-position showed a measurable inhibition. The competitive inhibition constants (Kic) were lower for theaflavins (TFs) than catechins, with the lowest value recorded for TFDG, suggesting that TFs and catechins bound more tightly with free PPA than with the PPA-starch complex. A 3 and/or 3'-galloyl moiety in catechin and TF structures was consistently found to increase the inhibition effect on PPA by enhancing association with the enzyme activation site. Various catechins showed different inhibitory effects on PPA, with IC_{50} being 2.514 mg/mL for EGCG, 1.729 mg/mL for ECG, 0.412 mg/mL for TF, 0.244 mg/mL for TFG, and 0.130 mg/mL for TFDG [55].

3.2. Preventing Protein Misfolding and Aβ-Induced Membrane Damages

Misfolded Aβ peptides self-assemble into higher-order oligomers that compromise membrane integrity, leading to synaptic degeneration and neuronal cell death. The misfolding of the Aβ peptide is one of the pathological hallmarks of AD. Aβ(1–42) peptides aggregated into a range of oligomers that efficiently permeabilized small unilamellar liposomes that were used to assess the ability of tea extracts to antagonize liposome permeabilization by the Aβ(1–42) oligomers. The dihydroxyphenyl ring structure of tea catechins, alone or as part of a flavanol scaffold, is particularly effective in protecting against membrane damage induced by the Aβ(1–42) oligomers [56]. Given the critical role of membrane perforation in the neurodegenerative cascade, these could guide the design and development of novel therapeutic drugs for the treatment of AD. EGCG plays special role in protein-misfolding diseases because of its potent anti-amyloid activity against Aβ, α-synuclein and huntingtin. EGCG redirected the aggregation of these polypeptides to a disordered off-folding pathway that results in the formation of non-toxic amorphous aggregates. EGCG also inhibits in vitro fibril formation via reduced and carboxymethylated kappa-casein (RCMkappa-CN), by preventing RCMkappa-CN fibril formation by stabilizing RCMkappa-CN in its native-like state. EGCG was proposed to be directed to the amyloidogenic sheet-turn-sheet motif of monomeric RCMkappa-CN with high affinity by strong non-specific hydrophobic associations, with non-covalent pi-pi stacking interactions between the polyphenolic and aromatic residues on the amyloidogenic sequence [57].

The chelating ability of EGCG also plays a role in reducing fibril formation. Observations using square wave voltammetry and transmission electron microscopy showed that the interaction of Cu(II) ions with the Tyr-10 residue of Aβ was affected by the surrounding His residues. With only Cu(II) present, the Aβ(1–40) aggregates showed a dense structure due to possible interactions within the metal binding region of Aβ(1–40) peptides. However, unstructured aggregates were observed when both EGCG and Cu(II) ions were incubated with Aβ(1–40), demonstrating that the chelating ability of EGCG impeded the formation of the Cu(II)-His complex, resulting in reduced fibril formation [58]. Both unoxidized and oxidized EGCG are active in inhibiting fibril formation, but the in vitro EGCG amyloid remodeling activity was dependent on auto-oxidation of the EGCG. Tests showed that the oxidized and unoxidized EGCG bound to amyloid fibrils, preventing the binding of thioflavin T. The hydrophobic binding sites were in A1–40, IAPP8–24, or Sup35NMAc7–16 Y→F amyloid fibrils. The oxidized EGCG molecules reacted with free amines within the amyloid fibril through the formation of Schiff bases, cross-linking the fibrils, which may prevent dissociation and toxicity [59].

3.3. Mitigating Aβ-Induced Oxidative Stress

Aβ peptides play a bilateral role in neuronal cell oxidative stress. Reactive oxygen species (ROS) induce formation of Aβ, which stimulates oxidative stress and neuronal toxicity. This process is typically attenuated by antioxidants and free radical scavengers. Tea catechins are a group of natural antioxidants that have protective effects against Aβ-induced neuronal apoptosis by scavenging ROS. One study recorded marked hippocampal neuronal injuries and increases in malondialdehyde (MDA) levels and caspase activity after the hippocampal neuronal cells were exposed to Aβ for 48 h. However, co-treatment of cells with EGCG to Aβ exposure increased the cell survival rate and decreased the levels of MDA and caspase activity. Proapoptotic (p53 and Bax), Bcl-XL, and cyclooxygenase (COX) proteins have been implicated in Aβ-induced neuronal death. The protective effects of EGCG are considered to be independent of the regulation of p53, Bax, Bcl-XL, and COX proteins. This suggests that EGCG has protective effects against Aβ-induced neuronal apoptosis by scavenging ROS, which is beneficial for the prevention and slowing of AD [60]. Aβ and pro-oxidant evoked neurotoxicity in PC12 cells, which resulted in a concentration-dependent reduction in viability of PC12 cell and human SH-SY5Y neuroblastoma cells via multiple protection mechanisms including the reduction of the pro-apoptotic proteins and Bax, the decrease in apoptosis-associated Ser139 phosphorylated H2A.X, and inhibition of the cleavage and activation of caspase-3. EGCG significantly reduced Aβ-evoked neurotoxicity [61,62].

EGCG may have preventive and/or therapeutic potential in AD patients by augmenting cellular antioxidant defense capacity and attenuating Aβ-mediated oxidative and/or nitrosative cell death. Aβ-induced damage of the neurons and glia are mediated via nitrosative and oxidative stress. BV2 cells exposed to Aβ underwent nitrosative stress, as shown by the increased expression of inducible nitric oxide synthase (iNOS) and subsequent production of nitric oxide (NO) and peroxynitrite, which were effectively suppressed by EGCG pretreatment. The mechanism considered to be at work is EGCG treatment fortifying the cellular GSH pool through elevated mRNA expression of γ-glutamylcysteine ligase, a rate limiting enzyme in glutathione biosynthesis [63]. Tea polyphenols EGCG, EC, and TF suppressed oxidative stress-induced BACE-1 mRNA upregulation in neuronal cells, resulting in the reduction of amyloidogenic cleavage of APP and Aβ production [3,64]. Green tea extracts protected neuronal dPC12 cells from H_2O_2-induced and Aβ-induced cytotoxicity at concentration ranges of 0.3–10 µg/mL and 0.03–0.125 µg/mL, respectively [65].

Aβ fragment individuals caused neurotoxicity through oxidative stress. Partial tea components and/or their complexes with Aβ fragments showed antioxidative activity. Injection of Aβ(25–35) (100 µM/µL) into the CA1 hippocampal region of mice caused a significant increase in lipid peroxidation and ROS, resulting in a decrease in memory skills. Hippocampal tissues from Aβ(25–35)-treated mice showed an increased immune reactivity against glial-fibrillar acidic protein. In contrast, mice pretreated with green tea EC (30 mg/kg) had a significant decrease in lipid peroxidation and ROS, as well as an improvement in memory skills. This result shows that Aβ(25–35)-caused oxidative damage in the hippocampus was blocked by the administration of EC [66]. CA-Aβ(38–42), a complex of the antioxidant caffeic acid (CA) and Aβ, exhibited potent inhibitory activity against Aβ(1–42) aggregation and scavenged Aβ(1–42)-induced intracellular oxidative stress. CA-Aβ(38–42) also significantly protected human neuroblastoma SH-SY5Y cells against Aβ(1–42)-induced cytotoxicity, with an IC_{50} of 4 µM, suggesting that CA-Aβ(38–42) has potential for AD prevention [67].

3.4. Suppressing Aggregation of Aβ Oligomers and Formation of Aβ Fibrils

One of the key factors in the development of AD is the conversion of Aβ from its soluble random coil form into various aggregated forms. EGCG may play an important role in APP secretion and protection against toxicity induced by Aβ. EGCG enhanced the release of the non-amyloidogenic soluble amyloid precursor protein (sAPPα) into the conditioned media of human SH-SY5Y neuroblastoma cells and rat pheochromocytoma PC12 cells. Treatment with EGCG reduced the Aβ levels by enhancing endogenous APP nonamyloidogenic proteolytic processing. EGCG also decreased nuclear translocation of c-Abl and blocked the amyloid precursor protein fragment (APP-C99)-dependent GSK3 β activation. These inhibitory effects occurred via the interruption of c-Abl/Fe65 interaction [68].

Islet amyloid polypeptide (IAPP, amylin) lacks a well-defined structure in its monomeric state, but readily assembles to form amyloid. Amyloid fibrils formed from IAPP, intermediates generated in the assembly of IAPP amyloid, or both, are toxic to β-cells. EGCG inhibited unseeded amyloid fibril formation and disaggregated IAPP amyloid, which protected cultured rat INS-1 cells against IAPP-induced toxicity [69]. EGCG effectively reduced the cytotoxicity of Aβ by remodeling seeding-competent Aβ oligomers into off-pathway seeding-incompetent Aβ assemblies.

During the initial EGCG-Aβ interactions, EGCG interfered with the aromatic hydrophobic core of Aβ and the EGCG-induced Aβ oligomers adopted a well-defined structure. The C-terminal part of the Aβ peptide (residues 22–39) adopted a β-sheet conformation, whereas the N-terminus (residues 1–20) was unstructured. The characteristic salt bridge involving residues D23 and K28 is present in the structure of these oligomeric Aβ aggregates [70]. The remodeling adhered to a Hill-Scatchard model where by the Aβ(1–40) self-association occurred cooperatively and generated Aβ(1–40) oligomers with multiple independent binding sites for EGCG with a Kd 10-fold lower than that for the Aβ(1–40) monomers. Upon binding to EGCG, the Aβ(1–40) oligomers were less exposed to solvents, and the β-regions, which were involved in direct monomer-protofibril contacted intheabsence of EGCG, underwent a direct-to-tethered contact shift. This switch toward less engaged monomer-protofibril contacts explained the seeding incompetency observed upon EGCG remodeling and suggested that EGCG interferes with secondary nucleation events known to generate toxic Aβ assemblies. The N-terminal residues experienced an opposite EGCG-induced shift from tethered to direct contacts, explaining why EGCG remodeling occurred without release of Aβ(1–40) monomers. Upon binding Aβ(1–40) oligomers, the relative positions of the B and D rings of EGCG changed with respect to that of ring A [71]. The binding stoichiometry N is linearly related to the EGCG/Aβ42 ratio. Hydrophobic interaction and hydrogen bonding are both essential in the binding process, but the extent of their contributions changes with experimental conditions. Namely, the predominant interaction gradually shifts from a hydrogen bonding to a hydrophobic interaction with the increase in the EGCG/Aβ42 ratio, resulting in a transition of the binding from enthalpy-driven to entropy-driven. The binding of EGCG to Aβ42 can be promoted by increasing temperature and salt concentration as well as changing pH away from Aβ42's pI [72].

L-theanine, an amide found in tea, inhibited Aβ(1–42)-induced generation of ROS and activation of extracellular signal-regulated kinase and p38 mitogenic activated protein kinase, as well as the activity of nuclear factor kappa-B. L-theanine (10–50 μg/mL) concomitantly decreased Aβ(1–42)-induced neurotoxicity in SK-N-MC and SK-N-SH human neuroblastoma cells, indicating that L-theanine prevented oxidative damages of neuronal cells and Aβ-induced neurotoxicity, which may be useful in the prevention and treatment of neurodegenerative disease like AD [73].

TFs (TF, TFG, and TFDG) had suppressive effects on Aβ aggregation, but compared to catechins, they showed different inhibitory capabilities at different mechanistic steps of the Aβ aggregation pathway. Catechins only affect the later stages of aggregation, in which catechins may bind a specific structure present in aggregates. Conversely, TFs show inhibitory capabilities at every stage of aggregation, alluding to a sequence-specific recognition. The number of gallate groups was positively correlated with inhibitory capabilities [74]. Solution-state nuclear magnetic resonance (NMR) showed that EGCG nonspecifically bound to the Aβ monomers [75]. Black tea polyphenolic component TF is a potent inhibitor of Aβ and α-synuclein (αS) fibrillogenesis. The binding regions of TFDG, congo red, and EGCG bound to two regions of the Aβ peptides, amino acids 12–23 and 24–36, albeit with different specificities. However, their mechanisms of amyloid inhibition differ. Like EGCG but unlike congo red, TFs stimulate the assembly of Aβ and αS into nontoxic, spherical aggregates that are incompetent in seeding amyloid formation and remodel Aβ fibrils into nontoxic aggregates. Compared to EGCG, TFDG was less susceptible to air oxidation and had an increased efficacy under oxidizing conditions [76].

3.5. Regulating Signaling Pathways Involving Aβ Generation

The EGCG-induced sAPPα secretion is blocked by the inhibition of protein kinase C (PKC). Therefore, the secretion process is considered to be PKC-dependent. EGCG shows protective effects against Aβ-induced neurotoxicity and regulates secretory processing of sAPPα via the PKC pathway. Administration of EGCG (2 mg/kg) to mice for 7 or 14 days significantly decreased membrane-bound holoprotein APP levels, with a concomitant increase in sAPPα levels in the hippocampus. EGCG markedly increased PKCα and PKε in the membrane and the cytosolic fractions of mice hippocampus. Here, EGCG was not only able to protect but also rescue PC12 cells against the Aβ toxicity in a dose-dependent manner [77]. EGCG markedly strengthened activation of α7 nicotinic acetylcholine receptor (α7nAChR) as well as its downstream pathway signaling molecules PI3K and Akt, subsequently leading to suppression of Bcl-2 downregulation in Aβ-treated neurons. Administration of α7nAChR antagonist methyllycaconitine (MLA, 20 μM) to neuronal cultures significantly attenuated the neuroprotection of EGCG against Aβ-induced neurotoxicity.

The α7nAChR activity, together with PI3K/Akt transduction signaling, may contribute to the molecular mechanism underlying the neuroprotective effects of EGCG against Aβ-induced cell death [78]. The deposition of Aβ peptides is closely correlated with the balance of nerve growth factor (NGF)-related TrkA/p75(NTR) signaling. In APP/PS1 mice, EGCG treatment (2 mg/kg·day) dramatically improved the CoI, reduced the over expression of Aβ(1–40) and APP, and inhibited neuronal apoptosis. EGCG also enhanced the relative expression level of NGF by increasing the NGF/proNGF ratio in APP/PS1 mice. After EGCG treatment, TrkA signaling was activated by increasing the phosphorylation of TrkA following the increased phosphorylation of the c-Raf, ERK1/2, and cAMP response to element-binding protein (CREB). Simultaneously, p75(NTR) signaling was significantly inhibited by decreasing the p75(ICD) expression, JNK2 phosphorylation, and cleaved-caspase 3 expression, resulting in inhibition of the Aβ deposits and neuronal apoptosis in the hippocampus [79].

Neprilysin (NEP) is an important Aβ-degrading enzyme in the brain; thus, defective enzyme expression may facilitate Aβ deposition in sporadic late onset AD patients. Treatment of cultured rat astrocytes with EGCG significantly reduced the expression of NEP in a concentration- and time-dependent manner. NEP expression in cultured astrocytes was suppressed by activation of extracellular signal-regulated kinase (ERK) and PI3K. Reduced NEP expression was accompanied by an increase in NEP release into the extracellular medium. The culture medium from EGCG-treated astrocytes facilitated the degradation of exogenous Aβ, suggesting that EGCG may have a beneficial effect on persons with AD by activating ERK- and PI3K-mediated pathways in astrocytes, thereby increasing astrocyte secretion of NEP and facilitating degradationofAβ [80].

L-theanine in tea also plays a role in regulating the signaling pathway related to Aβ deposits. Oral administration of L-theanine (2 and 4 mg/kg) to mice for five weeks in the drinking water, followed by injection of Aβ(1–42) (2 μg/mouse, i.c.v.), significantly alleviated Aβ(1–42)-induced memory impairment. L-theanine decreased Aβ(1–42) levels and the accompanying Aβ(1–42)-induced neuronal cell death in the cortex and hippocampus regions of the brain. L-theanine also inhibited Aβ(1–42)-induced ERK and p38 mitogen-activated protein kinase along with the activity of nuclear factor kappa B (NF-kappa B), togethershowing that the positive effects of L-theanine on memory might be mediated by suppression of ERK/p38 and NF-kappa B, as well as through the reduction of macromolecular oxidative damage [81].

3.6. Alleviating Aβ-Induced Mitochondria Disfunction

L-theanine (a special amide found in tea leaf), EGCG, and rutin from green and black tea extracts showed protective effects against mitochondrial impairment, a very early event in AD pathogenesis. As a result, therapeutics targeting improved mitochondrial function could be beneficial. L-theanine significantly affected regulating mitochondrial fusion proteins in SH-SY5Y (APP(sw)) cells. Its possible molecular mechanism might be via its suppression of the abnormal expression of Mfn1 and Mfn2 caused by excessive intracellular Aβ [82].

Aβ induces mitochondrial dysfunction and synaptic impairments via production of ROS, which plays a role in the onset and progression ofAD. EGCG was identified as a mitochondrial restorative compound. EGCG treatment in an Aβ PP/PS-1 (presenilin 1) double mutant transgenic mice with AD restored mitochondrial respiratory rates, MMP, ROS production, and ATP levels by 50–85% in mitochondria isolated from the hippocampus, cortex, and striatum [83]. Aβ treatment increased Bax and intracytoplasmic cytochrome C, a protein associated with the mitochondria-dependent pathway. EGCG blocked the effect of Aβ-induced Bax increase, showing a protective effect against Aβ-induced neurotoxicity via inhibition of the expression of the protein associated with the mitochondria-dependent cell death pathway [84]. EGCG has the potential to protect neuronal mitochondrial function in AD.

Rutin is a component in green tea that can mitigate mitochondrial damage by alleviating oxidative stress and modulate the production of proinflammatory cytokines by decreasing TNF-α and IL-1β generation in microglia [85]. Black tea extract inhibited permeation of mitochondrial membranes induced by aggregate complexes of Aβ(42) and α-syn [86].

3.7. Inhibiting Hyperphosphorylation of TAU Protein

The accumulation of Aβ and TAU (a highly soluble microtubule-associated protein on the chromosome) aggregates is another pathological hallmark of AD. These polypeptides form fibrillar deposits and toxic oligomeric aggregation intermediates. Depleting these structures could therefore be a powerful therapeutic strategy for AD. GTP pretreatment reduced the hyperphosphorylated TAU protein in mice, showing neuroprotection against OA-induced neurotoxicity [36]. EGCG enhanced the clearance of phosphorylated TAU species in a highly specific manner byincreasing adaptor protein expression [87]. Both i.p. and orally-treated Tg mice were found to have modulated TAU profiles, with markedly suppressed sarkosyl-soluble phosphorylated TAU isoforms [37]. A test on a sporadic AD transgenic mouse model, known as senescence accelerated mouse prone 8 (SAMP8), showed that administration of EGCG could improve recognition and memory function by reducing Aβ and TAU hyperphosphorylation. Long-term oral consumption of EGCG at a relatively high dose (15 mg/kg) improved memory function in the SAMP8 mice in the Y-maze and Morris water maze. EGCG treatment also prevented the hyperphosphorylation of TAU and reversed the decreased synaptic protein marker synaptophysin and postsynaptic density protein 95 in the FC and hippocampus (Hip) of SAMP8 mice, accompanied by a significant decrease in the levels of Aβ(1–42) and BACE-1 activity. Long-term oral administration of EGCG may reduce the impairments in spatial learning and memory and decrease the reduction in synaptic proteins observed in an AD mouse mode [88].

TAU fragments (His-K18 δK280) formed toxic oligomeric aggregation intermediates individually or by interaction with Aβ. EGCG inhibited the aggregation of TAU (His-K18 δK280) into toxic oligomers at ten- to hundred-fold sub-stoichiometric concentrations, resulting in rescuing toxicity in neuronal model cells [89].

4. Conclusion and Future Challenges

In the beginning half of this review, we outlined the epidemiological evidence showing how tea consumption in many different regions of the world has been associated with either a decreased risk of neurodegenerative disease AD or an improvement in cognitive function in older populations. In the second half of this review, we discussed the numerous mechanisms by which the bioactive components in tea (EGCG, ECG, EGC, EC, L-theanine, and rutin) have anti-amyloid effects, thereby resulting in protection against AD. The anti-amyloid mechanisms of these bioactive compounds include: (1) inhibiting APP cleavage by regulating the activity of related enzymes, (2) preventing protein misfolding and membrane damage induced by Aβ, (3) mitigating Aβ-induced oxidative stress, (4) suppressing the aggregation of Aβ oligomers, (5) regulating signaling pathways involving Aβ generation, (6) reducing Aβ-induced mitochondria disfunction, and (7) inhibiting hyperphosphorylation of TAU protein (Figure 1).

Additional research will be required before we can affirmatively support a link between tea consumption and the prevention of cure for AD. Specifically, more clinical studies are needed to help clarify inconsistent epidemiological results [17,31,34]. Factors causing inconsistencies include poor stability of tea bioactive components [90], dosage differences between in vitro and in vivo tests [91], low bioavailability [92], and conversion of bioactivities in the gastrointestinal track [93,94]. In-depth studies on these factors will be of significance for bridging the gap between in vitro studies and clinical applications.

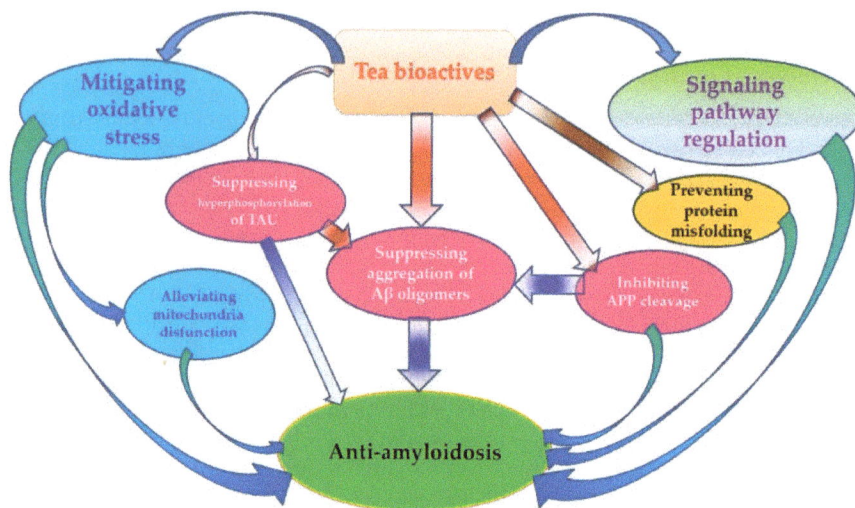

Figure 1. Anti-amyloidosis effects of tea.

Author Contributions: C.A.P.: Section 1. Introduction; English polishing and grammar correction; Z.-Y.C. & Y.-L.S.: Section 2; X.-M.L. & R.Y.: Section 3.1.; M.S.: Section 3.2.; Q.-S.L.: Section 3.3.; S.-C.M.& L.-P.X.: Section 3.4; K.-R.W.: Figure 1; J.-H.Y.: Section 3.5.; J.-L.L.: Section 3.6.; Y.-R.L.: Project design, literature search, Table 1 & Section 4; X.-Q.Z.: literature search, Abstract, Section 3.7.

Acknowledgments: The authors acknowledge the Science Technology Department of Zhejiang Province for financial support to this work (Project No. 2016C02053-5). This work was also financially supported by the China Agriculture Research System (Tea) (CARS-19).

Conflicts of Interest: The authors declare no conflict of interest.

References

1. Kou, X.; Chen, N. Resveratrol as a natural autophagy regulator for prevention and treatment of Alzheimer's disease. *Nutrients* **2017**, *9*, 927. [CrossRef]

2. Swaminathan, N. How to save your brain. *Psychol. Today* **2012**, *45*, 74–79.

3. Geiser, R.J.; Chastain, S.E.; Moss, M.A. Regulation of Bace1 mRNA expression in Alzheimer's disease by green tea catechins and black tea theaflavins. *Biophys. J.* **2017**, *112* (Suppl. 3), 362a. [CrossRef]

4. Hwang, S.; Lim, J.W.; Kim, H. Inhibitory effect of lycopene on amyloid-β-induced apoptosis in neuronal cells. *Nutrients* **2017**, *9*, 883. [CrossRef] [PubMed]

5. Ribarič, S. Peptides as potential therapeutics for Alzheimer's disease. *Molecules* **2018**, *23*, 283. [CrossRef] [PubMed]

6. Ding, D.; Zhao, Q.; Guo, Q.; Meng, H.; Wang, B.; Yu, P.; Luo, J.; Zhou, Y.; Yu, L.; Zheng, L.; Chu, S.; et al. The Shanghai aging study: Study design, baseline characteristics, and prevalence of dementia. *Neuroepidemiology* **2014**, *43*, 114–122. [CrossRef] [PubMed]

7. Javier, O.P.; Carmelo, P.V. Dietary supplements for cognitive impairment. *Actas Esp. Psiquiatr.* **2017**, *45*, 37–47.

8. Rubio-Perez, J.M.; Albaladeo, M.D.; Zafrilla, P.; Vidal-Guevara, M.L.; Morillas-Ruiz, J.M. Effects of an antioxidant beverage on biomarkers of oxidative stress in Alzheimer's patients. *Eur. J. Nutr.* **2016**, *55*, 2105–2116. [CrossRef] [PubMed]

9. Kesse-Guyot, E.; Fezeu, L.; Andreeva, V.A.; Touvier, M.; Scalbert, A.; Hercberg, S.; Galan, P. Total and specific polyphenol intakes in midlife are associated with cognitive function measured 13 years later. *J. Nutr.* **2012**, *142*, 76–83. [CrossRef] [PubMed]

10. Feng, L.; Chong, M.S.; Lim, W.S.; Lee, T.S.; Kua, E.H.; Ng, T.P. Tea for Alzheimer prevention. *J. Prev. Alzheimer Dis.* **2015**, *2*, 136–141.

11. Liu, K.; Liang, X.; Kuang, W. Tea consumption maybe an effective active treatment for adult attention deficit hyperactivity disorder (ADHD). *Med. Hypotheses* **2011**, *76*, 461–463. [CrossRef] [PubMed]

12. Weinreb, O.; Amit, T.; Mandel, S.; Youdim, M.B.H. Neuroprotective molecular mechanisms of (−)-epigallocatechin-3-gallate: A reflective outcome of its antioxidant, iron chelating and neuritogenic properties. *Genes Nutr.* **2009**, *4*, 283–296. [CrossRef] [PubMed]

13. Singh, N.A.; Mandal, A.K.A.; Khan, Z.A. Potential neuroprotective properties of epigallocatechin-3-gallate (EGCG). *Nutr. J.* **2016**, *15*, 60. [CrossRef] [PubMed]

14. Fernando, W.; Somaratne, G.; Goozee, K.G.; Williams, S.; Singh, H.; Martins, R.N. Diabetes and Alzheimer's Disease: Can Tea Phytochemicals Play a Role in Prevention? *J. Alzheimer Dis.* **2017**, *59*, 481–501. [CrossRef] [PubMed]

15. Rusted, J.; Sheppard, L. Action-based memory in Alzheimer's disease: A longitudinal look at tea making. *Neurocase* **2002**, *8*, 111–126. [CrossRef] [PubMed]

16. Kuriyama, S.; Hozawa, A.; Ohmori, K.; Shimazu, T.; Matsui, T.; Ebihara, S.; Awata, S.; Nagatomi, R.; Arai, H.; Tsuji, I. Green tea consumption and cognitive function: A cross-sectional study from the Tsurugaya Project. *Am. J. Clin. Nutr.* **2006**, *83*, 355–361. [CrossRef] [PubMed]

17. Tomata, Y.; Kakizaki, M.; Nakaya, N.; Tsuboya, T.; Sone, T.; Kuriyama, S.; Hozawa, A.; Tsuji, I. Green tea consumption and the risk of incident functional disability in elderly Japanese: The Ohsakicohort 2006 study. *Am. J.Clin. Nutr.* **2012**, *95*, 732–739. [CrossRef] [PubMed]

18. Noguchi-Shinohara, M.; Yuki, S.; Dohmoto, C.; Ikeda, Y.; Samuraki, M.; Iwasa, K.; Yokogawa, M.; Asai, K.; Komai, K.; Nakamura, H.; et al. Consumption of green tea, but not black tea or coffee, is associated with reduced risk of cognitive decline. *PLoS ONE* **2014**, *9*, E96013. [CrossRef] [PubMed]

19. Kitamura, K.; Watanabe, Y.; Nakamura, K.; Sanpei, K.; Wakasugi, M.; Yokoseki, A.; Onodera, O.; Ikeuchi, T.; Kuwano, R.; Momotsu, T.; et al. Modifiable factors associated with cognitive impairment in 1143 Japanese outpatients: The project in Sado for total health (PROST). *Dement.Geriatr. Cogn. Disord. Extra* **2016**, *6*, 341–349. [CrossRef] [PubMed]

20. Ide, K.; Yamada, H.; Takuma, N.; Kawasaki, Y.; Harada, S.; Nakase, J.; Ukawa, Y.; Sagesaka, Y.M. Effects of green tea consumption on cognitive dysfunction in an elderly population: A randomized placebo controlled study. *Nutr. J.* **2016**, *15*, 49. [CrossRef] [PubMed]

21. Ng, T.P.; Feng, L.; Niti, M.; Kua, E.H.; Yap, K.B. Tea consumption and cognitive impairment and decline in older Chinese adults. *Am. J. Clin. Nutr.* **2008**, *88*, 224–231. [CrossRef] [PubMed]

22. Feng, L.; Gwee, X.; Kua, E.H.; Ng, T.P. Cognitive function and tea consumption in community dwelling older Chinese in Singapore. *J. Nutr. Health Aging* **2010**, *14*, 433–438. [CrossRef] [PubMed]

23. Feng, L.; Li, J.L.; Kua, E.K.; Lee, T.S.; Yap, K.B.; Rush, A.J.; Ng, T.P. Association between tea consumption and depressive symptoms in older Chinese adults. *J. Am. Geriatr. Soc.* **2012**, *60*, 2358–2360. [CrossRef] [PubMed]

24. Chan, S.P.; Yong, P.Z.; Sun, Y.; Mahendran, R.; Wong, J.C.M.; Qiu, C.; Ng, T.P.; Kua, E.H.; Feng, L. Associations of long-term tea consumption with depressive and anxiety symptoms in community-living elderly: Findings from the diet and healthy aging study. *J. Prev. Alzheimer Dis.* **2018**, *5*, 21–25.

25. Huang, C.Q.; Dong, B.R.; Zhang, Y.L.; Wu, H.M.; Liu, Q.X. Association of cognitive impairment with smoking, alcohol consumption, tea consumption, and exercise among Chinese nonagenarians/centenarians. *Cogn. Behav. Neurol.* **2009**, *22*, 190–196. [CrossRef] [PubMed]

26. Chen, X.; Huang, Y.; Cheng, H.G. Lower intake of vegetables and legumes associated with cognitive decline among illiterate elderly Chinese: A 3-year cohort study. *J. Nutr. Health Aging* **2012**, *16*, 549–552. [CrossRef] [PubMed]

27. Gu, Y.J.; He, C.H.; Li, S.; Zhang, S.Y.; Duan, S.Y.; Sun, H.P.; Shen, Y.P.; Xu, Y.; Yin, J.Y.; Pan, C.W. Tea consumptionis associated with cognitive impairment in older Chinese adults. *Aging Ment. Health* **2017**. [CrossRef] [PubMed]

28. Feng, L.; Yan, Z.R.; Sun, B.L.; Cai, C.Z.; Jiang, H.; Kua, E.H.; Ng, T.P.; Qiu, C.X. Tea consumption and depressive symptoms in older people in rural China. *J. Am. Geriatr. Soc.* **2013**, *61*, 1943–1947. [CrossRef] [PubMed]

29. Shen, W.; Xiao, Y.; Ying, X.; Li, S.; Zhai, Y.; Shang, X.; Li, F.; Wang, X.; He, F.; Lin, J. Tea consumption and cognitive impairment: A cross-sectional study among Chinese elderly. *PLoS ONE* **2015**, *10*, e0137781. [CrossRef] [PubMed]

30. Yang, L.; Jin, X.Q.; Yan, J.; Jin, Y.; Yu, W.; Wu, H.B.; Xu, S.H. Prevalence of dementia, cognitive status and associated risk factors among elderly of Zhejiang province, China in 2014. *Age Ageing* **2016**, *45*, 707–711. [CrossRef] [PubMed]

31. Qiu, L.; Sautter, J.; Gu, D. Associations between frequency of tea consumption and health and mortality: Evidence from old Chinese. *Br. J. Nutr.* **2012**, *108*, 1686–1697. [CrossRef] [PubMed]

32. Feng, L.; Li, J.; Ng, T.P.; Lee, T.S.; Kua, E.H.; Zeng, Y. Tea drinking and cognitive function in oldest-old Chinese. *J. Nutr. Health Aging* **2012**, *16*, 754–758. [CrossRef] [PubMed]

33. Yang, Y.H.; Cheng, G.W.; Rong, S.; Zhu, H.L.; Chen, D.; Yang, B.; Li, W.F. A cross-sectional study on mild cognitive impairment among the elderly in communities of Huangshi City. *Chin. J. Dis. Control Prev.* **2017**, *21*, 767–771.

34. Wang, Z.; Dong, B.; Zeng, G.; Li, J.; Wang, W.; Wang, B.; Yuan, Q. Is there an association between mild cognitiveimpairment and dietary pattern in Chineseelderly? Results from a cross-sectional population study. *BMC Public Health* **2010**, *10*, 595. [CrossRef] [PubMed]

35. Nurk, E.; Refsum, H.; Drevon, C.A.; Tell, G.S.; Nygaard, H.A.; Engedal, K.; Smith, A.D. Intake of flavonoid-rich wine, tea, and chocolate by elderly men and women is associated with better cognitive test performance. *J. Nutr.* **2009**, *139*, 120–127. [CrossRef] [PubMed]

36. Beking, K.; Vieira, A. Flavonoid intake and disability-adjusted life years due to Alzheimer's and related dementias: A population-based study involving twenty-three developed countries. *Public Health Nutr.* **2010**, *13*, 1403–1409. [CrossRef] [PubMed]

37. Ma, Q.P.; Huang, C.; Cui, Q.Y.; Yang, D.J.; Sun, K.; Chen, X.; Li, X.H. Meta-analysis of the association between tea intake and the risk of cognitive disorders. *PLoS ONE* **2016**, *11*, e0165861. [CrossRef] [PubMed]

38. Ono, K.; Yoshiike, Y.; Takashima, A.; Hasegawa, K.; Naiki, H.; Yamada, M. Potent anti-amyloidogenic and fibril-destabilizing effects of polyphenols in vitro: Implications for the prevention and therapeutics of Alzheimer's disease. *J. Neurochem.* **2003**, *87*, 172–181. [CrossRef] [PubMed]

39. Li, H.Y.; Wu, X.K.; Wu, Q.; Gong, D.Z.; Shi, M.J.; Guan, L.L.; Zhang, J.; Liu, J.; Yuan, B.; Han, G.Z.; Zou, Y. Green tea polyphenols protect against okadaic acid-induced acute learning and memory impairments in rats. *Nutrition* **2014**, *30*, 337–342. [CrossRef] [PubMed]

40. Rezai-Zadeh, K.; Arendash, G.W.; Hou, H.Y.; Fernandez, F.; Jensen, M.; Runfeldt, M.; Shytle, R.D.; Tan, J. Green tea epigallocatechin-3-gallate (EGCG) reduces beta-amyloid mediated cognitive impairment and modulates tau pathology in Alzheimer transgenic mice. *Brain Res.* **2008**, *1214*, 177–187. [CrossRef] [PubMed]

41. Rezai-Zadeh, K.; Shytle, D.; Sun, N.; Mori, T.; Hou, H.Y.; Jeanniton, D.; Ehrhart, J.; Townsend, K.; Zeng, J.; Morgan, D.; Hardy, J.; et al. Green Tea epigallocatechin-3-gallate (EGCG) modulates amyloid precursor protein cleavage and reduces cerebral amyloidosis in Alzheimer transgenic mice. *J. Neurosci.* **2005**, *25*, 8807–8814. [CrossRef] [PubMed]

42. Omar, S.H. Biophenols pharmacology against the amyloidogenic activity in Alzheimer's disease. *Biomed. Pharmacother.* **2017**, *89*, 396–413. [CrossRef] [PubMed]

43. Zhang, Z.X.; Li, Y.B.; Zhao, R.P. Epigallocatechingallate attenuates beta-amyloid generation and oxidative stress involvement of PPAR gamma in N2a/APP695 cells. *Neurochem. Res.* **2017**, *42*, 468–480. [CrossRef] [PubMed]

44. Obregon, D.F.; Rezai-Zadeh, K.; Bai, Y.; Sun, N.; Hou, H.Y.; Ehrhart, J.; Zeng, J.; Mori, T.; Arendash, G.W.; Shytle, D.; et al. ADAM10 activation is required for green tea (−)-epigallocatechin-3-gallate-induced α-secretase cleavage of amyloid precursor protein. *J. Biol. Chem.* **2006**, *281*, 16419–16427. [CrossRef] [PubMed]

45. Fernandez, J.W.; Rezai-Zadeh, K.; Obregon, D.; Tan, J. EGCG functions through estrogen receptor-mediated activation of ADAM10 in the promotion of non-amyloidogenic processing of APP. *FEBS Lett.* **2010**, *584*, 4259–4267. [CrossRef] [PubMed]

46. Cox, C.J.; Choudhry, F.; Peacey, E.; Perkinton, M.S.; Richardson, J.C.; Howlett, D.R.; Lichtenthaler, S.F.; Francis, P.T.; Williams, R.J. Dietary (−)-epicatechin as a potent inhibitor of β γ-secretase amyloid precursor protein processing. *Neurobiol. Aging* **2015**, *36*, 178–187. [CrossRef] [PubMed]

47. Rennex, D.; Hemmings, B.A.; Hofsteenge, J.; Stone, S.R. cDNA cloning of porcine brain prolylendopeptidase and identification of the active-site seryl residue. *Biochemistry* **1991**, *30*, 2195–2203. [CrossRef] [PubMed]
48. Aoyagi, T.; Nagai, M.; Ogawa, K.; Gojima, F.; Okada, M.; Ikeda, T.; Hamada, M.; Takeuchi, T. Poststatin, a new inhibitor of prolylendopeptidase, produced by streptomycesviridochromogens MH534-30F3. I. Taxonomy, production, isolation, physico-chemical properties and biological activities. *J. Antibiot.* **1991**, *44*, 949–955. [CrossRef] [PubMed]
49. Ishiura, S.; Tsukahara, T.; Tabira, T.; Shimizu, T.; Arahata, K.; Sugita, H. Identification of a putative amyloid A4-generating enzyme as a prolylendopeptidase. *FEBS Lett.* **1990**, *260*, 131–134. [CrossRef]
50. Kim, J.H.; Kim, S.I.; Song, K.S. Prolylendopeptidaseinhibitors from green tea. *Arch. Pharm. Res.* **2001**, *24*, 292–296. [CrossRef] [PubMed]
51. Yuksel, M.; Biberoglu, K.; Onder, S.; Akbulut, K.G.; Tacal, O. Effects of phenothiazine-structured compounds on APP processing in Alzheimer's disease cellular model. *Biochimie* **2017**, *138*, 82–89. [CrossRef] [PubMed]
52. Ali, B.; Jamal, Q.M.S.; Shams, S.; Al-Wabel, N.A.; Siddiqui, M.U.; Alzohairy, M.A.; Al Karaawi, M.A.; Kesari, K.K.; Mushtaq, G.; Kamal, M.A. In Silico Analysis of Green Tea Polyphenols as Inhibitors of AChE and BChE Enzymes in Alzheimer's Disease Treatment. *CNS Neurol. Disord.-Drug* **2016**, *15*, 624–628. [CrossRef]
53. Ayoub, S.; Melzig, M.F. Induction of neutral endopeptidase (NEP) activity of SK-N-SH cells by natural compounds from green tea. *J. Pharm. Pharmacol.* **2006**, *58*, 495–501. [CrossRef] [PubMed]
54. Lee, Y.K.; Yuk, D.Y.; Lee, J.W.; Lee, S.Y.; Ha, T.Y.; Oh, K.W.; Yun, Y.P.; Hong, J.T. Epigallocatechin-3-gallate prevents lipopolysaccharide-induced elevation of beta-amyloid generation and memory deficiency. *Brain Res.* **2009**, *1250*, 167–174. [CrossRef] [PubMed]
55. Sun, L.J.; Warren, F.J.; Netzel, G.; Gidley, M.J. 3 or 3′-Galloyl substitution plays an important role in association of catechins and theaflavins with porcine pancreatic α-amylase: The kinetics of inhibition of α-amylase by tea polyphenols. *J. Funct. Foods* **2016**, *26*, 144–156. [CrossRef]
56. Gauci, A.J.; Caruana, M.; Giese, A.; Scerri, C.; Vassallo, N. Identification of polyphenolic compounds and black tea extract as potent inhibitors of lipid membrane destabilization by Aβ(42) aggregates. *J. Alzheimers Dis.* **2011**, *27*, 767–779. [CrossRef] [PubMed]
57. Hudson, S.A.; Ecroyd, H.; Dehle, F.C.; Musgrave, I.F.; Carver, J. (−)-Epigallocatechin-3-gallate (EGCG) maintains k-casein in its pre-fibrillar state without redirecting its aggregation pathway. *J. Mol. Biol.* **2009**, *392*, 689–700. [CrossRef] [PubMed]
58. Zhang, B.A.; Cheng, X.R.; da Silva, I.S.; Hung, V.W.S.; Veloso, A.J.; Angnes, L.; Kerman, K. Electroanalysis of the interaction between (−)-epigallocatechin-3-gallate (EGCG) and amyloid-beta in the presence of copper. *Metallomics* **2013**, *5*, 259–264. [CrossRef] [PubMed]
59. Palhano, F.L.; Lee, J.; Grimster, N.P.; Kelly, J.W. Toward the molecular mechanism(s) by which EGCG treatment remodels mature amyloid fibrils. *J. Am. Chem. Soc.* **2013**, *135*, 7503–7510. [CrossRef] [PubMed]
60. Choi, Y.T.; Jung, C.H.; Lee, S.R.; Bae, J.H.; Baek, W.K.; Suh, M.H.; Park, J.; Park, C.W.; Suh, S.I. The green tea polyphenol (−)-epigallocatechingallate attenuates β-amyloid-induced neurotoxicity in cultured hippocampal neurons. *Life Sci.* **2001**, *70*, 603–614. [CrossRef]
61. Harvey, B.S.; Musgrave, I.F.; Ohlsson, K.S.; Fransson, A.; Smid, S.D. The green tea polyphenol (−)-epigallocatechin-3-gallate inhibits amyloid-β evoked fibril formation and neuronal cell death in vitro. *Food Chem.* **2011**, *129*, 1729–1736. [CrossRef]
62. Avramovich-Tirosh, Y.; Rezrlichenko, D.; Amit, T.; Zheng, H.; Fridkin, M.; Weinreb, O.; Mandel, S.; Youdim, M.B.H. Neurorescue activity, APP regulation and amyloid-β peptide reduction by novel multi-functional brain permeable iron- chelating- antioxidants, m-30 and green tea polyphenol, EGCG. *Curr. Alzheimer Res.* **2007**, *4*, 403–411. [CrossRef] [PubMed]
63. Kim, C.Y.; Lee, C.; Park, G.H.; Jang, J.H. Neuroprotective effect of epigallocatechin-3-gallate against β-amyloid-induced oxidative and nitrosative cell death via augmentation of antioxidant defense capacity. *Arch. Pharm. Res.* **2009**, *32*, 869–881. [CrossRef] [PubMed]
64. Shimmyo, Y.; Kihara, T.; Akaike, A.; Niidome, T.; Sugimoto, H. Epigallocatechin-3-gallate and curcumin suppress amyloid beta-induced beta-site APP cleaving enzyme-1 upregulation. *Neuroreport* **2008**, *19*, 1329–1333. [CrossRef] [PubMed]
65. Okello, E.J.; McDougall, G.J.; Kumar, S.; Seal, C.J. In vitro protective effects of colon-available extract of *Camellia sinensis* (tea) against hydrogen peroxide and beta-amyloid (A beta((1-42))) induced cytotoxicity in differentiated PC12 cells. *Phytomedicine* **2011**, *18*, 691–696. [CrossRef] [PubMed]

66. Cuevas, E.; Limon, D.; Perez-Severiano, F.; Diaz, A.; Ortega, L.; Zenteno, E.; Guevara, J. Antioxidant effects of epicatechin on the hippocampal toxicity caused by amyloid-beta 25–35 in rats. *Eur. J. Pharmacol.* **2009**, *616*, 122–127. [CrossRef] [PubMed]
67. Arai, T.; Ohno, A.; Mori, K.; Kuwata, H.; Mizuno, M.; Imai, K.; Hara, S.; Shibanuma, M.; Kurihara, M.; Miyata, N.; et al. Inhibition of amyloid fibril formation and cytotoxicity by caffeic acid-conjugated amyloid-beta C-terminal peptides. *Bioorg. Med. Chem. Lett.* **2016**, *26*, 5468–5471. [CrossRef] [PubMed]
68. Lin, C.L.; Chen, T.F.; Chiu, M.J.; Way, T.D.; Lin, J.K. Epigallocatechingallate (EGCG) suppresses beta-amyloid-induced neurotoxicity through inhibiting c-Abl/FE65 nuclear translocation and GSK3 beta activation. *Neurobiol. Aging* **2009**, *30*, 81–92. [CrossRef] [PubMed]
69. Meng, F.; Abedini, A.; Plesner, A.; Verchere, C.B.; Raleigh, D.P. The flavanol (−)-epigallocatechin 3-gallate inhibits amyloid formation by islet amyloid polypeptide, disaggregates amyloid fibrils and protects cultured cells against IAPP induced toxicity. *Biochemistry* **2010**, *49*, 8127–8133. [CrossRef] [PubMed]
70. Lopez del Amo, J.M.; Fink, U.; Dasari, M.; Grelle, G.; Wanker, E.E.; Bieschke, J.; Reif, B. Structural properties of EGCG-induced, nontoxic Alzheimer's disease A β oligomers. *J. Mol. Biol.* **2012**, *421*, 517–524. [CrossRef] [PubMed]
71. Ahmed, R.; VanSchouwen, B.; Jafari, N.; Ni, X.D.; Ortega, J.; Melacini, G. Molecular mechanism for the (−)-epigallocatechingallate-induced toxic to nontoxic remodeling of A beta oligomers. *J. Am. Chem. Soc.* **2017**, *139*, 13720–13734. [CrossRef] [PubMed]
72. Wang, S.H.; Liu, F.F.; Dong, X.Y.; Sun, Y. Thermodynamic analysis of the molecular interactions between amyloid β-peptide 42 and (−)-epigallocatechin-3-gallate. *J. Phys. Chem. B* **2010**, *114*, 11576–11583. [CrossRef] [PubMed]
73. Jo, M.; Park, M.H.; Choi, D.Y.; Yuk, D.Y.; Lee, Y.M.; Lee, J.M.; Jeong, J.H.; Oh, K.W.; Lee, M.S.; Han, S.B.; et al. Neuroprotective effect of L-theanine on A β-induced neurotoxicity through anti-oxidative mechanisms in SK-N-SH and SK-N-MC cells. *Biomol. Ther.* **2011**, *19*, 288–295. [CrossRef]
74. Chastain, S.E.; Moss, M. Green and black tea polyphenols mechanistically inhibit the aggregation of amyloid-β in Alzheimer's disease. *Biophys. J.* **2015**, *108*, 357a. [CrossRef]
75. Sinha, S.; Du, Z.M.; Maiti, P.; Klärner, F.G.; Schrader, T.; Wang, C.Y.; Bitan, G. Comparison of three amyloid assembly inhibitors: The sugar scyllo-inositol, the polyphenol epigallocatechingallate, and the molecular Tweezer CLR01. *ACS Chem. Neurosci.* **2012**, *3*, 451–458. [CrossRef] [PubMed]
76. Grelle, G.; Otto, A.; Lorenz, M.; Frank, R.F.; Wanker, E.E.; Bieschke, J. Black tea theaflavins inhibit formation of toxic amyloid-β and α-synuclein fibrils. *Biochemistry* **2011**, *50*, 10624–10636. [CrossRef] [PubMed]
77. Levites, Y.; Amit, T.; Mandel, S.; Youdim, M.B.H. Neuroprotection and neurorescue against A beta toxicity and PKC-dependent release of non-amyloidogenic soluble precursor protein by green tea polyphenol (−)-epigallocatechin-3-gallate. *FASEB J.* **2003**, *17*, 952–954. [CrossRef] [PubMed]
78. Zhang, X.J.; Wu, M.M.; Lu, F.; Luo, N.; He, Z.P.; Yang, H. Involvement of α7 nAChR signaling cascade inepigallocatechingallate suppression of β-amyloid-induced apoptotic cortical neuronal insults. *Mol. Neurobiol.* **2014**, *49*, 66–67. [CrossRef] [PubMed]
79. Liu, M.Y.; Chen, F.J.; Sha, L.; Wang, S.; Tao, L.; Yao, L.T.; He, M.; Yao, Z.M.; Liu, H.; Zhu, Z.; et al. (−)-Epigallocatechin-3-gallate ameliorates learning and memory deficits by adjusting the balance of TrkA/p75(NTR) signaling in *APP/PS1* transgenic Mice. *Mol. Neurobiol.* **2014**, *49*, 1350–1363. [CrossRef] [PubMed]
80. Yamamoto, N.; Shibata, M.; Ishikuro, R.; Tanida, M.; Taniguchi, Y.; Ikeda-Matsuo, Y.; Sobue, K. Epigallocatechingallate induces extracellular degradation of amyloid beta-protein by increasing neprilysin secretion from astrocytes through activation of ERK and PI3K pathways. *Neuroscience* **2017**, *362*, 70–78. [CrossRef] [PubMed]
81. Il Kim, T.; Lee, Y.K.; Park, S.G.; Choi, I.S.; Ban, J.O.; Park, H.K.; Nam, S.Y.; Yun, Y.W.; Han, S.B.; Oh, K.W.; et al. L-Theanine, an amino acid in green tea, attenuates beta-amyloid-induced cognitive dysfunction and neurotoxicity: Reduction in oxidative damage and inactivation of ERK/p38 kinase and NF-kappa B pathways. *Free Radic. Biol. Med.* **2009**, *47*, 1601–1610. [CrossRef] [PubMed]
82. Wu, Z.F.; Zhu, Y.S.; Cao, X.S.; Sun, S.F.; Zhao, B.L. Mitochondrial toxic effects of a beta through mitofusins in the early pathogenesis of Alzheimer's disease. *Mol. Neurobiol.* **2014**, *50*, 986–996. [CrossRef] [PubMed]

83. Dragicevic, N.; Smith, A.; Lin, X.Y.; Yuan, F.; Copes, N.; Delic, V.; Tan, J.; Cao, C.H.; Shytle, R.D.; Bradshaw, P.C. Green tea epigallocatechin-3-gallate (EGCG) and other flavonoids reduce Alzheimer's amyloid-induced mitochondrial dysfunction. *J. Alzheimers Dis.* **2011**, *26*, 507–521. [CrossRef] [PubMed]

84. Kim, M.S.; Jung, J.Y.; Kim, E.C.; Kim, H.J.; Kim, W.J.; Lee, E.J.; Kim, S.H. Inhibition of amyloid β peptide-induced neuronal cytotoxicity by EGCG. *Korean J. Phys. Anthropol.* **2005**, *18*, 139–147. [CrossRef]

85. Wang, S.W.; Wang, Y.J.; Su, Y.J.; Zhou, W.W.; Yang, S.G.; Zhang, R.; Zhao, M.; Li, Y.N.; Zhang, Z.P.; Zhan, D.W.; et al. Rutin inhibits beta-amyloid aggregation and cytotoxicity, attenuates oxidative stress, and decreases the production of nitric oxide and proinflammatory cytokines. *Neurotoxicology* **2012**, *33*, 482–490. [CrossRef] [PubMed]

86. Camilleri, A.; Zarb, C.; Caruana, M.; Ostermeier, U.; Ghio, S.; Högen, T.; Schmidt, F.; Giese, A.; Vassallo, N. Mitochondrial membrane permeabilisation by amyloid aggregates and protection by polyphenols. *BBA-Biomembr.* **2013**, *1828*, 2532–2543. [CrossRef] [PubMed]

87. Chesser, A.S.; Ganeshan, V.; Yang, J.; Johnson, G.V.W. Epigallocatechin-3-gallate enhances clearance of phosphorylated tau in primary neurons. *Nutr. Neurosci.* **2016**, *19*, 21–31. [CrossRef] [PubMed]

88. Guo, Y.F.; Zhao, Y.; Nan, Y.; Wang, X.; Chen, Y.L.; Wang, S. (−)-Epigallocatechin-3- gallate ameliorates memory impairment and rescues the abnormal synaptic protein levels in the frontal cortex and hippocampus in a mouse model of Alzheimer's disease. *Neuroreport* **2017**, *28*, 590–597. [CrossRef] [PubMed]

89. Wobst, H.J.; Sharma, A.; Diamond, M.I.; Wanker, E.E.; Bieschke, J. The green tea polyphenol (−)-epigallocatechingallate prevents the aggregation of tau protein into toxic oligomers at substoichiometric ratios. *FEBS Lett.* **2015**, *589*, 77–83. [CrossRef] [PubMed]

90. Xiang, L.P.; Wang, A.; Ye, J.H.; Zheng, X.Q.; Polito, C.A.; Lu, J.L.; Li, Q.S.; Liang, Y.R. Suppressive effects of tea catechins on breast cancer. *Nutrients* **2016**, *8*, 458. [CrossRef] [PubMed]

91. Du, L.L.; Fu, Q.Y.; Xiang, L.P.; Zheng, X.Q.; Lu, J.L.; Ye, J.H.; Li, Q.S.; Polito, C.A.; Liang, Y.R. Tea polysaccharides and their bioactivities. *Molecules* **2016**, *21*, 1449. [CrossRef] [PubMed]

92. Fu, Q.Y.; Li, Q.S.; Lin, X.M.; Qiao, R.Y.; Yang, R.; Li, X.M.; Dong, Z.B.; Xiang, L.P.; Zheng, X.Q.; Lu, J.L.; et al. Antidiabetic effects of tea. *Molecules* **2017**, *22*, 849. [CrossRef] [PubMed]

93. Shi, M.; Shi, Y.L.; Li, X.M.; Yang, R.; Cai, Z.Y.; Li, Q.S.; Ma, S.C.; Ye, J.H.; Lu, J.L.; Liang, Y.R.; et al. Food-grade encapsulation systems for (−)-epigallocatechingallate. *Molecules* **2018**, *23*, 445. [CrossRef] [PubMed]

94. Ye, J.H.; Augustin, M.A. Nano- and micro-particles for delivery of catechins: Physical and biological performance. *Crit. Rev. Food Sci.* **2018**. [CrossRef] [PubMed]

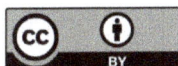

nutrients

MDPI

Article

Epigallocatechin-3-gallate and 6-OH-11-O-Hydroxyphenanthrene Limit BE(2)-C Neuroblastoma Cell Growth and Neurosphere Formation In Vitro

Fulvia Farabegoli [1,*], Marzia Govoni [2], Enzo Spisni [3] and Alessio Papi [3]

[1]   Department of Pharmacy and Biotechnology (FaBiT), University of Bologna, 40126 Bologna, Italy
[2]   Department of Experimental, Diagnostic and Specialty Medicine (DIMES), University of Bologna, 40138 Bologna, Italy; marzia.govoni@unibo.it
[3]   Department Biological, Geological, and Environmental Sciences (BiGeA), University of Bologna, 40126 Bologna, Italy; enzo.spisni@unibo.it (E.S.); alessio.papi2@unibo.it (A.P.)
*   Correspondence: fulvia.farabegoli@unibo.it; Tel.: +39-0512094717

Received: 9 July 2018; Accepted: 20 August 2018; Published: 22 August 2018

Abstract: We conducted an in vitro study combining a rexinoid, 6-OH-11-O-hydroxyphenanthrene (IIF), and epigallocatechin-3-gallate (EGCG), which is the main catechin of green tea, on BE(2)-C, a neuroblastoma cell line representative of the high-risk group of patients. Neuroblastoma is the most common malignancy of childhood: high-risk patients, having N-MYC over-expression, undergo aggressive therapy and show high mortality or an increased risk of secondary malignancies. Retinoids are used in neuroblastoma therapy with incomplete success: the association of a second molecule might improve the efficacy. BE(2)-C cells were treated by EGCG and IIF, individually or in combination: cell viability, as evaluated by 3-(4,5-dimethylthiazol-2-yl)-2,5-diphenyl tetrazolium bromide (MTT) assay, was reduced, EGCG+IIF being the most effective treatment. Apoptosis occurred and the EGCG+IIF treatment decreased N-MYC protein expression and molecular markers of invasion (MMP-2, MMP-9 and COX-2). Zymography demonstrated nearly 50% inhibition of MMP activity. When BE(2)-C cells were grown in non-adherent conditions to enrich the tumor-initiating cell population, BE(2)-C-spheres were obtained. After 48 h and 72 h treatment, EGCG+IIF limited BE(2)-C-sphere formation and elicited cell death with a reduction of N-MYC expression. We concluded that the association of EGCG to IIF might be applied without toxic effects to overcome the incomplete success of retinoid treatments in neuroblastoma patients.

Keywords: EGCG; 6-OH-11-O-hydroxyphenanthrene; neuroblastoma; BE(2)-C; N-MYC; neuro-sphere

1. Introduction

Neuroblastoma is the most common malignancy of childhood, arising from embryonic sympathetic neural cell precursors and accounting 12% of cancer deaths in children younger than 15 years of age. Neuroblastoma is a heterogeneous disease: patients belonging to low- or intermediate-risk groups have excellent long-term survival, whereas patients harboring a high-risk phenotype, which are characterized by widespread disease dissemination, show long-term survival rates below 50%. In high-risk patients, complete clinical remission is often followed by relapse and fatal outcome, possibly because of the persistence of neoplastic cells (minimal residual disease). Furthermore, high-risk patients are treated aggressively with chemotherapy, radiation, surgery, and myeloablative and immunotherapies, thus giving rise to short- and long-term toxicity. The current intensive therapeutic strategy is associated with an 18-fold increased risk of secondary neoplastic disease, mainly acute myelogenous leukemia [1,2]. For these reasons, more effective and less toxic treatments are needed in addition to the development of targeted therapies [3].

Retinoids are Vitamin A derivatives that include all-*trans*-retinoic acid (ATRA), 13-*cis*-retinoic acid, (13cRA), and fenretinide (4-HPR). Retinoic acid is one of the most effective differentiation inducers of neuroblastoma cells in vitro. Both ATRA and 13cRA can cause the arrest of cell growth and induce morphological differentiation of human neuroblastoma cell lines [4]. Clinical trials also demonstrated significantly improved survival in high-risk neuroblastoma patients. To control minimal residual disease, high-risk neuroblastoma patients are currently treated with the differentiating agent 13cRA at the completion of cytotoxic therapy (myeloablative therapy, followed by autologous hematopoietic stem cell transplantation), leading to a three-year disease-free survival rate in nearly 50% of patients [5,6]. Differences in the pharmacokinetic properties of 13cRA and ATRA (higher peak levels and a much longer half life for 13cRA with respect to ATRA) make 13cRA the best molecule for use in high-risk neuroblastoma [6].

Retinoids are usually well tolerated with minimal side-effects. However, certain high-risk cohorts, such as patients with N-MYC-amplified neuroblastoma, are innately resistant to retinoid therapy [7]. N-MYC is a neuronal-specific member of the MYC proto-oncogene family, which is expressed during normal neural crest development. Under normal regulation, N-MYC does not prevent terminal differentiation of neuroblasts, whereas aberrant N-MYC signaling alone is sufficient to induce neuroblastoma in animal models [8]. N-MYC amplification occurs in over 20% of neuroblastomas: both copy number increase and overexpression are the strongest negative prognostic factors in neuroblastoma [9]. N-MYC amplification contributes to metastasis, chemoresistance, and resistance to retinoic acid (RA) therapy [10]. The reasons for resistance are unknown, but recent results demonstrated that N-MYC and retinoic acid (RA) are antagonist regulators, with N-MYC overexpression preventing the normal transcriptional response to RA [7].

Preclinical and clinical data support the use of single drugs inhibiting multiple molecular targets or combination therapies involving multiple drugs to achieve greater antineoplastic activity and overcome drug resistance [11]: inhibition of multiple signaling pathways is emerging as a new paradigm for anticancer treatment. Our previous studies on human carcinoma cell lines demonstrated that when the synthetic retinoid 6-OH-11-O-hydroxyphenanthrene (IIF) was associated with epigallocatechin-3-gallate (EGCG), the most active catechin being present in green tea, cytotoxicy increased and molecules that were related to invasion were downregulated [12–14]. IIF was more effective than ATRA in arresting cell growth and differentiation in neuroblastoma cells [15]. As retinoid treatments were found to be synergistic with flavonoids, including EGCG [16,17], we investigated the cytotoxic effects of the EGCG plus IIF combination and the molecular network underlying the cytotoxic effects in a neuroblastoma cell line BE(2)-C, a clone of the SK-N-BE(2) neuroblastoma cell line having N-MYC amplification and p53 mutation and isolated from a bone marrow biopsy that was taken in a neuroblastoma patient after repeated courses of chemotherapy and radiotherapy. We also investigated the effects of EGCG and IIF on neurosphere formation. The neurosphere is considered a subpopulation of tumor-initiating cells (also called cancer stem cells) showing the capacity for self-renewal, multipotency, and tumor maintenance [18]. These cells are thought to play a central role in tumor initiation and progression, resistance to therapy, and metastasis formation, and to be primarily responsible for relapse and poor outcome.

2. Materials and Methods

2.1. Cell Lines

BE(2)-C cell line was purchased from the American Type Culture Collection (Rockville, MD, USA) and grown in Dulbecco's modified Eagle's medium (DMEM) (Sigma-Aldrich, St. Louis, MO, USA), supplemented with 10% fetal calf serum (FCS, Euroclone, Milan, Italy), 2 mM L-glutamine, 50 U/mL penicillin, and 50 µg/mL streptomycin in a humidified atmosphere with 5% CO_2.

Cell lines were routinely tested for mycoplasma infection by fluorescence microscope inspection after 4′,6-diamidino-2-phenylindole (DAPI) staining.

2.2. Neurosphere Formation Assay

The neurosphere assay is the gold standard method for studying normal and cancer stem cells. BE(2)-C cells (1×10^5) were grown in low attachment 24-well plates in DMEM/F12, supplemented with 40 ng/mL FGF, 20 ng/mL GF, B27 and 500 U/mL of penicillin/streptomycin. EGCG (20 µg/mL, corresponding to 43.6 µM) or IIF (10 µM) or the EGCG + IIF combination were dissolved in the medium to evaluate sphere formation. After 48 h and 72 h, the spheres were mechanically disaggregated and the cells were collected, centrifuged, stained by trypan blue, and then counted. Some cells were also used for RNA isolation and RT-PCR.

2.3. Reagents

EGCG, ʟ-glutamine, penicillin-streptomycin, 3-(4,5-dimethylthiazol-2-yl)-2,5-diphenyl tetrazolium bromide (MTT), 4′,6-diamidino-2-phenylindole (DAPI), 1,4-diazabicyclo(2.2.2)ctane (DABCO), basic fibroblast growth factor (bFGF), and epidermal growth factor (EGF) were all purchased by Sigma-Aldrich, St. Louis, MO, USA. B27 was provided by Thermo-Fisher, Waltham, MA, USA. 6-OH-11-O-hydroxyphenanthrene (IIF) (pat. WIPO W0 00/17143) was provided by K. Ammar, Houston, TX USA. E-MEM, Dulbecco's modified Eagle's medium (D-MEM), D-MEM/nutrient mixture F-12 (DMEM/F12), and FBS were purchased by Euroclone, Milan, Italy. Formalin (40%) was from Carlo Erba, Milan, Italy. Antibodies: anti-RARα and anti-RXRγ (Tema Ricerca, Bologna, Italy), anti-EGFR (Thermo Scientific, Waltham, MA, USA), anti-p1068EGFR (Novex, Life Technologies, Carlsbad, CA, USA), anti-Bcl-2 (Sigma-Aldrich, St. Louis, MO, USA), anti-Bax (Applied Biosystem, Monza, Italy) anti-PARP (Santa Cruz Biotechnology, Dallas, TX, USA), anti-COX-2 (Sigma-Aldrich, St. Louis, MO, USA), anti-N-MYC, anti MMP-2, MMP-9, and anti-TIMP-1 (all from Santa Cruz Biotechnology, Dallas, TX, USA), anti-β-tubulin (Sigma-Aldrich, St. Louis, MO, USA), anti-rabbit, and anti-mouse peroxidase conjugated antibodies (GE Healthcare, Milan, Italy).

2.4. EGCG and IIF Treatments

EGCG (10 mg/mL tock solution, stored at −20 °C) and IIF (780 µM in polyethylene glycol, stored at 4 °C) were dissolved in complete DMEM medium before treatments. EGCG concentrations from 5 to 20 µg/mL (corresponding to 10.9 µM−43.6 µM) and IIF 5−20 µM were used.

2.5. MTT Assay

Cells (20,000/well) were plated in triplicate in a 96-well plate and then incubated with EGCG and IIF, alone and in combination at the defined concentrations for 24, 48, and 72 h. The medium was removed and cells were washed with phosphate buffered saline (PBS). MTT (dissolved in PBS) was diluted in fresh complete medium to a final concentration of 0.5 mg/mL and then incubated at 37 °C. After 3 h, the medium was removed and 100 µL dimethyl sulfoxide (DMSO) was added. After 1 h (at room temperature) the purple formazan crystals were dissolved and the plates were read in a microplate reader (Bio-Rad, Hercules, CA, USA). Absorbance was set at 570 nm. The results were expressed as a percentage of treated on control samples (untreated cells).

2.6. Combination Index (CI)

Synergistic, additive, or antagonistic effects after EGCG and IIF treatments were evaluated by the combination index (CI) method, as previously reported [13]. Briefly, C > 1 indicates Antagonism, C = 1 indicates Additivity and C < 1 indicates Synergism.

2.7. RNA Isolation

RNA was isolated with PureZOL™ RNA Isolation Reagent (Bio-Rad laboratories, Berkeley, CA, USA), according to the manufacturer's specifications.

2.8. Reverse Transcriptase-Polymerase Chain Reaction (RT-PCR)

RT-PCR was performed by one-step RT-PCR kit from Thermo Fisher Scientific (Waltham, MA, USA), which enables retrotranscription and cDNA amplification to occur in a single step. β-actin was used as a housekeeping gene and the primers were added to the target gene primers in the same tube. The primer sequences are reported in Table S1. PCR products were loaded onto a 2% agarose gel, run in an electrophoresis chamber, stained by ethidium bromide, and visualized with a UV transilluminator. Bands were analyzed by Kodak Electrophoresis Detection and Analysis System (EDAS 290) (Eastman Kodak Company, Rochester, NY, USA).

2.9. Quantitative Polymerase Chain Reaction (qPCR)

Real Time Quantitative analysis of cDNA was performed using a fluorescent nucleic acid dye that was similar to SYBR Green (SsoFast™ EvaGreen Supermix, BioRad Laboratories Inc., Hercule, CA, USA) in a CFX96 system (BioRad Laboratories Inc., Hercule, CA, USA). Primer sequences are reported in Table S2. We used the $2^{-\Delta\Delta Ct}$ method for relative quantification of gene expression.

2.10. Western Blot

The cells were treated with EGCG and/or IIF for 24 h or 48 h and then dissolved in lysis buffer as previously described [19]. Cell lysates were size-fractioned in 10–12% SDS-polyacrylamide before transfer to Hybond TM-C Extra membranes (GE Healthcare, Buckinghamshire, UK). Membranes were blocked and incubated overnight at 4 °C with the antibodies. Anti-EGFR, anti-p 1068EGFR, anti-Bax, anti-Bcl2, anti-PARP, anti-RARα and anti-RXRγ, anti-MMP2, anti-MMP9, anti-COX-2, and anti-TIMP1 were diluted 1:500 and the anti-rabbit/mouse peroxidase conjugated antibodies (GE Healthcare, Buckinghamshire, UK) were diluted 1:1000. Bands were quantified by using densitometric image analysis software (Image Master VDS, Pharmacia Biotech, Sweden). Protein loading was controlled by anti-actin or anti-tubulin (1:1000) (both from Sigma-Aldrich, St. Louis, MO, USA) detection. Experiments were performed in triplicate, normalized against actin or tubulin control, and statistically evaluated. Stripping solution (Pierce, Waltham, MA, USA) was used to reprobe the same membranes.

2.11. Zymography

Cells were seeded and after 18 h were placed in serum-free medium (D-MEM) with EGCG or IIF or both for 24 h. MMP2 and MMP9 activity was determined by gelatine zymography, as previously described [12]. The MMP activities, indicated by clear bands of gelatin digestion on a blue background, were quantified by using densitometric image analysis software (Image Lab Master, Hercules, CA, USA).

2.12. Statistical Analysis

Statistical significance was assessed by ANOVA multiple comparison test with standard deviation (SD), as appropriate, while using PRISM 5.1 (GraphPad, La Jolla, CA, USA). The level for accepted statistical significance was $p < 0.05$.

3. Results

3.1. RAR and RXR Expression Changed after EGCG and IIF Treatments

Initiation of the retinoid signal is believed to require the formation of RAR-RXR protein heterodimers in the promoter regions of the retinoid target genes. We examined RAR and RXR mRNA expression and protein changes after individual and combined treatments. EGCG alone did not elicit any change in RARα, β or γ in BE(2)-C cells, whereas IIF, alone and/or in combination with EGCG, raised RARα, β or γ mRNA expression a hundredfold. As RARα was the main RAR isoform expressed in BE(2)-C cells (about 80%, data not shown) and mRNA expression was so greatly increased, we only investigated RARα protein expression by Western blot. We found that RARα protein expression nearly doubled in EGCG+IIF-treated samples (Figure 1B). RXR and particularly RXRγ are the main targets of IIF: as we found that RXRγ mRNA was hardly detectable (data not shown), we used a primer couple that is able to cover a homology region in RXRβ and γ genes, a strategy that we already applied elsewhere [12]. As expected, RXRα and βγ RNA expression augmented after IIF treatment and RXRγ protein expression increased significantly after all treatments (Figure 2). Interestingly, EGCG individual treatment significantly enhanced RXRγ protein expression (Figure 2C). PPARs are potential RXR ligands that are able to elicit a response in neuronal cells, including neuroblastoma cells: EGCG+IIF treatment increased PPARβ expression in BE(2)-C cells (Figure S1). In addition, the retinoid-dependent signaling was triggered by IIF when it was given alone and/or in combination with EGCG.

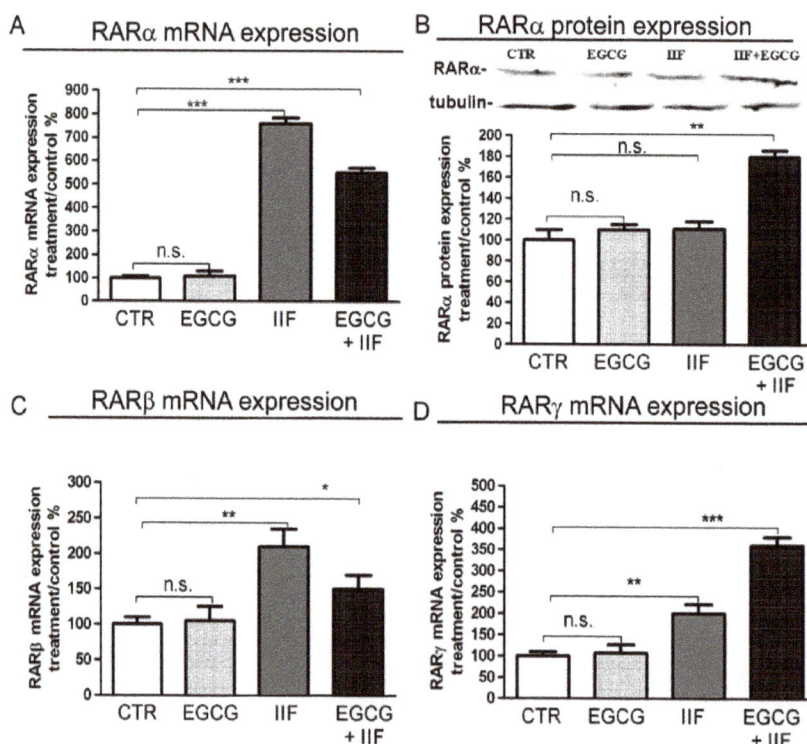

Figure 1. RARα β and γ mRNA expression and RARα protein expression in BE(2)-C neuroblastoma cells. Cells were treated with 20 µg/mL epigallocatechin-3-gallate (EGCG) and 10 µM 6-OH-11-O-hydroxyphenanthrene (IIF), individually and in combination for 24 h. (**A,C,D**) RARα β and γ mRNA expression as detected by qPCR in control (CTR) and treated samples. (**B**) RARα protein expression. Proteins (50 µg) from total cell lysates were subjected to Sodium Dodecyl Sulphate-PolyAcrylamide Gel Electrophoresis SDS–PAGE and Western blot analysis. The values were normalized to the untreated controls. β-tubulin was used as a loading control. The results are expressed as the average ± standard errors (SE) of three independent experiments. * $p < 0.05$; ** $p < 0.01$; *** $p < 0.001$. n.s.: not significant.

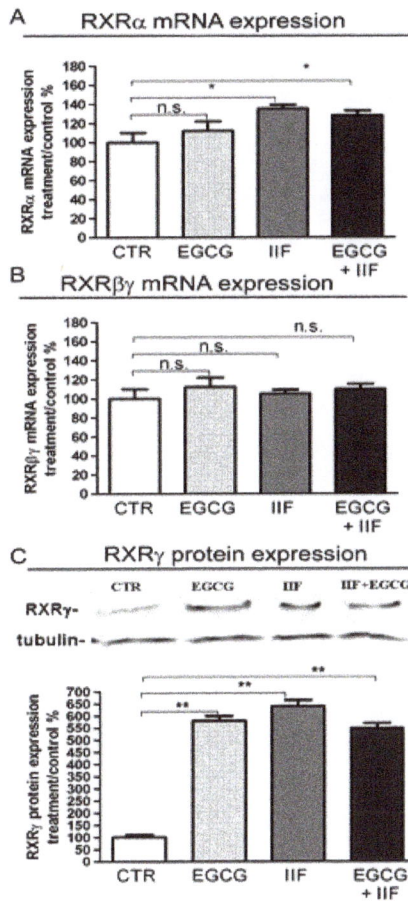

Figure 2. RARα β and γ mRNA expression and RXRγ protein expression in BE(2)-C neuroblastoma cells. Cells were treated with 20 μg/mL l EGCG and 10 μM 6-OH-11-O-hydroxyphenanthrene (IIF), individually and in combination for 24 h. RXRα (**A**) and RXRβγ (**B**) mRNA expression as detected by qPCR in control (CTR) and treated samples. (**C**) RXRγ protein expression. Proteins (50 μg) from total cell lysates were subjected to SDS–PAGE and Western blot analysis. The values were normalized to the untreated controls. β-tubulin was used as a loading control. The results are expressed as the average ± SE of three independent experiments. * $p < 0.05$; ** $p < 0.01$. n.s.: not significant.

3.2. Synergistic Effect of EGCG and IIF in Combination Enhanced Cytotoxicity and Activated Apoptosis in BE(2)-C Cells

After 72 h exposure to individual IIF and EGCG doses, the cell viability decreased to 62% (20 μg/mL EGCG) and 52% (20 μM IIF), respectively (Figure 3A,B). Combination treatments resulted in greater cytotoxicity, even using lower IIF concentrations: 10 μM IIF and 20 μg/mL EGCG given in combination to BE(2)-C cells for 72 h lowered cell viability to 26% (Figure 3C). Synergism was found using 10 μM IIF and 20 μg/mL EGCG: these concentrations were used for all of the subsequent experiments (Table S3). Increased cytotoxicity and inhibition of cell proliferation were associated with apoptosis, as demonstrated by Bax, Bcl-2, and PARP Western blot analysis. In our hands, Bax was nearly undetectable (data not shown), possibly related to apoptosis pathway dysregulation [20] or p53 missense mutation at codon 135 found in the BE(2)-C cell line [21,22]. A Bcl-2 decrease was clearly detected and it was primarily achieved by IIF activity, whereas PARP cleavage was mainly due to the EGCG effect (Figure 4), a finding that does not reflect synergism but diverse activity on the apoptosis pathway.

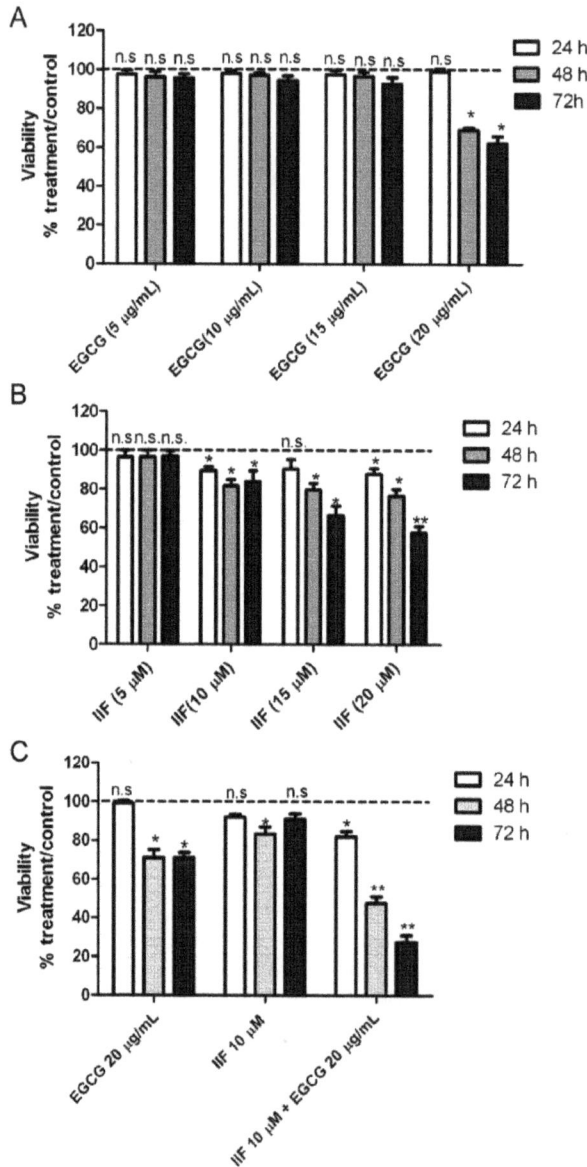

Figure 3. Inhibitory effects of EGCG and IIF treatments on BE(2)-C neuroblastoma cell growth as evaluated by 3-(4,5-dimethylthiazol-2-yl)-2,5-diphenyl tetrazolium bromide (MTT) assay. (**A**) EGCG cytotoxicity time-course (24 h–48 h–72 h) at different concentrations (5, 10, 15, 20 µg/mL). (**B**) IIF cytotoxicity time-course (24 h–48 h–72 h) at different concentrations (5, 10, 15, 20 µM). (**C**) EGCG (20 µg/mL) and IIF (10 µM) (EGCG+IIF) combination. The results are expressed as the average ± SE of three independent experiments. * $p < 0.05$; ** $p < 0.01$. n.s.: not significant.

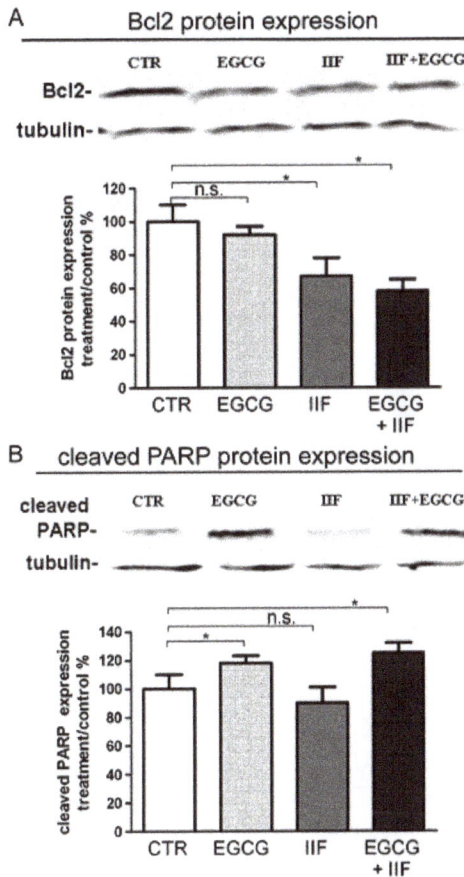

Figure 4. Effect of EGCG and IIF treatments on apoptosis-related proteins in BE(2)-C neuroblastoma cells. Modulation of Bcl-2 and cleaved PARP levels after 24 h individual and combined 20 μg/mL EGCG and 10 μM IIF treatments. Proteins (50 μg) from total cell lysates were subjected to SDS–PAGE and Western blot analysis while using Bcl-2 (**A**) and cleaved PARP antibodies (**B**). The values were normalized to the untreated controls. β-tubulin was used as a loading control. The results are expressed as the average ± SE of three independent experiments. * $p < 0.05$. n.s.: not significant.

3.3. EGCG and IIF Downregulated N-MYC Expression

N-MYC amplification and overexpression is the best-characterized genetic marker of risk in neuroblastoma. N-MYC is expressed in neural cells during development and is downregulated along with differentiation. In neuroblastoma, N-MYC amplification and/or overexpression play multiple roles in malignancy and maintenance of a stem-like state, as they can activate the transcription of genes that are involved in metastasis, survival, proliferation, pluripotency, self-renewal, and angiogenesis. We treated BE(2)-C cells with EGCG and IIF, evaluating N-MYC expression by q-PCR and Western blot. A significant mRNA N-MYC decrease was only found after 4 h EGCG+IIF treatment (Figure 5A,B). In contrast, N-MYC protein expression was dramatically reduced after combined treatment for 24 h (Figure 5C), a finding that might be due to synergism. Therefore, EGCG+IIF treatment was effective in reducing the N-MYC protein level in BE(2)-C cells.

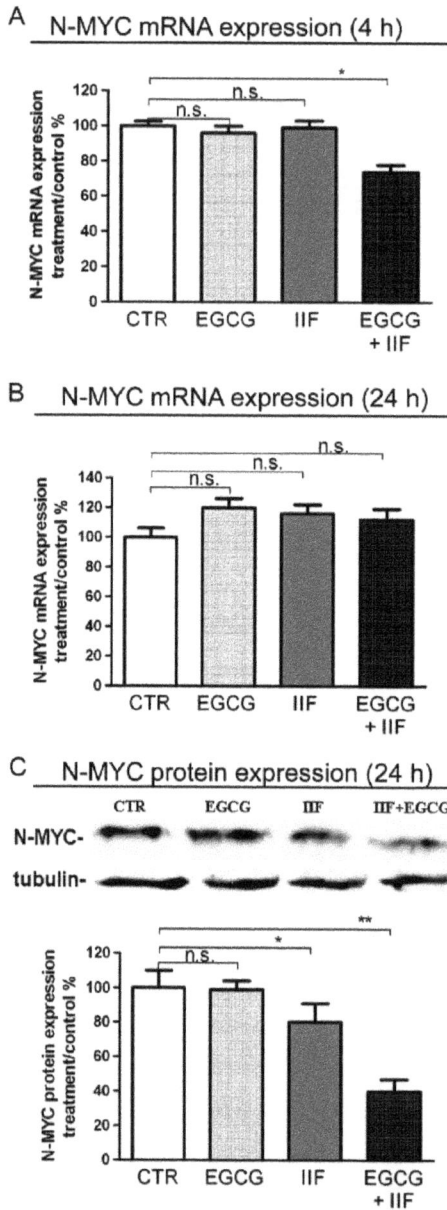

Figure 5. Downregulation of N-MYC expression by EGCG and IIF treatments in BE(2)-C neuroblastoma cells. Cells were treated with 20 μg/mL EGCG and 10 μM IIF, individually and in combination. N-MYC qPCR analysis in control and treated cells after 4 h (**A**) and 24 h (**B**). GAPDH was used as a control. (**C**) Proteins (50 μg) from total cell lysates were subjected to SDS–PAGE and Western blot analysis of N-MYC expression after 24 h treatments. The values were normalized to the untreated controls. β-tubulin was used as a loading control. The results are expressed as the average ± SE of three independent experiments. * $p < 0.05$; ** $p < 0.01$. n.s.: not significant. GAPDH: Glyceraldehyde 3-phosphate dehydrogenase.

3.4. Molecular Targets of EGCG and IIF and N-MYC Downregulation

EGFR is a gene that is directly downregulated by N-MYC [23], which is often overexpressed in neuroblastoma, and previously demonstrated to be a molecular target of both EGCG and IIF [12,14]. EGFR expression was detected in control BE(2)-C cells: protein expression was reduced as was p1068 phosphorylation (Figure 6A) in keeping with a significant decrease of RNA expression after both individual and combined treatments (Figure 6B). N-MYC and EGFR expression are reciprocally related with N-MYC downregulated gene 1 (NDRG1). NDRG1 is a transcription factor that is implicated in growth arrest, cell differentiation, and response to hypoxia, and it is regarded as an anti-metastatic molecule in prostate carcinoma [24]. Furthermore, NDRG1 can be upregulated by retinoic acid. N-MYC downregulation was found to induce re-expression of NDRG1 that, in turn, can repress the HER family oncogenes, including EGFR [25]. We found that NDRG1 was expressed in untreated BE(2)-C cells: after 24 h, treatments no significant change was detected (Figure 6C).

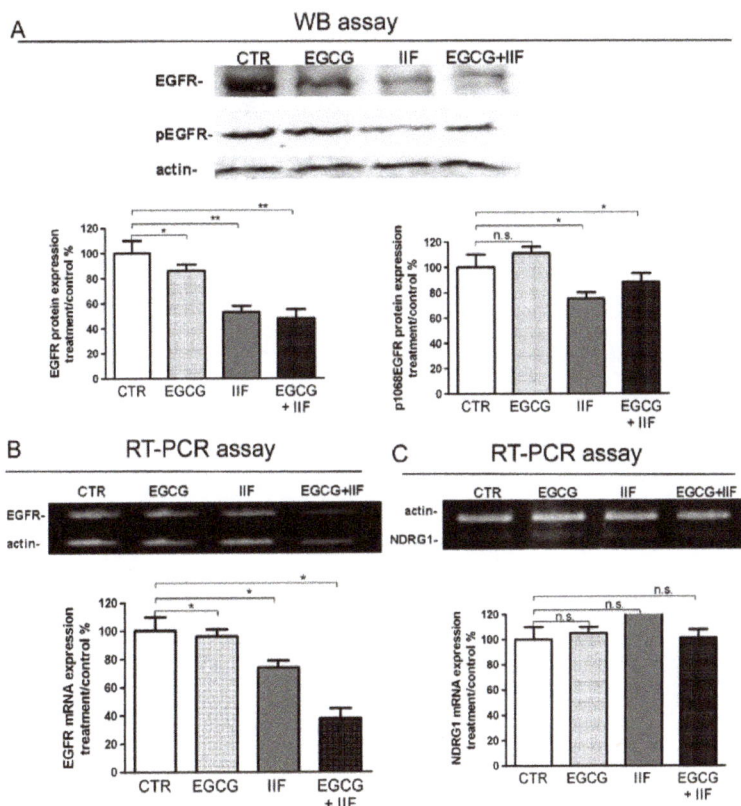

Figure 6. Downregulation of EGFR and p1068EGFR expression by EGCG and IIF treatments in BE(2)-C neuroblastoma cells. Cells were treated with 20 µg/mL EGCG and 10 µM IIF, individually and in combination for 24 h. (**A**) Proteins (50 µg) from total cell lysate were subjected to SDS–PAGE and Western blot analysis of EGFR and p1068EGFR expression after 24 h treatments. Actin was used as a loading control. RT-PCR analysis of EGFR (**B**) and NDRG1 (**C**) in control and treated cells. β-actin was used as a control. The values were normalized to the untreated controls. The results are expressed as the average ± SE of three independent experiments. $* p < 0.05$; $** p < 0.01$. n.s.: not significant. WB: western blot; RT-PCR: reverse transcriptase-polymerase chain reaction.

3.5. EGCG and IIF Limited Invasion and Metastatic Capability

N-MYC overexpression contributes to all phases, leading to metastasis: loss of cell adhesion, increased motility, invasion, and degradation of surrounding matrices. Our previous studies on human carcinoma demonstrated that the EGCG+IIF combination was very effective in decreasing the expression of MMP-2 and MMP-9, which are molecular markers of invasion.

MMP-2 and MMP-9 qPCR showed that MMP-2 mRNA and protein expression were significantly lowered by EGCG+IIF treatments (Figure 7A,B). To further investigate the functional activity of MMP-2 and 9, we turned to zymography, which detects MMP activity. We found that both EGCG and EGCG+IIF-treated samples showed around 50% MMP-2 and MMP-9 inhibition (Figure 7C): so EGCG resulted more active than IIF in inhibiting MMP activity. In parallel, TIMP-1, which negatively regulates MMP-9, was upregulated (Figure 8C). We investigated the effects on COX-2, a molecule that is associated with osteolytic bone metastasis in neuroblastoma [26], which promotes MMP expression. We observed that COX2 mRNA and protein expression were also downregulated (Figure 8A,B): in this case, a synergistic effect may be speculated. We concluded that, in addition to N-MYC downregulation, EGCG+IIF treatment attenuated the biopathological features of metastatic potential.

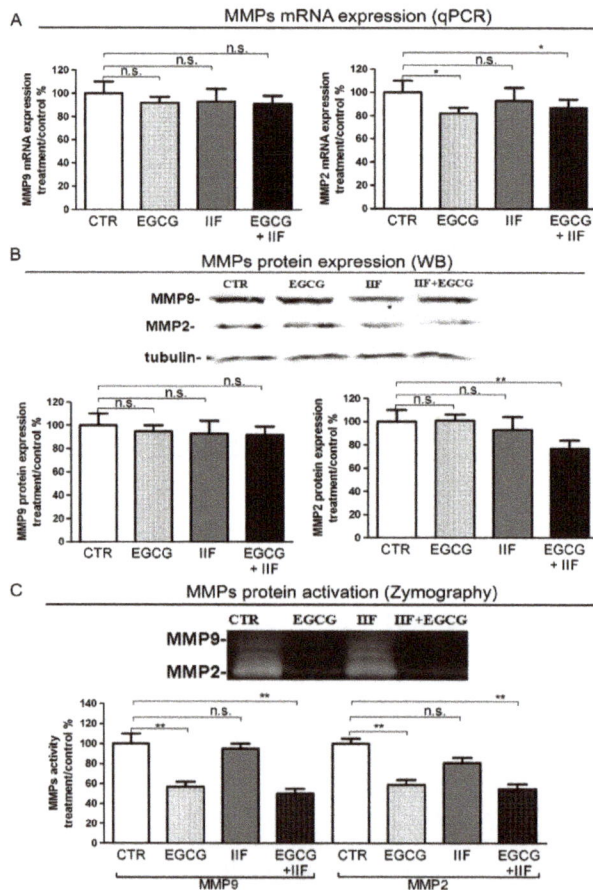

Figure 7. MMP-2 and MMP-9 expression and activity after EGCG and IIF treatments in BE(2)-C neuroblastoma cells. Cells were treated with 20 μg/mL EGCG and 10 μM IIF, individually and in combination for 24 h. (**A**) MMP-2 and MMP-9 qPCR was performed after RNA isolation and GAPDH

was used as an internal control. (**B**) Western blot analysis of MMP-2 and MMP-9. The values were normalized to the untreated controls. β-tubulin was used as a loading control. (**C**) Zymography analysis of MMP-2 and MMP-9. Cells were seeded and after 18 h placed in serum-free medium with EGCG (20 μg/mL) or IIF (10 μM) or both for 24 h. MMP activity is indicated by clear bands. The results are expressed as the average ± SE of three independent experiments. * $p < 0.05$; ** $p < 0.01$. n.s.: not significant. MMP-2: Metalloproteinase-2 (MMP-2); MMP-9: Metalloproteinase-9.

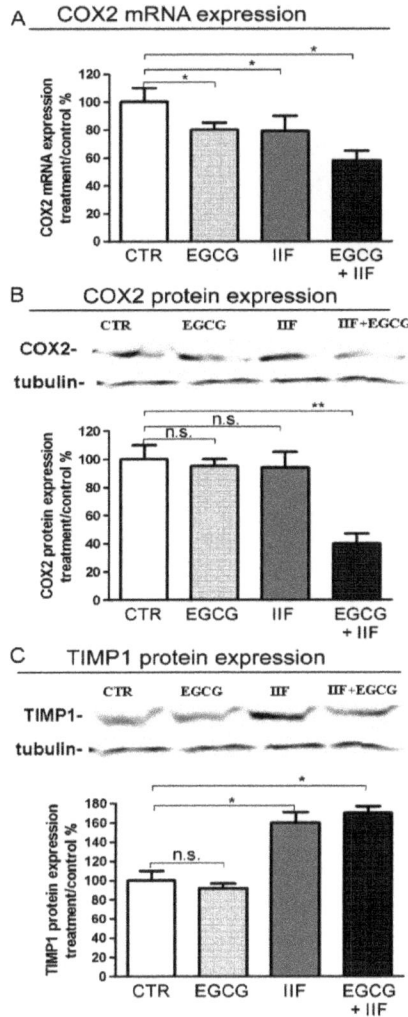

Figure 8. COX-2 and TIMP-1 expression after EGCG and IIF treatments in BE(2)-C neuroblastoma cells. (**A**) Cells were treated with 20 μg/mL EGCG and 10 μM IIF, individually and in combination for 24 h. (**A**) qPCR of COX-2 expression was performed after RNA isolation. GAPDH was used as an internal control. Western blot analysis of COX-2 (**B**) and TIMP-1 (**C**). The values were normalized to the untreated controls. β-tubulin was used as a loading control. The results are expressed as the average ± SE of three independent experiments. * $p < 0.05$; ** $p < 0.01$. n.s.: not significant.

3.6. EGCG and IIF Impaired Sphere Formation in BE(2)-C Cells

Neuroblastoma is a stem-like cell disease: neuroblastoma cancer cells can undergo tumor sphere transformation when grown under serum-free conditions. We investigated the effects of EGCG and IIF treatments on BE(2)-C sphere formation and viability, as evaluated by Trypan blue assay. In the control samples, spheres were clearly detected after 48 h. Incubation with EGCG and IIF at 48 h and 72 h reduced the sphere number and size (Figure 9A). Trypan blue assay demonstrated a cytotoxic effect: after 72 h treatment viability decreased to 50%. N-MYC gene expression significantly decreased after all the treatments (Figure 9B). We therefore concluded that individual and combined treatments with EGCG and IIF impaired sphere formation and increased cytotoxicity: a synergistic effect was detected after 48 h of treatment (Table S4).

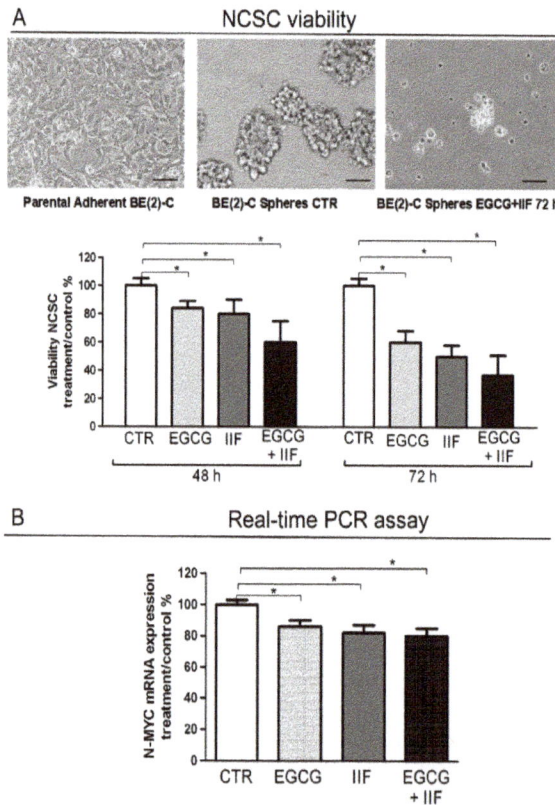

Figure 9. EGCG and IIF treatments limited sphere formation and N-MYC expression in BE(2)-C neuroblastoma cells. (**A**) Neural cancer stem cells (NCSC). Parental adherent BE(2)-cells were grown in non-adherent serum-free conditions to develop spheres for 72 h (CTR) and treated with 20 µg/mL EGCG and 10 µM IIF, individually and in combination for 72 h. Viability was evaluated by Trypan blue assay. (**B**) N-MYC mRNA expression was evaluated by qPCR in control (CTR) and treated cells. GAPDH was used as a loading control. The results are expressed as the average ± SE of three independent experiments. * $p < 0.05$. n.s.: not significant.

4. Discussion

We studied the effects of EGCG and IIF on BE(2)-C, a neuroblastoma cell line representative of high-risk neuroblastoma patients, and on BE(2)-C-spheres, which is a derivative BE(2)-C subpopulation, grown in low attachment conditions and serum-free medium, thought to correspond to cancer stem cells. We found a significant arrest of cell growth together with downregulation of N-MYC expression and molecular markers of invasion. Furthermore, the EGCG and IIF combination was cytotoxic: sphere formation was impaired and cell death occurred in a significant percentage of cells after 48 and 72 h. Overall, these findings demonstrated the efficacy of EGCG and IIF to limit neuroblastoma cell growth.

EGCG and green tea catechins are considered powerful antioxidant and chemopreventive molecules. They have been found to serve as antioxidants and improve the detoxification system, thereby inhibiting carcinogen metabolism and cancerogenesis. Furthermore, they limit cancer cell proliferation and tumor-initiating cell self-renewal by modulating the numerous molecules fundamental for cancer onset and progression [27]. Retinoids are used in neuroblastoma therapy: high-risk neuroblastoma patients are treated with 13cRA in postconsolidation therapy after autologous hematopoietic stem cell transplantation [5]. Retinoids are capable of inducing differentiation at low doses, but many high-risk neuroblastoma patients do not respond to 13cRA treatment [4]. Adverse effects were not severe, but better results were achieved while combining 13cRA with immunotherapy [28] or the histone deacetylase inhibitor Vorinostat [6]. The combination of ATRA, 13-cRA, and 4-HPR with EGCG was investigated on SH-SY5Y cells, which is a neuroblastoma cell line lacking N-MYC amplification and overexpression, resulting in cell growth inhibition, apoptosis and N-MYC protein decrease [16]. IIF is a synthetic and safe derivative of Vitamin A, used as a food supplement, which demonstrated enhanced anti-neoplastic effects in neuroblastoma and various cancer cell lines [29]. When IIF was given in combination with EGCG to breast and colorectal carcinoma cell lines, cytotoxicity increased with downregulation of the molecular markers of neoplastic progression [12–14]. In BE(2)-C cells, EGCG+IIF treatment downregulated N-MYC protein expression, whereas mRNA was reduced only after 4h EGCG+IIF treatment. N-MYC is considered to be the most prominent molecular marker in neuroblastoma therapy, but it is not a directly targetable molecule [30]. N-MYC expression is high during early developmental stages then gradually subsides as the neural crest precursors differentiate into sympathetic neurons. Aberrantly high N-MYC is thought to contribute to neuroblastoma development, at least in part, by promoting a persistent mesenchymal phenotype within neuroblastoma cells. Strategies to circumvent N-MYC activity include the targeting regulators of N-MYC mRNA and protein stability, and differentiation agents [10]. We found that EGCG and IIF decreased N-MYC protein expression, with a modest impact on mRNA expression after 4h treatment, in keeping with data obtained using other molecules regulating N-MYC protein stability by different mechanisms (LY294002, BEZ235, AURAKA ligands) [10]. Indeed, a significant inhibition of N-MYC mRNA expression was found after 72 h EGCG and IIF treatments of the BE(2)-C sphere. This discrepancy might be attributed to different treatment time and cell population analyzed. NSCS is a minority subset of the tumor cell population, which is thought to be rich in tumor-initiating cells [31] considered responsible for drug resistance, local relapse and metastatic spread. N-MYC promotes a stem-like state by impairing the differentiation pathways and supporting self-renewal and pluripotency. N-MYC-amplified neuroblastoma cell lines, including BE(2)-C cells, form spheres more frequently than non-N-MYC-amplified cell lines and sphere formation is sensitive to cellular differentiation status [32]. In the present study, BE(2)-C sphere formation was reduced and associated with cell death after EGCG and IIF treatments. In addition, the EGCG and IIF combination was effective in limiting cell growth in both adherent BE(2)-C cells and the BE(2)-C sphere, possibly by downregulation of N-MYC. We cannot exclude that EGCG and IIF treatments might act in adherent and sphere BE(2)-C cells by different mechanisms: N-MYC acts in the context of a large protein network. A specific subset of genes might regulate N-MYC in the stem-like or lineage committed pattern. This point needs to be clarified and it goes beyond the aim of the present study, but this finding makes EGCG and IIF molecules potentially useful in patients in the remission phase, as they might limit and kill the tumor-initiating cells that are responsible for relapse and therapeutic failure.

The efficacy of EGCG and IIF treatments against BE-(2)-C cells extended beyond their cytotoxic activity to include changes and downregulation of molecules that are associated with the invasive

Nutrients **2018**, *10*, 1141

phenotype. In some cases, this effect was clearly synergistic (MTT, N-MYC, and COX2 protein downregulation); in others, the individual effects of EGCG or IIF predominated. Whereas, IIF belongs to class of molecules that are known to target a specific signaling pathway, EGCG is a polytarget molecule that is able to down or upregulate numerous different molecules. We can speculate that, in some cases, the final effects resulted from an independent regulation of different molecules. In human neuroblastoma cells, N-MYC and Bcl-2 co-expression induced MMP-2 secretion and activation [33]. In the present study, zymography demonstrated significant inactivation of both MMP-2 and MMP-9. The EGCG+IIF treatment was not more effective than individual EGCG treatments, as IIF did not significantly reduce MMP-2 and -9 activity. Likewise, the expression of TIMP-1, which is a negative regulator of MMP-9, increased after IIF and EGCG+IIF treatments, a finding that explains the downregulation of MMP-9 activity. The combined EGCG+IIF treatment also downregulated COX-2, which is a strong pro-inflammatory molecule that enhances MMP expression and activity.

The major signaling pathways leading to uncontrolled tumor growth and aggressive behavior in high-risk neuroblastoma patients are related to a small number of altered genes, N-MYC being one of the most important. With respect to many solid tumors, primary neuroblastoma shows an unexpectedly low genetic complexity [34], but the outcome in high-risk patients remains dismal. EGFR is often expressed in neuroblastoma, but there is no consensus on its role and prognostic impact [35]. In mice, EGF (and EGFR) is a key molecule in sympathoadrenal progenitor migration to either the analogue of the paravertebral sympathetic ganglia or adrenal medulla/suprarenal sympathetic ganglia. Different cell origin might explain the distinct worse clinical presentations of adrenal neuroblastoma when compared to non-adrenal derivative neoplasm [36]. A few neuroblastoma patients proved responsive to EGFR inhibitors such as Gefitinib, but only in association with other drugs [37]. In breast carcinoma, we demonstrated that EGFR is a molecular target of both EGCG and IIF, but the present study failed to find a relation between N-MYC and EGFR in BE(2)-C cells. Although IIF induced a significant increase in mRNA NDRG1 expression and EGFR (mRNA, total protein, and p1068EGFR) decreased, the real meaning and role of EGFR activity in neuroblastoma require further investigation.

In conclusion, an RXR agonist (IIF) that is associated with a polytarget molecule (EGCG) might be a promising adjunct to improve the outcome of retinoid treatment. Both of the molecules are used as food supplements, lack side-effects, and are considered beneficial for human health. EGCG, in particular, has been widely investigated in healthy volunteers ruling out toxic effects. Our previous study also found no cytotoxic effect on normal human peripheral blood lymphocytes after EGCG treatments [12]. IIF was not toxic in animals [38] and it is now sold as a food supplement in the USA. High-risk neuroblastoma patients who survive and do not relapse may experience long-term toxic effects, chronic diseases and increased risk of tumor recurrence. In the search for less aggressive but efficient therapies, the EGCG and IIF combination is a promising candidate.

Supplementary Materials: The following are available online at http://www.mdpi.com/2072-6643/10/9/1141/s1, Table S1. Primer sequences for RT-PCR. Table S2. Primer sequences for qPCR. Figure S1: PPAR and PPAR mRNA expression in BE(2)-C neuroblastoma cells. Table S3. Combination Index (CI). Table S4. Combination index (CI).

Author Contributions: F.F. and A.P. designed the study. F.F., A.P. and M.G. contributed with their expertise to provide and elaborate data for the study. A.P. carried out the statistical evaluation. F.F. drafted the manuscript. A.P., M.G. and E.S. revised the manuscript. All authors approved the final version of manuscript.

Funding: This research received no external funding.

Acknowledgments: This work was supported by the University of Bologna (RFO grant to Fulvia Farabegoli and Enzo Spisni). We are grateful to Anne Collins for editing the English text.

Conflicts of Interest: The authors declare they have no conflict of interest.

References

1. Speleman, F.; Park, J.R.; Henderson, T.O. Neuroblastoma: A Tough Nut to Crack. *Am. Soc. Clin. Oncol. Educ. Book* **2016**, *35*, e548–e557. [CrossRef] [PubMed]

2. Applebaum, M.A.; Desai, A.V.; Glade Bender, J.L.; Cohn, S.L. Emerging and investigational therapies for neuroblastoma. *Expert Opin. Orphan Drugs* **2017**, *5*, 355–368. [CrossRef] [PubMed]
3. Maris, J.M. Recent advances in neuroblastoma. *N. Engl. J. Med.* **2010**, *362*, 2202–2211. [CrossRef] [PubMed]
4. Reynolds, C.P.; Matthay, K.K.; Villablanca, J.G.; Maurer, B.J. Retinoid therapy of high-risk neuroblastoma. *Cancer Lett.* **2003**, *197*, 185–192. [CrossRef]
5. Peinemann, F.; van Dalen, E.C.; Enk, H.; Berthold, F. Retinoic acid postconsolidation therapy for high-risk neuroblastoma patients treated with autologous haematopoietic stem cell transplantation. *Cochrane Database Syst. Rev.* **2017**, *8*, CD010685. [CrossRef] [PubMed]
6. Masetti, R.; Biagi, C.; Zama, D.; Vendemini, F.; Martoni, A.; Morello, W.; Gasperini, P.; Pession, A. Retinoids in pediatric onco-hematology: The model of acute promyelocytic leukemia and neuroblastoma. *Adv. Ther.* **2012**, *29*, 747–762. [CrossRef] [PubMed]
7. Duffy, D.J.; Krstic, A.; Halasz, M.; Schwarzl, T.; Konietzny, A.; Iljin, K.; Higgins, D.G.; Kolch, W. Retinoic acid and TGF-β signalling cooperate to overcome MYCN-induced retinoid resistance. *Genome Med.* **2017**, *9*, 15. [CrossRef] [PubMed]
8. Schulte, J.H.; Lindner, S.; Bohrer, A.; Maurer, J.; De Preter, K.; Lefever, S.; Heukamp, L.; Schulte, S.; Molenaar, J.; Versteeg, R.; et al. MYCN and ALKF1174L are sufficient to drive neuroblastoma development from neural crest progenitor cells. *Oncogene* **2013**, *32*, 1059–1065. [CrossRef] [PubMed]
9. Brodeur, G.M. Neuroblastoma: Biological insights into a clinical enigma. *Nat. Rev. Cancer* **2003**, *3*, 203–216. [CrossRef] [PubMed]
10. Huang, M.; Weiss, W.A. Neuroblastoma and MYCN. *Cold Spring Harb. Perspect. Med.* **2013**, *3*, a014415. [CrossRef] [PubMed]
11. Faivre, S.; Djelloul, S.; Raymond, E. New paradigms in anticancer therapy: Targeting multiple signaling pathways with kinase inhibitors. *Semin. Oncol.* **2006**, *33*, 407–420. [CrossRef] [PubMed]
12. Farabegoli, F.; Govoni, M.; Ciavarella, C.; Orlandi, M.; Papi, A. A RXR ligand 6-OH-11-O-hydroxyphenanthrene with antitumour properties enhances (-)-epigallocatechin-3-gallate activity in three human breast carcinoma cell lines. *BioMed Res. Int.* **2014**, *2014*, 853086. [CrossRef] [PubMed]
13. Papi, A.; Govoni, M.; Ciavarella, C.; Spisni, E.; Orlandi, M.; Farabegoli, F. Epigallocatechin-3-gallate Increases RXRγ-mediated Pro-apoptotic and Anti-invasive Effects in Gastrointestinal Cancer Cell Lines. *Curr. Cancer Drug Targets* **2016**, *16*, 373–385. [CrossRef] [PubMed]
14. Farabegoli, F.; Govoni, M.; Spisni, E.; Papi, A. EGFR inhibition by (-)-epigallocatechin-3-gallate and IIF treatments reduces breast cancer cell invasion. *Biosci. Rep.* **2017**, *37*, BSR20170168. [CrossRef] [PubMed]
15. Bartolini, G.; Orlandi, M.; Ammar, K.; Magrini, E.; Ferreri, A.M.; Rocchi, P. Effect of a new derivative of retinoic acid on proliferation and differentiation in human neuroblastoma cells. *Anticancer Res.* **2003**, *23*, 1495–1499. [PubMed]
16. Das, A.; Banik, N.L.; Ray, S.K. Retinoids induce differentiation and downregulate telomerase activity and N-MYC to increase sensitivity to flavonoids for apoptosis in human malignant neuroblastoma SH-SY5Y cells. *Int. J. Oncol.* **2009**, *34*, 757–765. [CrossRef] [PubMed]
17. Chakrabarti, M.; Khandkar, M.; Banik, N.L.; Ray, S.K. Alterations in expression of specific microRNAs by combination of 4-HPR and EGCG inhibited growth of human malignant neuroblastoma cells. *Brain Res.* **2012**, *1454*, 1–13. [CrossRef] [PubMed]
18. Garner, E.F.; Beierle, E.A. Cancer Stem Cells and Their Interaction with the Tumor Microenvironment in Neuroblastoma. *Cancers* **2015**, *8*, 5. [CrossRef] [PubMed]
19. Papi, A.; Ferreri, A.M.; Rocchi, P.; Guerra, F.; Orlandi, M. Epigenetic modifiers as anticancer drugs: Effectiveness of valproic acid in neural crest-derived tumor cells. *Anticancer Res.* **2010**, *30*, 535–540. [PubMed]
20. Goldsmith, K.C.; Lestini, B.J.; Gross, M.; Lp, L.; Bhumbla, A.; Zhang, X.; Zhao, H.; Liu, X.; Hogarty, M.D. Mitochondrial Bcl-2 family dynamics define therapy response and resistance in neuroblastoma. *Cell Death Differ.* **2010**, *17*, 872–882. [CrossRef] [PubMed]
21. Keshelava, N.; Zuo, J.J.; Chen, P.; Waidyaratne, S.N.; Luna, M.C.; Gomer, C.J.; Triche, T.J.; Reynolds, C.P. Loss of p53 function confers high-level multidrug resistance in neuroblastoma cell lines. *Cancer Res.* **2001**, *61*, 6185–6193. [PubMed]
22. McCurrach, M.E.; Connor, T.M.; Knudson, C.M.; Korsmeyer, S.J.; Lowe, S.W. *bax*-deficiency promotes drug resistance and oncogenic transformation by attenuating p53-dependent apoptosis. *Proc. Natl. Acad. Sci. USA* **1997**, *94*, 2345–2349. [CrossRef] [PubMed]

23. Perini, G.; Diolaiti, D.; Porro, A.; Della Valle, G. In vivo transcriptional regulation of N-MYC target genes is controlled by E-box methylation. *Proc. Natl. Acad. Sci. USA* **2005**, *102*, 12117–12122. [CrossRef] [PubMed]

24. Sharma, A.; Mendonca, J.; Ying, J.; Kim, H.S.; Verdone, J.E.; Zarif, J.C.; Carducci, M.; Hammers, H.; Pienta, K.J.; Kachhap, S. The prostate metastasis suppressor gene NDRG1 differentially regulates cell motility and invasion. *Mol. Oncol.* **2017**, *11*, 655–669. [CrossRef] [PubMed]

25. Kovacevic, Z.; Menezes, S.V.; Sahni, S.; Kalinowski, D.S.; Bae, D.H.; Lane, D.J.; Richardson, D.R. The Metastasis Suppressor, N-MYC Downstream-regulated Gene-1 (NDRG1), Down-regulates the ErbB Family of Receptors to Inhibit Downstream Oncogenic Signaling Pathways. *J. Biol. Chem.* **2016**, *291*, 1029–1052. [CrossRef] [PubMed]

26. Tsutsumimoto, T.; Williams, P.; Yoneda, T. The SK-N-AS human neuroblastoma cell line develops osteolytic bone metastases with increased angiogenesis and COX-2 expression. *J. Bone Oncol.* **2014**, *3*, 67–76. [CrossRef] [PubMed]

27. Sur, S.; Panda, C.K. Molecular aspects of cancer chemopreventive and therapeutic efficacies of tea and tea polyphenols. *Nutrition* **2017**, *43–44*, 8–15. [CrossRef] [PubMed]

28. Handgretinger, R.; Schlegel, P. Emerging role of immunotherapy for childhood cancers. *Chin. Clin. Oncol.* **2018**, *7*, 14. [CrossRef] [PubMed]

29. Papi, A.; Orlandi, M. Role of nuclear receptors in breast cancer stem cells. *World J. Stem Cells* **2016**, *8*, 62–72. [CrossRef] [PubMed]

30. Fletcher, J.I.; Ziegler, D.S.; Trahair, T.N.; Marshall, G.M.; Haber, M.; Norris, M.D. Too many targets, not enough patients: Rethinking neuroblastoma clinical trials. *Nat. Rev. Cancer* **2018**, *18*, 389–400. [CrossRef] [PubMed]

31. Nishimura, N.; Hartomo, T.B.; Pham, T.V.; Lee, M.J.; Yamamoto, T.; Morikawa, S.; Hasegawa, D.; Takeda, H.; Kawasaki, K.; Kosaka, Y.; et al. Epigallocatechin gallate inhibits sphere formation of neuroblastoma BE(2)-C cells. *Environ. Health Prev. Med.* **2012**, *17*, 246–251. [CrossRef] [PubMed]

32. Craig, B.T.; Rellinger, E.J.; Alvarez, A.L.; Dusek, H.L.; Qiao, J.; Chung, D.H. Induced differentiation inhibits sphere formation in neuroblastoma. *Biochem. Biophys. Res. Commun.* **2016**, *477*, 255–259. [CrossRef] [PubMed]

33. Noujaim, D.; van Golen, C.M.; van Golen, K.L.; Grauman, A.; Feldman, E.L. N-MYC and Bcl-2 coexpression induces MMP-2 secretion and activation in human neuroblastoma cells. *Oncogene* **2002**, *21*, 4549–4557. [CrossRef] [PubMed]

34. Uryu, K.; Nishimura, R.; Kataoka, K.; Sato, Y.; Nakazawa, A.; Suzuki, H.; Yoshida, K.; Seki, M.; Hiwatari, M.; Isobe, T.; et al. Identification of the genetic and clinical characteristics of neuroblastomas using genome-wide analysis. *Oncotarget* **2017**, *8*, 107513–107529. [CrossRef] [PubMed]

35. Light, J.E.; Koyama, H.; Minturn, J.E.; Ho, R.; Simpson, A.M.; Iyer, R.; Mangino, J.L.; Kolla, V.; London, W.B.; Brodeur, G.M. Clinical significance of NTRK family gene expression in neuroblastomas. *Pediatr. Blood Cancer* **2012**, *59*, 226–232. [CrossRef] [PubMed]

36. Tsubota, S.; Kadomatsu, K. Origin and initiation mechanisms of neuroblastoma. *Cell Tissue Res.* **2018**, *372*, 211–221. [CrossRef] [PubMed]

37. Furman, W.L.; McGregor, L.M.; McCarville, M.B.; Onciu, M.; Davidoff, A.M.; Kovach, S.; Hawkins, D.; McPherson, V.; Houghton, P.J.; Billups, C.A.; et al. A single-arm pilot phase II study of gefitinib and irinotecan in children with newly diagnosed high-risk neuroblastoma. *Investig. New Drugs* **2012**, *30*, 1660–1670. [CrossRef] [PubMed]

38. Papi, A.; Tatenhorst, L.; Terwel, D.; Hermes, M.; Kummer, M.P.; Orlandi, M.; Heneka, M.T. PPARgamma and RXRgamma ligands act synergistically as potent antineoplastic agents in vitro and in vivo glioma models. *J. Neurochem.* **2009**, *109*, 1779–1790. [CrossRef] [PubMed]

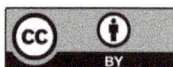

nutrients

MDPI

Article

Polyphenols in Liubao Tea Can Prevent CCl$_4$-Induced Hepatic Damage in Mice through Its Antioxidant Capacities

Yanni Pan [1,2,3,4,5], Xingyao Long [1,2,3,5], Ruokun Yi [1,2,3] and Xin Zhao [1,2,3,*]

1   Chongqing Collaborative Innovation Center for Functional Food, Chongqing University of Education, Chongqing 400067, China; panyanni@foods.ac.cn (Y.P.); longyaoyao@foods.ac.cn (X.L.); yirk@cque.edu.cn (R.Y.)
2   Chongqing Engineering Research Center of Functional Food, Chongqing University of Education, Chongqing 400067, China
3   Chongqing Engineering Laboratory for Research and Development of Functional Food, Chongqing University of Education, Chongqing 400067, China
4   College of Biological and Chemical Engineering, Chongqing University of Education, Chongqing 400067, China
5   Department of Food Science and Biotechnology, Cha University, Gyeongghi-do 487-010, South Korea
*   Correspondence: zhaoxin@cque.edu.cn; Tel.: +86-23-6265-3650

Received: 1 August 2018; Accepted: 7 September 2018; Published: 10 September 2018

Abstract: The present study investigated the preventive effect of polyphenols in Liubao tea (PLT) on carbon tetrachloride (CCl$_4$)-induced liver injury in mice. The mice were initially treated with PLT, followed by induction of liver injury using 10 mL/kg CCl$_4$. Then liver and serum indices, as well as the expression levels of related messenger RNAs (mRNAs) and proteins in liver tissues were measured. The results showed that PLT reduces the liver quality and indices of mice with liver injury. PLT also downregulates aspartate aminotransferase (AST), alanine aminotransferase (ALT), triglycerides (TGs), and malondialdehyde (MDA), and upregulates superoxide dismutase (SOD) and glutathione peroxidase (GSH-Px) in the sera of mice with liver injury. PLT also reduces serum levels of interleukin-6 (IL-6), interleukin-12 (IL-12), tumor necrosis factor-α (TNF-α), and interferon-γ (IFN-γ) cytokines in mice with liver injury. Pathological morphological observation also shows that PLT reduces CCl$_4$-induced central venous differentiation of liver tissues and liver cell damage. Furthermore, qPCR and Western blot also confirm that PLT upregulates the mRNA and protein expressions of Gu/Zn-SOD, Mn-SOD, catalase (CAT), GSH-Px, and nuclear factor of κ-light polypeptide gene enhancer in B-cells inhibitor-α (IκB-α) in liver tissues, and downregulates the expression of cyclooxygenase 2 (COX-2) and nuclear factor κ-light-chain-enhancer of activated B cells (NF-κB). Meanwhile, PLT also raised the phosphorylated (p)-NF-κB p65 and cytochrome P450 reductase protein expression in liver injury mice. The components of PLT include gallic acid, catechin, caffeine, epicatechin (EC), epigallocatechin gallate (EGCG), gallocatechin gallate (GCG), and epicatechin gallate (ECG), which possibly have a wide range of biological activities. Thus, PLT imparts preventive effects against CCl$_4$-induced liver injury, which is similar to silymarin.

Keywords: polyphenol; Liubao tea; hepatic damage; mRNA expression; protein expression

---

1. Introduction

Liubao tea is prepared from Wuzhou large tea leaves from China. It is a specialty tea generated through the processes of natural fermentation, pile fermentation, drying, autoclaving, aging, and other characteristics. Therefore, Liubao tea is a kind of black tea that is post-fermented [1]. This tea is named according to its geographical origin, namely, Liubao County, Wuzhou City, Guangxi

Province, China. Liubao tea was historically used as a preventive medicine [2]. The majority of research studies focus on Pu'er tea, Hunan black tea, and Fuzhuan tea, whereas investigations of relevant technology and functions of Liubao tea are limited [3]. Recent studies showed that Liubao tea imparts lipid-lowering effects, regulates glucose and lipid metabolism, possesses anti-oxidation activity, and regulates immune function and intestinal flora. These health benefits come from the components of Liubao tea, which include polyphenols, flavonoids, caffeine, free amino acids, and soluble sugars [4–6].

The liver is an important metabolic organ, and damage to this organ can cause severe harm to the human body, which includes liver injury due to chemicals such as higher alcohol intake, drug side effects, and environmental toxic chemicals, ultimately leading to cirrhosis and liver cancer [7]. Carbon tetrachloride (CCl_4) is a common chemical inducer of liver damage in the laboratory. CCl_4 triggers the production of high levels of inflammatory cytokines in liver cells during liver injury, which aggravates inflammation and liver damage. Simultaneously, CCl_4 can induce the formation of Cl^- and CCl_3^- in liver cell microsomes, leading to lipid peroxidation of liver microsomes, resulting in lipid peroxidation and destruction of cell membranes, and ultimately, liver damage [8].

Active oxygen free radicals cause oxidative stress, which is a common pathophysiological mechanism of liver diseases. Oxidative stress could cause hepatic damage by inducing membrane lipid peroxidation that changes biofilm function, as well as inducing covalent combinations with biological macromolecules, and destruction of enzyme activities (such as tumor necrosis factor-α (TNF-α) and nuclear factor κ-light-chain-enhancer of activated B cells (NF-κB)) [9]. Oxidative stress plays an important role in fatty liver, viral hepatitis, liver fibrosis, and other liver diseases [10]. Energy metabolism in organisms utilizes oxygen as an electronic acceptor in the process of aerobic metabolism, which inevitably produces reactive oxygen species (ROS). ROS has a dual effect, which is closely related to the regulation of some physiological active substances and the inflammatory immune process, but excessive ROS can easily lead to oxidative stress [11]. The mitochondrial respiratory chain complex uses electron transfer to produce ATP, which is the main source of ROS. The liver is rich in mitochondria, and is, therefore, the main organ susceptible to ROS attack, and oxidative stress has a close relationship with most liver damage [12]. ROS can also initiate a variety of cytokines such as transforming growth factor-beta (TGF-β), interleukin-8 (IL-8), and NF-κB. These cytokines can lead to infiltration of neutrophils, enhance inflammatory response, and ultimately lead to liver cell injury [13].

Tea polyphenols are a very important component of tea. Studies showed that tea polyphenols have a strong scavenging effect on oxygen free radicals [14,15]. Tea polyphenols can sequester lipid peroxidation free radicals during the peroxidation process, lower polyphenolic free-radical content, and interrupt free-radical oxidation chain reactions, thereby effectively removing free radicals [14]. Simultaneously, tea polyphenols can activate and enhance the activity of various antioxidant enzymes such as superoxide dismutase (SOD), glutathione peroxidase (GSH-Px), and catalase (CAT), as well as efficiently eliminate free radicals [16]. Tea polyphenols can prevent lipid peroxidation caused by CCl_4, as well as avoid the damage of the membrane structure and function of liver cells caused by the covalent binding of CCl_4 and liver microsomal lipids and proteins [17]. In addition, tea polyphenols impart a protective effect on obstructive jaundice liver injury caused by peroxidation, acute liver injury caused by cadmium poisoning, alcoholic liver injury, and liver cancer [18]. In addition, except for certain reports of catechins and other individual tea polyphenols on liver injury protective effects, the characteristics of the tea polyphenols and polyphenol composition analysis remain unclear, including those of Liubao tea [19].

This study utilized CCl_4 in establishing a chemical liver injury mouse model to investigate the preventive effect of PLT. We also employed molecular biology methods to test the indices of serum and liver tissue, and the preventive mechanism of PLT on liver injury was elucidated. The results of this study may facilitate the development and utilization of PLT in food processing and the manufacture of health products.

2. Materials and Methods

2.1. PLT Extraction

Approximately 150 g of Liubao tea (Guilin Lijiang Tea Factory Co. Ltd., Guilin, Guangxi, China), placed in a 15-L beaker, was mixed with 500 mL of boiling water, extracted in a 95 °C water bath, and after 1 h of filtration, the filtrate was collected. This process was repeated, and the two filtrates were pooled, and thoroughly mixed with 100 g of $ZnCl_2$, before the mixture's pH was adjusted to 7.5 using 2 mol/L ammonia. The mixture was then centrifuged at 3000 rpm for 10 min, and the supernatant was discarded and the precipitate containing the crude polyphenols was collected. Approximately 3 L of hydrochloric acid solution (2 mol/L) was added to the sediment, which was stirred to dissolve. Then, 2 mol/L ammonia was added to adjust the pH of the mixture to 4.0. After filtration, the filtrate was extracted with 4000 mL of ethyl acetate twice, and the extract was evaporated with a rotary evaporator to obtain the polyphenol extract [20].

2.2. Experimental Model in Kunming (KM) Mice

The male KM mice (eight weeks old) were divided into five groups (10 mice in each group), which included the normal group, control group, silymarin gavage group (silymarin, positive control group), low-dose PLT group via intragastric administration (LPLT group, 50 mg/kg), and high-dose PLT group via intragastric administration (HPLT group, 100 mg/kg). The mice were first allowed to acclimatize to the laboratory conditions for one week. The mice in the normal group and the control group were intragastrically given 2 mL of normal saline. The mice in the silymarin-instilled group were given 0.2 mL of silymarin solution daily at a dose of 100 mg/kg. The high-/low-dose PLT group mice were treated with PLT at 100 mg/kg and 50 mg/kg, respectively, daily for two weeks. All mice except for the normal group were intraperitoneally injected with CCl_4 inducer (2 mL/kg; CCl_4: olive oil = 1:1, v/v) on the 14th day, and then all mice were fasted, but allowed to drink water. The mice were sacrificed after fasting for 24 h, and their hearts were collected for dissection, whereas the livers were isolated for later use [21]. The liver index was calculated using the formula as liver weight/body weight × 100. This study was approved by the Animal Ethics Committee of Chongqing University of Education (Chongqing, China).

2.3. Measurement of Serum Indices

The mouse serum samples were separated by centrifugation at 4000 rpm for 10 min. The serum levels of aspartate aminotransferase (AST), alanine aminotransferase (ALT), triglycerides (TGs), SOD, GSH-Px, and malondialdehyde (MDA) were determined using assay kits (Nanjing Jiancheng Bioengineering Institute, Nanjing City, China).

2.4. Cytokine Levels in Serum

The serum samples were isolated by centrifugation and cytokine levels were assayed using IL-6 (ab46100), IL-12 (ab119531), TNF-α (ab100747), and interferon-γ (IFN-γ; ab100689) cytokine assay kits (Abcam, Cambridge, MA, USA).

2.5. Histopathological Analysis of Liver Tissues

Mouse liver tissue samples were fixed in 10% formalin solution for 24 h, followed by dehydration in 95% ethanol for 24 h. Then, the tissues were sectioned, stained with hematoxylin and eosin (H&E), and then assessed under a BX43 microscope (Olympus, Tokyo, Japan). The grading of liver injury is shown in Table 1.

Table 1. Pathological grading of liver injury.

Grade	Portal Area and Surrounding Area	Hepatic Lobule
0	No inflammation	No inflammation
1	Portal inflammation	Degeneration and few necrotic foci
2	Mild detrital necrosis	Degeneration, focal necrosis
3	Moderate detrital necrosis	Degeneration or necrosis, or bridge necrosis
4	Severe detrital necrosis	Bridge necrosis wide range, involving multiple lobules, leaflet structure disorder

2.6. qPCR Analysis

The messenger RNA (mRNA) expression of liver tissue in mice was determined by SYBR green assay. The liver tissues were homogenized, followed by total RNA extraction using TRIzol reagent (Thermo Fisher Scientific, Waltham, MA, USA). The concentration of RNA was detected using a micro-ultraviolet (UV) spectrophotometer (Nano 300, Aosheng, Hanzhou, Zhejiang, China). Approximately 1 μg of mRNA was reverse transcribed into complementary DNA (cDNA). The PCR conditions were as follows: pre-denaturation at 95 °C for 3 min, followed by 40 cycles of denaturation at 95 °C for 10 s, annealing at 57 °C for 30 s, and extension at 72 °C for 15 s [22]. The primers in this study are shown in Table 2. The relative transcription levels of the mRNAs were calculated using the $2^{-\Delta\Delta Cr}$ method.

Table 2. qPCR assay sequences.

Gene	Forward Sequence	Reverse Sequence
COX-2	5′–GGTGCCTGGTCTGATGATG–3′	5′–TGCTGGTTTGGAATAGTTGCT–3′
iNOS	5′–GTTCTCAGCCCAACAATACAAGA–3′	5′–GTGGACGGGTCGATGTCAC–3
NF-κB	5′–ATGGCAGACGATGATCCCTAC–3′	5′–CGGAATCGAAATCCCCTCTGTT–3′
IκB-α	5′–TGAAGGACGAGGAGTACGAGC–3′	5′–TGCAGGAACGAGTCTCCGT–3′
Cu/Zn-OD	5′–AACCAGTTGTGTTGTCAGGAC–3′	5′–CCACCATGTTTCTTAGAGTGAGG–3′
Mn-SOD	5′–CAGACCTGCCTTACGACTATGG–3′	5′–CTCGGTGGCGTTGAGATTGTT–3′
GSH-Px	5′–CCACCGTGTATGCCTTCTCC–3′	5′–AGAGAGACGCGACATTCTCAAT–3′
CAT	5′–GGAGGCGGGAACCCAATAG–3′	5′–GTGTGCCATCTCGTCAGTGAA–3′
GAPDH	5′–AGGTCGGTGTGAACGGATTTG–3′	5′–GGGGTCGTTGATGGCAACA–3′

2.7. Western Blot Analysis

The 100-mg liver tissue samples were homogenized with 1 mL of radio immunoprecipitation assay (RIPA) and 10 μL of phenylmethanesulfonyl fluoride (PMSF); then, they were centrifuged at 12,000 rpm (5 min, 4 °C), the hepatocytes were lysed, and the lysate was kept on ice for 30 min. The bicinchoninic acid (BCA) method was used to determine the protein concentration. The sample was mixed with an equal volume of 5× loading buffer and then placed in a water bath at 100 °C for 5 min. The hepatocytes were then sonicated by SJIALAB for 2 min (10% ultrasound intensity), and centrifuged (4500 rpm) for 10 min to separate the supernatant. The extracted protein was then subjected to polyacrylamide gel electrophoresis (80–120 V), and transferred onto a polyvinylidene fluoride (PVDF) membrane, sealed, and incubated overnight at 4 °C with the corresponding primary antibodies, namely, cyclooxygenase 2 (COX-2; MA514568, Thermo Fisher Scientific), inducible nitric oxide synthase (iNOS) (PA1036), NF-κB (PA1186), phosphorylated (p)-NF-κB p65 (MA515160), nuclear factor of κ-light polypeptide gene enhancer in B-cells inhibitor-α (IκB-α; 397700), Cu/Zn-SOD (PA5270240), Mn-SOD (PA530604), GSH-Px (PA540504), CAT (PA259183), cytochrome P450 reductase (PA577820), and β-actin (MA5157739), incubated at 37 °C with the second antibody (A21241) for 1 h, followed by colorimetric detection and chemiluminescence imaging (iBright FL1000, Thermo Fisher Scientific) [23].

2.8. High-Performance Liquid Chromatography (HPLC) Assay

The standard products of gallic acid, catechin, caffeine, epicatechin (EC), epigallocatechin gallate (EGCG), gallocatechin gallate (GCG), and epicatechin gallate (ECG) were weighed accurately, and the standard products were placed in 50-mL volumetric flasks, to the appropriate amount of methanol. The mixture was vortexed to dissolve, and diluted to scale with methanol, i.e., to obtain the standard stock solution. One milliliter of gallic acid, catechin, caffeine, EC, EGCG, GCG, and ECG stock solutions were each placed into 10-mL volumetric flasks and mixed with an equal volume of methanol to obtain a mixed standard solution. The PLT extract was extracted with precision, and a 0.5 mg/mL solution was prepared using methanol. PLT components were detected (UltiMate3000 HPLC System, Thermo Fisher Scientific) using the following chromatographic conditions: Accucore perfluorophenyl (PFP) column (4.6 mm × 150 mm, 2.6 μm, Thermo Fisher Scientific); flow rate of 0.6 mL/min; detection wavelength of 280 nm; injection volume of 10 L; column temperature of 30 °C; collection time of 20 min; and mobile phases A for acetonitrile, and B for 0.1% formic acid solution. The gradient elution conditions are shown in Table 3 [24].

Table 3. Flow phase gradient elution program.

t/min	A/%	B/%
0	10	90
6.5	18.5	81.5
20	29.5	70.5

2.9. Statistical Analysis

The data are expressed as the mean ± standard deviation (SD). Differences between mean values for each group were assessed by one-way ANOVA with Duncan's new multiple-range test (MRT). Differences with a $p < 0.05$ were considered statistically significant. The SAS v9.1 statistical software package (SAS Institute, Cary, NC, USA) was used for these analyses.

3. Results

3.1. Body Weight, Liver Weight, and Liver Indices of the Experimental Mice

As shown in Table 4, on the first day, there was no significant difference ($p > 0.05$) in body weight across all mice. On the 14th day, the body weight of the control group was significantly higher ($p < 0.05$) than that of the other groups because of individual differences, while the mice in the Liupao tea treatment group had lower body weight gain than that of the other groups probably because of the lipid-reducing effect of Liupao tea. After being treated with CCl_4, the body weight of mice in the control group was the heaviest, whereas that of the other groups was lower than that of the control mice. The liver weight and liver indices of mice in control group were also the highest, while the liver weight and liver indices of mice in the normal group were the lowest. Because of the treatment with PLT, the liver indices of the hepatic damage-induced mice decreased compared to those of the control group, and the HPLT group exhibited lower liver indices than the LPLT group. The indices of the HPLT group were also roughly similar to the silymarin group.

Table 4. Body weight, liver weight, and liver indices in experimental mice with CCl_4-induced hepatic damage.

Group	1st Day Body Weight (g)	14th Day Body Weight (g)	15th Day Body Weight (g)	Liver Weight (g)	Liver Index
Normal	35.17 ± 0.32 [a]	42.66 ± 1.59 [b]	42.12 ± 1.96 [b]	1.57 ± 0.07 [b]	3.73 ± 0.18 [e]
Control	35.53 ± 0.28 [a]	48.22 ± 2.62 [a]	46.64 ± 1.38 [a]	2.41 ± 0.18 [a]	5.15 ± 0.23 [a]
Silymarin	35.06 ± 0.22 [a]	41.43 ± 0.55 [b]	40.35 ± 0.84 [b]	1.58 ± 0.08 [b]	3.92 ± 0.19 [d]
LPLT	35.19 ± 0.26 [a]	36.62 ± 1.45 [c]	35.61 ± 1.81 [c]	1.61 ± 0.12 [b]	4.51 ± 0.11 [b]
HPLT	35.41 ± 0.20 [a]	36.63 ± 2.41 [c]	35.84 ± 3.70 [c]	1.48 ± 0.15 [b]	4.14 ± 0.03 [c]

Values presented are the means ± standard deviation ($N = 10$/group). [a-e] Mean values with different letters in the same column are significantly different ($p < 0.05$) and those with the same letter in the same column are not significantly different ($p > 0.05$) according to Duncan's new multiple-range test (MRT). Silymarin group: 50 mg/kg body weight (b.w.) silymarin treatment dose; LPLT group: 50 mg/kg b.w. polyphenols of Liubao tea (PLT) low (L) treatment dose; HPLT group: 100 mg/kg b.w. polyphenols of Liubao tea (PLT) high (H) treatment dose.

3.2. Serum AST, ALT, and TG Levels

Table 5 shows that the serum AST, ALT, and TG levels of mice in the normal group were the lowest, whereas those of the control group were the highest. The serum AST, ALT, and TG serum levels of mice in the HPLT group were significantly higher ($p < 0.05$) than those of the silymarin group, but were significantly lower ($p < 0.05$) than those of the LPLT group.

Table 5. Serum aspartate aminotransferase (AST), alanine aminotransferase (ALT), and triglyceride (TG) levels in experimental mice with CCl_4-induced hepatic damage.

Group	AST (U/L)	ALT (U/L)	TG (pg/mL)
Normal	6.20 ± 0.43 [e]	1.54 ± 0.22 [e]	150.00 ± 26.15 [e]
Control	21.13 ± 0.93 [a]	17.98 ± 1.53 [a]	563.75 ± 16.18 [a]
Silymarin	12.13 ± 0.35 [d]	4.09 ± 0.44 [d]	208.75 ± 20.06 [d]
LPLT	17.75 ± 0.57 [b]	12.36 ± 2.23 [b]	385.00 ± 57.72 [b]
HPLT	13.85 ± 0.55 [c]	8.45 ± 0.64 [c]	273.75 ± 32.89 [c]

Values presented are the means ± standard deviation ($N = 10$/group). [a–e] Mean values with different letters in the same column are significantly different ($p < 0.05$) and those with the same letter in the same column are not significantly different ($p > 0.05$) according to Duncan's new MRT. Silymarin group: 50 mg/kg b.w. silymarin treatment dose; LPLT group: 50 mg/kg b.w. polyphenols of Liubao tea (PLT) low (L) treatment dose; and HPLT group: 100 mg/kg b.w. polyphenols of Liubao tea (PLT) high (H) treatment dose.

3.3. Serum SOD, GSH-Px, and MDA Levels

Table 6 shows that the serum SOD and GSH-Px levels of mice in the normal group were the highest, whereas the SOD and GSH-Px levels of those in the HPLT group were significantly higher ($p < 0.05$) than those in the LPLT and control groups, but lower than those in the silymarin group. However, the MDA levels in mice of the HPLT group were significantly lower ($p < 0.05$) than those of the LPLT and control groups, but significantly higher ($p < 0.05$) than those of the silymarin and normal groups.

Table 6. Serum superoxide dismutase (SOD), glutathione peroxidase (GSH-Px), and malondialdehyde (MDA) levels in experimental mice with CCl_4-induced hepatic damage.

Group	SOD (U/mL)	GSH-Px (U/mL)	MDA (nmol/mL)
Normal	121.38 ± 4.88 [a]	85.92 ± 1.83 [a]	2.24 ± 0.06 [e]
Control	58.56 ± 2.42 [d]	5.52 ± 1.02 [e]	5.93 ± 0.45 [a]
Silymarin	107.11 ± 1.77 [b]	63.94 ± 3.20 [b]	2.89 ± 0.16 [d]
LPLT	78.44 ± 8.35 [c]	25.35 ± 1.03 [d]	4.44 ± 0.21 [b]
HPLT	106.12 ± 1.37 [b]	53.49 ± 2.84 [c]	3.34 ± 0.26 [c]

Values presented are the means ± standard deviation ($N = 10$/group). [a–e] Mean values with different letters in the same column are significantly different ($p < 0.05$) and those with the same letter in the same column are not significantly different ($p > 0.05$) according to Duncan's new MRT. Silymarin group: 50 mg/kg b.w. silymarin treatment dose; LPLT group: 50 mg/kg b.w. polyphenols of Liubao tea (PLT) low (L) treatment dose; and HPLT group: 100 mg/kg b.w. polyphenols of Liubao tea (PLT) high (H) treatment dose.

3.4. Serum IL-6, IL-12, TNF-α, and IFN-γ Cytokine Levels

Table 7 shows that the serum IL-6, IL-12, TNF-α, and IFN-γ cytokine levels of mice in the normal group were lowest; these levels were lower than those of the silymarin, HPLT, LPLT, and control groups in decreasing order.

Table 7. Cytokine interleukin (IL)-6, IL-12, tumor necrosis factor-α (TNF-α), and interferon-γ (IFN-γ) levels in experimental mice with CCl$_4$-induced hepatic damage.

Group	IL-6 (pg/mL)	IL-12 (pg/mL)	TNF-α (pg/mL)	IFN-γ (pg/mL)
Normal	31.11 ± 1.84 [d]	26.17 ± 3.06 [d]	365.40 ± 16.75 [e]	32.32 ± 0.59 [d]
Control	64.33 ± 3.80 [a]	56.68 ± 6.98 [a]	718.76 ± 40.28 [a]	77.94 ± 1.60 [a]
Silymarin	41.02 ± 3.01 [c]	34.50 ± 1.90 [c]	467.22 ± 38.47 [d]	39.07 ± 0.27 [c]
LPLT	54.27 ± 6.05 [b]	42.46 ± 4.92 [b]	622.90 ± 50.68 [b]	44.61 ± 0.79 [b]
HPLT	45.19 ± 1.24 [c]	36.69 ± 0.55 [bc]	547.63 ± 26.83 [c]	39.10 ± 0.56 [c]

Values presented are the means ± standard deviation ($N = 10$/group). [a–e] Mean values with different letters in the same column are significantly different ($p < 0.05$) and those with the same letter in the same column are not significantly different ($p > 0.05$) according to Duncan's new MRT. Silymarin group: 50 mg/kg b.w. silymarin treatment dose; LPLT group: 50 mg/kg b.w. polyphenols of Liubao tea (PLT) low (L) treatment dose; and HPLT group: 100 mg/kg b.w. polyphenols of Liubao tea (PLT) high (H) treatment dose.

3.5. Histopathological Assessment of the Liver

CCl$_4$ induced liver injury in mice of the control, silymarin, LPLT, and HPLT groups; the observed histopathological changes included degeneration and necrosis of the centrilobular cells. Normally, the central veins of the liver are rounded, the hepatocytes are uniform in size, and they are evenly arranged in a radial pattern around the central veins. The liver tissues of mice in the control group showed the most severe damage (Grade 4, Figure 1). Silymarin (Grade 1) and PLT reduced these hepatic injury changes, and silymarin facilitated the reduction in damage incurred by the hepatic tissues. HPLT (Grade 2) imparted effects similar to that observed with silymarin, and only a few liver cells demonstrated hemorrhage in the area around the centrilobular vein.

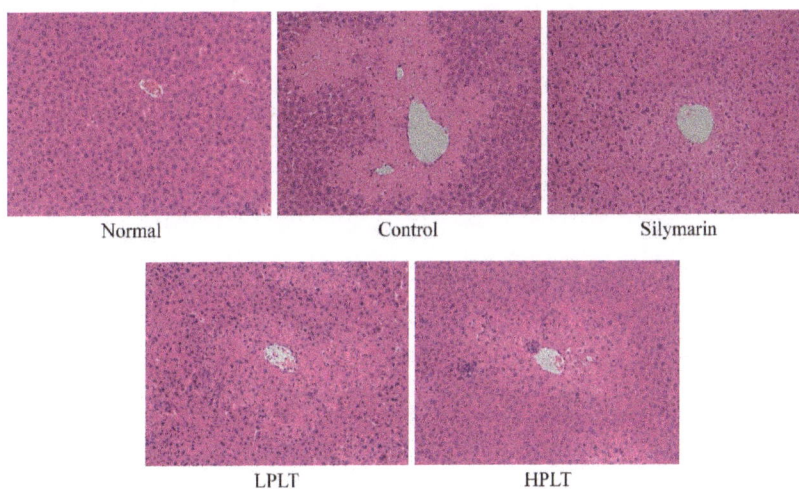

Normal   Control   Silymarin

LPLT   HPLT

Figure 1. Hematoxylin and eosin (H&E) pathological observation of hepatic tissue in experimental mice with CCl$_4$-induced hepatic damage. Magnification: 100×. Silymarin group: 50 mg/kg body weight (b.w.) silymarin treatment dose; LPLT group: 50 mg/kg b.w. polyphenols of Liubao tea (PLT) low (L) treatment dose; HPLT group: 100 mg/kg b.w. polyphenols of Liubao tea (PLT) high (H) treatment dose.

3.6. mRNA and Protein Expression of Cu/Zn-SOD, Mn-SOD, GSH-Px, and CAT in Mouse Hepatic Tissues

The mRNA and protein expressions of Cu/Zn-SOD (27.13-fold (mRNA) and 5.79-fold (protein) increase relative to control group), Mn-SOD (23.30-fold (mRNA) and 5.47-fold (protein) increase relative to control group), GSH-Px (18.43-fold (mRNA) and 153.10-fold (protein) increase relative to control group), and CAT (17.80-fold (mRNA) and 8.63-fold (protein) increase relative to control group) in the hepatic tissues of mice in the normal group were the highest, whereas those of the control group were the lowest (Figures 2 and 3). After treatment with silymarin and PLT, the Cu/Zn-SOD, Mn-SOD, GSH-Px, and CAT expressions of liver in CCl_4-treated mice were reduced; the HPLT-treated mice exhibited higher Cu/Zn-SOD (16.46-fold (mRNA) and 3.11-fold (protein) increase relative to control group), Mn-SOD (13.31-fold (mRNA) and 2.47-fold (protein) increase relative to control group), GSH-Px (9.85-fold (mRNA) and 33.52-fold (protein) increase relative to control group), and CAT (9.53-fold (mRNA) and 4.74-fold (protein) increase relative to control group) expressions than the LPLT-treated mice (8.71-, 5.71-, 7.11-, and 5.10-fold (mRNA) and 2.87-, 1.81-, 7.52-, and 3.74-fold (protein) increase, respectively, relative to control group), but weaker than the silymarin-treated (22.18-, 17.33-, 14.92-, and 13.27-fold (mRNA) and 3.78-, 3.02-, 97.47-, and 6.40-fold (protein) increase, respectively, relative to control group) mice.

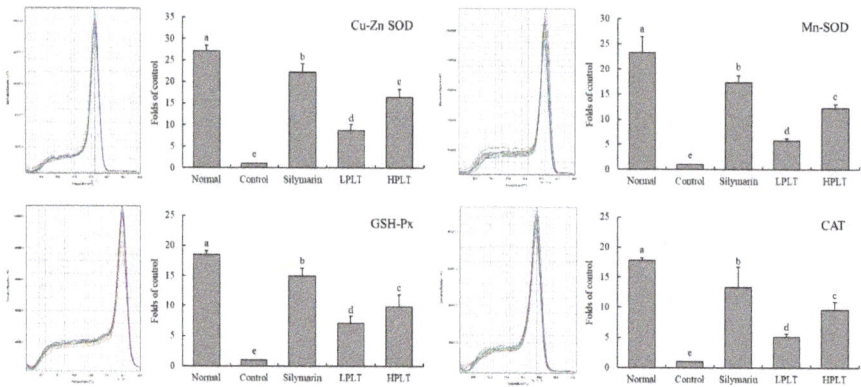

Figure 2. Cu/Zn- superoxide dismutase (SOD), Mn-SOD, glutathione peroxidase (GSH-Px), and catalase (CAT) messenger RNA (mRNA) expressions in hepatic tissue of experimental mice with CCl_4-induced hepatic damage. Values presented are the means ± standard deviation ($N = 3$/group). [a–e] Mean values with different letters in the same bars are significantly different ($p < 0.05$) and those with the same letter in the same column are not significantly different ($p > 0.05$) according to Duncan's new multiple-range test (MRT). Silymarin group: 50 mg/kg b.w. silymarin treatment dose; LPLT group: 50 mg/kg b.w. polyphenols of Liubao tea (PLT) treatment dose; and HPLT group: 100 mg/kg b.w. polyphenols of Liubao tea (PLT) treatment dose.

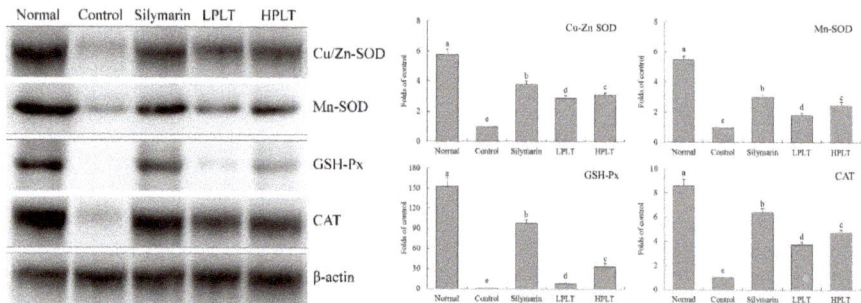

Figure 3. Cu/Zn-SOD, Mn-SOD, GSH-Px, and CAT protein expressions in hepatic tissue of experimental mice with CCl_4-induced hepatic damage. Values presented are the means ± standard deviation ($N = 3$/group). [a–e] Mean values with different letters in the same bars are significantly different ($p < 0.05$) and those with the same letter in the same column are not significantly different ($p > 0.05$) according to Duncan's new MRT. Silymarin group: 50 mg/kg b.w. silymarin treatment dose; LPLT group: 50 mg/kg b.w. polyphenols of Liubao tea (PLT) treatment dose; and HPLT group: 100 mg/kg b.w. polyphenols of Liubao tea (PLT) treatment dose.

3.7. mRNA and Protein Expression of COX-2, iNOS, NF-κB, and IκB-α in Mouse Hepatic Tissues

The IκB-α mRNA (25.30-fold increase relative to control group) and protein (2.41-fold increase relative to control group) expressions of mice in the normal group were the highest, whereas the COX-2 (0.01-fold (mRNA) and 0.16-fold (protein) increase relative to control group), iNOS (0.03-fold (mRNA) and 0.27-fold (protein) increase relative to control group), and NF-κB (0.07-fold (mRNA) and 0.06-fold (protein) increase relative to control group) expressions in the normal group were the lowest (Figures 4 and 5). The IκB-α mRNA (15.38-fold increase relative to control group) and protein (1.74-fold increase relative to control group) expressions of mice in the HPLT group were only lower than those of the silymarin (17.80-fold (mRNA) and 2.15-fold (protein) increase relative to control group) and normal groups, but stronger than those of the LPLT (7.03-fold (mRNA) and 1.21-fold (protein) increase relative to control group) and control groups. The HPLT group showed lower COX-2 (0.28-fold (mRNA) and 0.52-fold (protein) increase relative to control group), iNOS (0.39-fold (mRNA) and 0.41-fold (protein) increase relative to control group), and NF-κB (0.33-fold (mRNA) and 0.38-fold (protein) increase relative to control group) expression levels than the LPLT (0.61-, 0.65-, and 0.74-fold (mRNA) and 0.85-, 0.57-, and 0.62-fold (protein) increase, respectively, relative to control group) and control groups, but only slightly stronger than the silymarin group (0.17-, 0.20-, and 0.15-fold (mRNA) and 0.24-, 0.35-, and 0.21-fold (protein) increase, respectively, relative to control group). Meanwhile, mice in the normal group showed the strongest p-NF-κB p65 protein expression (5.88-fold increase relative to control group), while silymarin-treated mice also showed stronger p-NF-κB p65 protein expression (4.74-fold increase relative to control group) than that of the LPLT- (1.59-fold increase relative to control group) and HPLT- (3.35-fold increase relative to control group) treated mice.

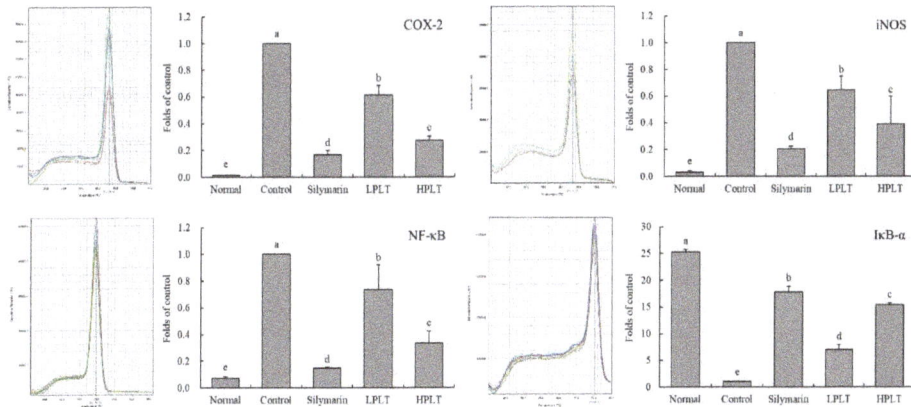

Figure 4. Cyclooxygenase 2 (COX-2), inducible nitric oxide synthase (iNOS), nuclear factor κ-light-chain-enhancer of activated B cells (NF-κB), and nuclear factor of κ-light polypeptide gene enhancer in B-cells inhibitor-α (IκB-α) mRNA expressions in hepatic tissue of experimental mice with CCl$_4$-induced hepatic damage. Values presented are the means ± standard deviation ($N = 3$/group). [a-e] Mean values with different letters in the same bars are significantly different ($p < 0.05$) and those with the same letter in the same column are not significantly different ($p > 0.05$) according to Duncan's new MRT. Silymarin group: 50 mg/kg b.w. silymarin treatment dose; LPLT group: 50 mg/kg b.w. polyphenols of Liubao tea (PLT) treatment dose; and HPLT group: 100 mg/kg b.w. polyphenols of Liubao tea (PLT) treatment dose.

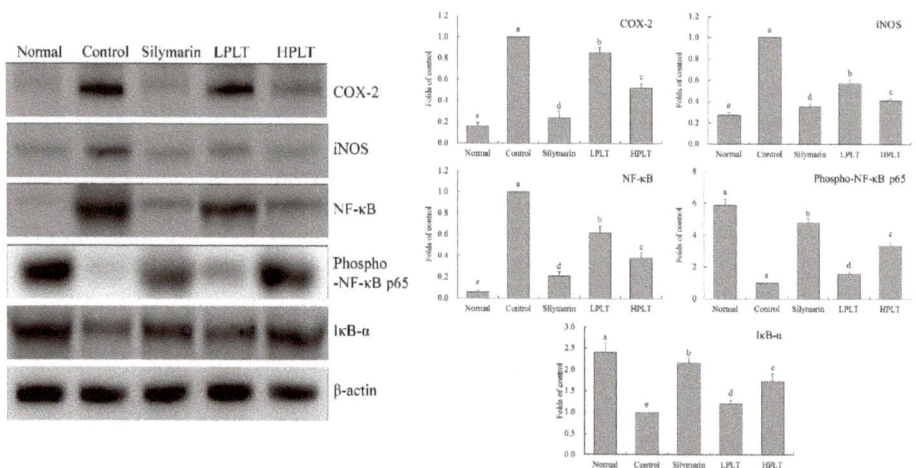

Figure 5. COX-2, iNOS, NF-κB, phosphorylated (p)-NF-κB p65, and IκB-α protein expressions in hepatic tissue of experimental mice with CCl$_4$-induced hepatic damage. Values presented are the means ± standard deviation (N = 3/group). [a–e] Mean values with different letters in the same bars are significantly different ($p < 0.05$) and those with the same letter in the same column are not significantly different ($p > 0.05$) according to Duncan's new MRT. Silymarin group: 50 mg/kg b.w. silymarin treatment dose; LPLT group: 50 mg/kg b.w. polyphenols of Liubao tea (PLT) treatment dose; and HPLT group: 100 mg/kg b.w. polyphenols of Liubao tea (PLT) treatment dose.

3.8. Protein Expression of Cytochrome P450 Reductase in Mouse Hepatic Tissues

The cytochrome P450 reductase protein (3.97-fold increase relative to control group) expression of mice in the normal group was highest (Figure 6), and HPLT-treated mice (2.8-fold increase relative to control group) also showed a higher expression than that of LPLT-treated mice (1.69-fold increase relative to control group), but it was lower than that of silymarin-treated mice (3.25-fold increase relative to control group).

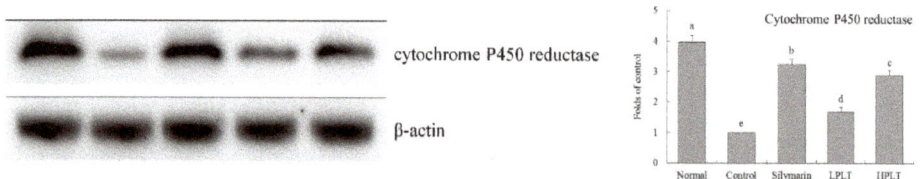

Figure 6. Cytochrome P450 reductase protein expression in hepatic tissue of experimental mice with CCl$_4$-induced hepatic damage. Values presented are the means ± standard deviation (N = 3/group). [a–e] Mean values with different letters in the same bars are significantly different ($p < 0.05$) and those with the same letter in the same column are not significantly different ($p > 0.05$) according to Duncan's new MRT. Silymarin group: 50 mg/kg b.w. silymarin treatment dose; LPLT group: 50 mg/kg b.w. polyphenols of Liubao tea (PLT) treatment dose; and HPLT group: 100 mg/kg b.w. polyphenols of Liubao tea (PLT) treatment dose.

3.9. Constituents of PTL

Figure 7 shows that PTL contains seven kinds of polyphenols, namely, gallic acid, catechin, caffeine, EC, EGCG, GCG, and ECG, with contents of 4.98%, 4.20%, 16.71%, 0.90%, 7.29%, 3.03%, and 34.44%, respectively.

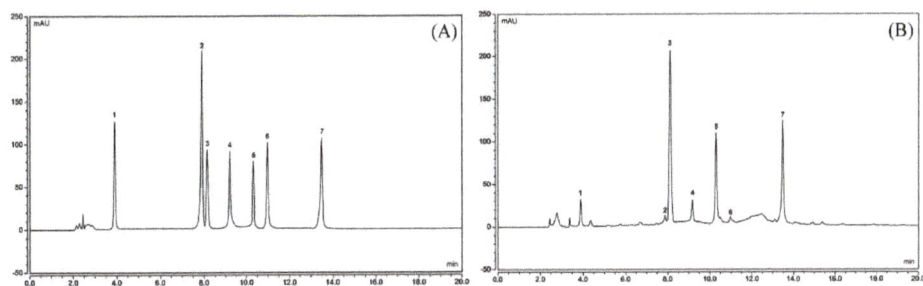

Figure 7. Polyphenol constituents of Liubao tea (PLT). (**A**) Standard chromatograms; (**B**) PLT chromatograms. 1: gallic acid; 2: catechin; 3: caffeine; 4: epicatechin (EC); 5: epigallocatechin gallate (EGCG); 6: gallocatechin gallate (GCG); 7: epicatechin gallate (ECG).

4. Discussion

Liubao tea is a non-toxic food and meets the requirements of food safety according to the standards of food toxicology [25]. Liupao tea was shown to have weight-loss effects [3], and Liupao tea polyphenols were also found to inhibit weight gain in mice in this study. Therefore, there were individual differences in the body weight of mice before carbon-tetrachloride (CTC) treatment. Liver injuries may result in harmful and sometimes life-threatening effects to the body. Liver quality and liver index, which are indices of CTC-induced liver injury, were used in the present study [26]. The results show that PLT can reduce the liver quality and liver indices of mice with liver injury, and these effects are similar to those using the liver injury drug, silymarin.

ALT and AST are expressed by hepatocytes; ALT is secreted into the cytoplasm, whereas AST is mainly produced in the mitochondria of hepatocytes. Damage to cells due to hepatitis, myocarditis, and pancreatitis induces ALT to enter the bloodstream. However, during severe damage, AST also enters the bloodstream [27]. Thus, a significant increase in ALT and AST levels indicates liver damage [28]. Liver injury can lead to the transfer of fatty acids to the liver, resulting in increased intrahepatic TG content, and TG levels also reflect the degree of liver lipid peroxidation [29]. In this study, PLT was found to inhibit the increase in ALT, AST, and TG levels caused by carbon tetrachloride liver injury. ALT, AST, and TG are the most typical clinical liver function indicators [27,28]. Observing the influence of these indicators can judge whether the liver function is normal or not. It could be seen that PLT had a certain effective role in restoring normal liver function.

CCl_4 will lead to the body's oxidation; the body utilizes two defenses, namely, non-enzymatic and enzymatic, to prevent oxidative damage, including regulation of SOD, CAT, and GSH-Px, which are the main mechanisms for enzymatic oxidation [30]. SOD catalyzes superoxide radicals and is capable of scavenging free radicals, whereas CAT and SOD synergistically enhance the role of free radicals [31]. GSH-Px is an important enzyme that catalyzes the decomposition of hydrogen peroxide, which in turn, protects cell membranes and prevents cell damage [32]. MDA is a metabolite of lipid peroxidation; a high content of MDA accumulates in the body after liver injury [33]. In this study, we found that PLT could significantly regulate the levels of SOD, GSH-Px, and MDA in the body caused by liver injury, thereby protecting the liver from the effects of carbon tetrachloride.

CCl_4 induces oxidization and liver inflammation, resulting in a significant increase in serum IL-6, IL-12, TNF-α, and IFN-γ levels in mice [21]. IL-6 is a factor secreted by T helper 2 (Th2) cells and is involved in the humoral immune response. An increase in Th2 levels may result in visceral dysfunction [34]. IL-6 promotes the differentiation, proliferation, and antibody production of T lymphocytes. It can also change intracellular G cell activity and upregulate neutrophil function, as well as enhance inflammatory reactions of the body [35]. IL-12 is an activating factor of natural killer (NK) cells, and its effect is the most intense. High rates of apoptosis in hepatocytes and excessive immune response during liver injury further aggravate the condition, which is related to the fact that

IL-12 increases the cytotoxicity of cluster of differentiation 8 (CD8)$^+$ T cells [36]. Binding of TNF-α and liver cell membrane TNF-α receptor 1 (TNF-αR1) can induce intracellular double-stranded DNA to fragment, thereby resulting in stem cell apoptosis. In addition, TNF-α triggers inflammatory responses by activating NF-κB, which exacerbates liver injury [37]. IFN-γ is a proinflammatory cytokine that increases the sensitivity of hepatocytes to TNF-α, rendering hepatocytes to further damage [38]. Oxidative stress after liver tissue damage can cause an imbalance in the level of inflammatory cytokines such as TNF-α, IL-1β, and IL-6, which increases in the levels of TNF-α, IL-1β, and IL-6 in the liver [39]. Through the detection of inflammatory cytokines, we also found that PLT could inhibit inflammation by reducing the level of inflammatory factors, thereby reducing liver injury.

Mn-SOD and Gu/Zn-SOD are SOD isomers [40]. Mn-SOD is an SOD radical scavenger in the mitochondria [41]. Gu/Zn-SOD is an SOD free radical scavenger in the cytoplasm and takes Cu^{2+} and Zn^{2+} as its active center [42]. The liver and heart are organs that are rich in mitochondria, and Mn-SOD activity markedly decreases after CCl_4-induced liver injury [43]. The same result was obtained in this study. Gu/Zn-SOD can purify the toxic effects of O^{2-} in the body, and protect the visceral tissues [44]. Studies showed that CCl_4 causes oxidative stress reactions in the body, resulting in the excessive production of free radicals. Mn-SOD and Gu/Zn-SOD can inhibit free radicals in the body, and play a preventive role in liver injury [45,46]. CAT is an important antioxidant enzyme in the body. CAT can eliminate H_2O_2 in the body, thereby inhibiting oxidative stress, reducing the body's oxidation caused by carbon tetrachloride, and inhibiting liver injury [47]. Through the detection of gene and protein expression, it was further found that PLT could regulate the expressions of oxidation-related proteins in tissues, thereby reducing the damage caused by oxidative stress to tissues, thus protecting the liver.

NF-κB is a key factor in the regulation of inflammatory response, including inflammation-related IL-6 and TNF-α; these are upregulated during inflammation. Under normal circumstances, NF-κB and IκB-α in the bound state show an inactivation of both. NF-κB and IκB-α in extrinsic inflammatory conditions lead to the inhibition of inflammation by binding to IκB-α to activate NF-κB [48]. Meanwhile, through phosphorylation of NF-κB, it can reduce the promotion of inflammation of NF-κB and alleviate tissue damage [49]. NO is a highly active oxidant that is produced in the liver by activated NOS in liver cells, and promotes the high expression of the *iNOS* gene upon liver damage progression. In liver injury, oxidative stress occurs in hepatocytes, and a large number of inflammatory factors are released [50]. iNOS is an important inflammatory factor, and iNOS is very active in inflammation. iNOS-induced NO also promotes further damage to the liver [51]. COX-2 is also an important inflammatory factor; the tissue is not expressed under normal conditions. COX-2 expression raises after liver injury, whereby Kupffer cells are activated, and COX-2 upregulation exacerbates the liver inflammation [52]. Further experiments showed that PLT could regulate the expressions of COX-2, iNOS, NF-κB, p-NF-κB p65, and IκB-α, alleviating the liver injury caused by inflammation and carbon tetrachloride.

Most foreign compounds depend on metabolism by P450 in the liver. When carbon tetrachloride induces acute liver injury, lipid peroxidation and a large number of free radicals are produced in the liver, resulting in a decrease in activity of cytochrome P450. At the same time, carbon tetrachloride directly inhibits the synthesis of the cytochrome P450 enzyme, and the decrease in cytochrome P450 enzyme activity directly or indirectly leads to a decrease in detoxification ability of the liver, thereby aggravating liver injury [53]. Upon carbon tetrachloride treatment, PLT could raise the activity of cytochrome P450 reductase, and inhibited the liver injury.

Gallic acid (GA) can inhibit oxidative stress and cytotoxicity to improve liver injury. The activation of hepatic stellate cells (HSCs) caused by liver injury is an important part of liver fibrosis [54]. GA can also induce HSCs to produce O^{2-}, OH^-, and H_2O_2, thereby inducing oxidative stress that selectively kills HSCs [55]. Catechin also affects free-radical scavenging by reducing the content of MDA and increasing the activity of SOD [56]. Catechin has inhibitory effects on chronic hepatitis [57]. IL-1β can induce hepatic acute-phase protein synthesis, thereby affecting normal liver activity [58], while caffeine suppresses the production of inflammatory molecules, thus preventing the activating of the immune system in IL-1β [59], which may play a role in liver protection. Animal model studies showed that caffeine could also inhibit acute alcoholic liver injury possibly by imparting antioxidant effects and inhibiting the expressions of IL-1β and TNF-α [60]. EC also has antioxidant effects that influence cardiovascular disease, hypertension, cancer, and obesity [61]. EC could reduce the inflammatory-related expression of NF-κB, iNOS, and TNF-α [62]. Oxidative stress is considered to be the main cause of CCl$_4$-induced liver damage. CCl$_4$ is metabolized by cytochrome P450 in hepatocytes to produce three chloromethyl radicals. These radicals cause lipid peroxidation and lipid peroxidation products, which cause liver cell damage and promote the formation of fibrous tissue. EGCG plays a role in anti-CCl$_4$-induced liver fibrosis in rats through its antioxidant capacity [63]. The effects of EGCG on anti-liver injury are also reflected in the inhibition of TNF-α and IFN-γ by EGCG expression, thus preventing further immune damage caused by TNF-α and IFN-γ [64]. GCG can inhibit oxidative damage to tissues and protect viscera from oxidative damage [65]. ECG has anti-cancer effects, possibly stronger than EGCG [66]. ECG has better melanin inhibition effects than EGCG, and ECG shows antioxidant effects, which are greater than EGCG [67]. These active components are combined together to form PLT, thereby strongly inhibiting liver injury. PLT is a mixture with substantial biological activity. Its action may be the combined action of many substances, and its specific mechanism needs further study.

In this study, toxic carbon tetrachloride was used to simulate chemical-induced liver injury, and the observed effects remained at the laboratory level. In order to better prove this study's argument, future research on the human body is expected. In addition, the role of PLT in liver injury needs to be further studied, which will be conducive to more obvious discoveries of the link between its active components and their mechanisms. At the same time, in view of the mechanism of PLT, it is necessary to verify the mechanism more accurately for the differences across PLT components in the future.

5. Conclusions

This study induced hepatic injury in mice, and the hepatic injury-reducing effects of PLT were determined. PLT reduced the liver weight and liver indices in hepatic injury mice. PLT also reduced serum AST, ALT, TG, and MDA levels and increased serum SOD and GSH-Px levels in hepatic injury mice. Meanwhile, PLT reduced serum IL-6, IL-12, TNF-α, and IFN-γ cytokine levels in mice with hepatic injury. Further investigation showed that PLT upregulates the mRNA and protein expressions of Mn-SOD, Gu/Zn-SOD, CAT, GSH-Px, and IκB-α, and downregulates COX-2, iNOS, and NF-κB in mice with hepatic injury. PLT contains gallic acid, catechin, caffeine, EC, EGCG, GCG, and ECG, and its effects are similar to the drug silymarin. PLT is a functional ingredient that may be used as a raw material in functional foods.

Author Contributions: Y.P. performed the majority of the experiments and wrote the manuscript; X.L. and R.Y. contributed to the data analysis; X.Z. designed and supervised the study, and checked the final manuscript.

Funding: This research was funded by [the Program for Innovation Team Building at Institutions of Higher Education in Chongqing] grant number [CXTDX201601040], [the Introduction of High-level Personnel Research Start-up Fund of Chongqing University of Education] grant number [2013BSRC001], [the Construction Program of Chongqing Engineering Research Center] grant number [cstc2015yfpt_gcjsyjzx0027], [the Scientific Research Foundation for Returned Overseas Chinese Scholars, and the State Education Ministry] grant number [Jiaowaisiliu (2014)1685], China.

Conflicts of Interest: The authors declare no conflict of interest.

References

1. Liu, X.L.; Li, Y.; Jiang, Y.X.; Yu, X. Analysis on feature composition of Guangxi Liubao tea. *J. Beijing Technol. Bus. Univ. (Nat. Sci. Ed.)* **2012**, *30*, 46–50.
2. Huang, L.; Peng, J.J.; Xia, N.; Teng, J.W.; Wei, B.Y. Effect on regulation of hyperlipidemia and anticoagulant for Liupu tea. *Food. Sci. Technol.* **2013**, *38*, 123–127.

3.   Liu, J.Q.; Shao, W.F.; Zhao, B.Q.; Zhao, B.; Wang, H.Q.; Ma, X.M.; Guo, T.; Hou, Y. Study of fermented pu-erh tea powder, dark tea powder and liupu tea on losing weight in hyperlipidemia model rats. *China J. Tradi. Chin. Med. Pharm.* **2014**, *29*, 108–112.

4.   Zhang, X.Y.; Huang, Y.S.; Liu, G.P.; Rao, W.Y.; Qin, L.; Deng, Y.Y. The effects of Liubao tea on blood lipid and antioxidation and hyperlipidemia mice. *J. Med. Theory Pract.* **2013**, *26*, 563–564.

5.   Zhao, Y.Y.; Huang, L.; Wei, B.Y.; Teng, J.W.; Xia, N. Effect of Liupao tea extract on fecal microbiota in hyperlipidemic mice. *Sci. Technol. Food Ind.* **2015**, *36*, 364–367.

6.   Teng, Q.Q.; Liu, Z.H.; Gong, S.J.; Peng, Y.X.; Ma, R. Effect of Liupao Tea on glucose and lipid metabolism in palmitate-induced insulin resistance 3T3-L1 adipocytes. *J. Tea Sci.* **2014**, *34*, 230–238.

7.   Xu, B.B.; Li, Y.L.; Wang, B.Y. Research advances in risk factors for alcoholic liver disease. *Zhonghua Gan Zang Bing Za Zhi* **2017**, *25*, 397–400. [PubMed]

8.   Burk, R.F.; Lane, J.M.; Patel, K. Relationship of oxygen and glutathione in protection against carbon tetrachloride-induced hepatic microsomal lipid peroxidation and covalent binding in the rat. Rationale for the use of hyperbaric oxygen to treat carbon tetrachloride ingestion. *J. Clin. Investig.* **1984**, *74*, 1996–2001. [CrossRef] [PubMed]

9.   Wu, N.; Cai, G.M.; He, Q. Oxidative stress and hepatic injury. *World Chin. J. Digestol.* **2008**, *16*, 3310–3315. [CrossRef]

10.   Kayesh, M.E.H.; Ezzikouri, S.; Sanada, T.; Chi, H.; Hayashi, Y.; Rebbani, K.; Kitab, B.; Matsuu, A.; Miyoshi, N.; Hishima, T.; et al. Oxidative stress and immune responses during hepatitis C virus infection in tupaia belangeri. *Sci. Rep.* **2017**, *7*, 9848. [CrossRef] [PubMed]

11.   Ali, N.; Rashid, S.; Nafees, S.; Hasan, S.K.; Shahid, A.; Majed, F.; Sultana, S. Protective effect of Chlorogenic acid against methotrexate induced oxidative stress, inflammation and apoptosis in rat liver: An experimental approach. *Chem. Biol. Interact.* **2017**, *272*, 80–91. [CrossRef] [PubMed]

12.   Du, J.; Zhang, X.; Han, J.; Man, K.; Zhang, Y.; Chu, E.S.; Nan, Y.; Yu, J. Pro-inflammatory CXCR3 impairs mitochondrial function in experimental non-alcoholic steatohepatitis. *Theranostics* **2017**, *7*, 4192–4203. [CrossRef] [PubMed]

13.   Choudhury, S.; Ghosh, S.; Mukherjee, S.; Gupta, P.; Bhattacharya, S.; Adhikary, A.; Chattopadhyay, S. Pomegranate protects against arsenic-induced p53-dependent ROS-mediated inflammation and apoptosis in liver cells. *J. Nutr. Biochem.* **2016**, *38*, 25–40. [CrossRef] [PubMed]

14.   Niedzwiecki, A.; Roomi, M.W.; Kalinovsky, T.; Rath, M. Anticancer efficacy of polyphenols and their combinations. *Nutrients* **2016**, *8*, E552. [CrossRef] [PubMed]

15.   Megow, I.; Darvin, M.E.; Meinke, M.C.; Lademann, J. A randomized controlled trial of green tea beverages on the in vivo radical scavenging activity in human skin. *Skin Pharmacol. Physiol.* **2017**, *30*, 225–233. [CrossRef] [PubMed]

16.   Yi, R.; Wang, R.; Sun, P.; Zhao, X. Antioxidant-mediated preventative effect of Dragon-pearl tea crude polyphenol extract on reserpine-induced gastric ulcers. *Exp. Ther. Med.* **2015**, *10*, 338–344. [CrossRef] [PubMed]

17.   Yuan, G.J.; Gong, Z.J.; Sun, X.M.; Zheng, S.H.; Li, X. Tea polyphenols inhibit expressions of iNOS and TNF-alpha and prevent lipopolysaccharide-induced liver injury in rats. *Hepatobiliary Pancreat. Dis. Int.* **2006**, *5*, 262–267. [PubMed]

18.   Salomone, F.; Godos, J.; Zelber-Sagi, S. Natural antioxidants for non-alcoholic fatty liver disease: Molecular targets and clinical perspectives. *Liver Int.* **2016**, *36*, 5–20. [CrossRef] [PubMed]

19.   Chen, X.Q.; Ye, Y.; Cheng, H.; Tang, D.D.; Su, L.H. Studies on physical and chemical properties of Liubao tea. *Chin. Agri. Sci. Bull.* **2008**, *24*, 77–80.

20.   Zhao, X.; Qian, Y. Preventive effects of Kuding tea crude polyphenols in DSS-induced C57BL/6J mice ulcerative colitis. *Sci. Technol. Food Ind.* **2017**, *38*, 357–362.

21.   Zhao, X.; Qian, Y.; Li, G.J.; Tan, J. Preventive effects of the polysaccharide of Larimichthys crocea swim bladder on carbon tetrachloride (CCl$_4$)-induced hepatic damage. *Chin. J. Nat. Med.* **2015**, *13*, 521–528. [CrossRef]

22.   Chen, X.; Zhao, X.; Wang, H.; Yang, Z.; Li, J.; Suo, H. Prevent effects of *Lactobacillus fermentum* HY01 on dextran sulfate sodium-induced colitis in mice. *Nutrients* **2017**, *9*, E545. [CrossRef] [PubMed]

23.   Zhao, X.; Cheng, Q.; Qian, Y.; Yi, R.K.; Gu, L.J.; Wang, S.S.; Song, J.L. Insect tea attenuates hydrochloric acid and ethanol-induced mice acute gastric injury. *Exp. Ther. Med.* **2017**, *14*, 5135–5142. [CrossRef] [PubMed]

24. Fan, D.M.; Fan, K.; Yu, C.P.; Lu, Y.T.; Wang, X.C. Tea polyphenols dominate the short-term tea (Camellia sinensis) leaf litter decomposition. *J. Zhejiang Univ. Sci. B* **2017**, *18*, 99–108. [CrossRef] [PubMed]

25. Wu, W.L.; Lin, Y.; Liu, Z.H.; Huang, J.A.; Long, Z.R.; Teng, C.Q.; Ma, S.C.; Qiu, R.J.; Cao, Z.H. Research on acute and subacute toxicity evaluation of Liupao tea. *J. Tea Sci.* **2017**, *37*, 173–181.

26. Wu, H.; Qiu, Y.; Shu, Z.; Zhang, X.; Li, R.; Liu, S.; Chen, L.; Liu, H.; Chen, N. Protective effect of Trillium tschonoskii saponin on CCl$_4$-induced acute liver injury of rats through apoptosis inhibition. *Can. J. Physiol. Pharmacol.* **2016**, *94*, 1291–1297. [CrossRef] [PubMed]

27. Ahmed, S.M.; Abdelrahman, S.A.; Salama, A.E. Efficacy of gold nanoparticles against isoproterenol induced acute myocardial infarction in adult male albino rats. *Ultrastruct. Pathol.* **2017**, *41*, 168–185. [CrossRef] [PubMed]

28. Maksymchuk, O.; Shysh, A.; Rosohatska, I.; Chashchyn, M. Quercetin prevents type 1 diabetic liver damage through inhibition of CYP2E1. *Pharmacol. Rep.* **2017**, *69*, 1386–1392. [CrossRef] [PubMed]

29. Mahmoodzadeh, Y.; Mazani, M.; Rezagholizadeh, L. Hepatoprotective effect of methanolic *Tanacetum parthenium* extract on CCl$_4$-induced liver damage in rats. *Pharmacol. Rep.* **2017**, *4*, 455–462. [CrossRef] [PubMed]

30. Zeng, B.; Su, M.; Chen, Q.; Chang, Q.; Wang, W.; Li, H. Protective effect of a polysaccharide from *Anoectochilus roxburghii* against carbon tetrachloride-induced acute liver injury in mice. *J. Ethnopharmacol.* **2017**, *200*, 124–135. [CrossRef] [PubMed]

31. Dreher, D.; Junod, A.F. Differential effects of superoxide, hydrogen peroxide, and hydroxyl radical on intracellular calcium in human endothelial cells. *J Cell Physiol.* **1995**, *162*, 147–153. [CrossRef] [PubMed]

32. Hou, J.; You, G.; Xu, Y.; Wang, C.; Wang, P.; Miao, L.; Dai, S.; Lv, B.; Yang, Y. Antioxidant enzyme activities as biomarkers of fluvial biofilm to ZnO NPs ecotoxicity and the Integrated Biomarker Responses (IBR) assessment. *Ecotoxicol. Environ. Saf.* **2016**, *133*, 10–17. [CrossRef] [PubMed]

33. Niu, C.; Ma, M.; Han, X.; Wang, Z.; Li, H. Hyperin protects against cisplatin-induced liver injury in mice. *Acta Cir. Bras.* **2017**, *32*, 633–640. [CrossRef] [PubMed]

34. Won, G.; Kim, T.H.; Lee, J.H. A novel Salmonella strain inactivated by a regulated autolysis system and expressing the B subunit of Shiga toxin 2e efficiently elicits immune responses and confers protection against virulent Stx2e-producing Escherichia coli. *BMC Vet. Res.* **2017**, *13*, 40. [CrossRef] [PubMed]

35. Kampan, N.C.; Madondo, M.T.; McNally, O.M.; Stephens, A.N.; Quinn, M.A.; Plebanski, M. Interleukin 6 present in inflammatory ascites from advanced epithelial ovarian cancer patients promotes tumor necrosis factor receptor 2-expressing regulatory T. cells. *Front. Immunol.* **2017**, *8*, 1482. [CrossRef] [PubMed]

36. Gil-Farina, I.; Di Scala, M.; Salido, E.; López-Franco, E.; Rodríguez-García, E.; Blasi, M.; Merino, J.; Aldabe, R.; Prieto, J.; Gonzalez-Aseguinolaza, G. Transient expression of transgenic IL-12 in mouse liver triggers unremitting inflammation mimicking human autoimmune hepatitis. *J. Immunol.* **2016**, *197*, 2145–2156. [CrossRef] [PubMed]

37. Erkasap, S.; Erkasap, N.; Bradford, B.; Mamedova, L.; Uysal, O.; Ozkurt, M.; Ozyurt, R.; Kutlay, O.; Bayram, B. The effect of leptin and resveratrol on JAK/STAT pathways and Sirt-1 gene expression in the renal tissue of ischemia/reperfusion induced rats. *Bratisl. Lek. Listy* **2017**, *118*, 443–448. [CrossRef] [PubMed]

38. Li, G.; Chen, M.J.; Wang, C.; Nie, H.; Huang, W.J.; Yuan, T.D.; Sun, T.; Shu, K.G.; Wang, C.F.; Gong, Q.; et al. Protective effects of hesperidin on concanavalin A-induced hepatic injury in mice. *Int. Immunopharmacol.* **2014**, *21*, 406–411. [CrossRef] [PubMed]

39. Ma, J.; Li, Y.; Duan, H.; Sivakumar, R.; Li, X. Chronic exposure of nanomolar MC-LR caused oxidative stress and inflammatory responses in HepG2 cells. *Chemosphere* **2018**, *192*, 305–317. [CrossRef] [PubMed]

40. Wu, S.X.; Han, X.M.; Jiang, X.W.; Tao, J. The Effects of two different multivitamins on aging mice. *Chin. J. Physiol.* **2017**, *60*, 284–292. [CrossRef] [PubMed]

41. Najafpour, M.M. A possible evolutionary origin for the Mn4 cluster in photosystem II: From manganese superoxide dismutase to oxygen evolving complex. *Orig. Life Evol. Biosph.* **2009**, *32*, 151–163. [CrossRef] [PubMed]

42. Suo, H.; Feng, X.; Zhu, K.; Wang, C.; Zhao, X.; Kan, J. Shuidouchi (fermented soybean) fermented in different vessels attenuates HCl/ethanol-induced gastric mucosal injury. *Molecules* **2015**, *20*, 19748–19763. [CrossRef] [PubMed]

43. Wang, M.; Zhang, X.J.; Feng, R.; Jiang, Y.; Zhang, D.Y.; He, C.; Li, P.; Wan, J.B. Hepatoprotective properties of *Penthorum chinense* Pursh against carbon tetrachloride-induced acute liver injury in mice. *Chin. Med.* **2017**, *12*, 32. [CrossRef] [PubMed]

44. Medeiros, M.H.; Wefers, H.; Sies, H. Generation of excited species catalyzed by horseradish peroxidase or hemin in the presence of reduced glutathione and H_2O_2. *Free Radic. Biol. Med.* **1987**, *3*, 107–110. [CrossRef]

45. Ma, Q.; Liu, C.M.; Qin, Z.H.; Jiang, J.H.; Sun, Y.Z. Ganoderma applanatum terpenes protect mouse liver against benzo(α)pyren-induced oxidative stress and inflammation. *Environ. Toxicol. Pharmacol.* **2011**, *31*, 460–468. [CrossRef] [PubMed]

46. Liu, C.M.; Zheng, Y.L.; Lu, J.; Zhang, Z.F.; Fan, S.H.; Wu, D.M.; Ma, J.Q. Quercetin protects rat liver against lead-induced oxidative stress and apoptosis. *Environ. Toxicol. Pharmacol.* **2010**, *29*, 158–166. [CrossRef] [PubMed]

47. Kaur, G.; Alam, M.S.; Jabbar, Z.; Javed, K.; Athar, M. Evaluation of antioxidant activity of Cassia siamea flowers. *J. Ethnopharmacol.* **2006**, *108*, 340–348. [CrossRef] [PubMed]

48. Chan, P.; Liu, C.; Chiang, F.Y.; Wang, L.F.; Lee, K.W.; Chen, W.T.; Kuo, P.L.; Liang, C.H. IL-8 promotes inflammatory mediators and stimulates activation of p38 MAPK/ERK-NF-κB pathway and reduction of JNK in HNSCC. *Oncotarget* **2017**, *8*, 56375–56388. [CrossRef] [PubMed]

49. Cai, L.; Chen, W.N.; Li, R.; Hu, C.M.; Lei, C.; Li, C.M. Therapeutic effect of acetazolamide, an aquaporin 1 inhibitor, on adjuvant-induced arthritis in rats by inhibiting NF-κB signal pathway. *Immunopharmacol. Immunotoxicol.* **2018**, *40*, 117–125. [CrossRef] [PubMed]

50. El-Gohary, A. Obestatin improves hepatic injury induced by ischemia/reperfusion in rats: Role of nitric oxide. *Gen. Physiol. Biophys.* **2017**, *36*, 109–115. [CrossRef] [PubMed]

51. Bachmann, M.; Waibler, Z.; Pleli, T.; Pfeilschifter, J.; Mühl, H. Type I interferon supports inducible nitric oxide synthase in murine hepatoma cells and hepatocytes and during experimental acetaminophen-induced liver damage. *Front. Immunol.* **2017**, *8*, 890. [CrossRef] [PubMed]

52. Araújo Júnior, R.F.; Garcia, V.B.; Leitão, R.F.; Brito, G.A.; Miguel Ede, C.; Guedes, P.M.; de Araújo, A.A. Carvedilol improves inflammatory response, oxidative stress and fibrosis in the alcohol-induced liver injury in rats by regulating Kuppfer cells and hepatic stellate cells. *PLoS ONE* **2016**, *12*, e0148868. [CrossRef] [PubMed]

53. Turesky, R.J.; Konorev, D.; Fan, X.; Tang, Y.; Yao, L.; Ding, X.; Xie, F.; Zhu, Y.; Zhang, Q.Y. Effect of cytochrome P450 reductase deficiency on 2-amino-9H-pyrido[2,3-b]indole metabolism and DNA adduct formation in liver and extrahepatic tissues of mice. *Chem. Res. Toxicol.* **2015**, *28*, 2400–2410. [CrossRef] [PubMed]

54. Hsieh, S.C.; Wu, C.H.; Wu, C.C.; Yen, J.H.; Liu, M.C.; Hsueh, C.M.; Hsu, S.L. Gallic acid selectively induces the necrosis of activated hepatic stellate cells via a calcium-dependent calpain I. activation pathway. *Life Sci.* **2014**, *102*, 55–64. [CrossRef] [PubMed]

55. Zheng, X.H.; Yang, J.; Yang, Y.H. Research progress on pharmacological effects of gallic acid. *Chin. Hosp. Pharm. J.* **2017**, *37*, 94–98.

56. Zhai, W.; Zheng, J.H.; Yao, X.D.; Peng, B.; Liu, M.; Huang, J.H.; Wang, G.C.; Xu, Y.F. Catechin prevents the calcium oxalate monohydrate induced renal calcium crystallization in NRK-52E cells and the ethylene glycol induced renal stone formation in rat. *BMC Complem. Altern. Med.* **2013**, *13*, 228. [CrossRef] [PubMed]

57. Suzuki, H.; Yamamoto, S.; Hirayama, C.; Takino, T.; Fujisawa, K.; Oda, T. Cianidanol therapy for HBe-antigen-positive chronic hepatitis: A multicentre, double-blind study. *Liver* **1986**, *6*, 35–44. [CrossRef] [PubMed]

58. Ramadori, G.; Sipe, J.D.; Dinarello, C.A.; Mizel, S.B.; Colten, H.R. Pretranslational modulation of acute phase hepatic protein synthesis by murine recombinant interleukin 1 (IL-1) and purified human IL-1. *J. Exp. Med.* **1995**, *162*, 930–942. [CrossRef]

59. Furman, D.; Chang, J.; Lartigue, L.; Bolen, C.R.; Haddad, F.; Gaudilliere, B.; Ganio, E.A.; Fragiadakis, G.K.; Spitzer, M.H.; Douchet, I.; et al. Expression of specific inflammasome gene modules stratifies older individuals into two extreme clinical and immunological states. *Nat. Med.* **2017**, *23*, 174–184. [CrossRef] [PubMed]

60. Chen, Z.; Lv, X.W.; Li, J.; Zhang, L.; Liu, H.F.; Huang, C.; Zhu, P.L. Protective effect of caffeine on alcohol-induce acute liver injury in mice. *Acta Univ. Med. Anhui* **2009**, *44*, 359–362.

61. Kim, A. Mechanisms underlying beneficial health effects of tea catechins to improve insulin resistance and endothelial dysfunction. *Endocr. Metab. Immune Disord. Drug Targets* **2008**, *8*, 82–88. [CrossRef] [PubMed]

62. Mohamed, R.H.; Karam, R.A.; Amer, M.G. Epicatechin attenuates doxorubicin-induced brain toxicity: Critical role of TNF-α, iNOS and NF-κB. *Brain Res. Bull.* **2011**, *86*, 22–28. [CrossRef] [PubMed]
63. Zhen, C.; Wang, X.M.; Yin, Z.Y.; Wang, Q.; Liu, P.G.; Wu, G.Y.; Yu, K.K.; Li, G.S. Effect of EGCG on expression of TGF-β1 and CTGF in rats with liver fibrosis. *World Chin. J. Digestol.* **2008**, *16*, 3828–3834. [CrossRef]
64. Liu, D.M.; Wang, X.F. EGCG influences the NF-κB and ICAM-I expression of ConA inducing liver injury. *Anat. Res.* **2014**, *36*, 27–30.
65. Ye, J.X.; Wang, L.; Liang, R.X.; Yang, B. Protection and its mechanism of catechin morphon on hypoxia-reoxynation induced in myocardial cells. *China J. Chin. Mater. Med.* **2008**, *33*, 801–805.
66. Huang, X.; Zhong, W.B.; Huang, S.L.; Hu, Y.H.; Wang, D.D.; Sun, Y. Anti-tumor activities of catechins EGCG and ECG against human hepatocarcinoma BEL-7402 cells. *J. Guangdong Pharm. Univ.* **2013**, *29*, 435–438.
67. Zhang, X.N.; Lin, Y.; Huang, J.A.; Liu, Z.H.; Liang, D.D. Inhibitory effects of tea extracts EGCG, GCG and ECG on the melanogenesis in melanoma cell B16. *J. Hunan Agric. Univ. (Nat. Sci.)* **2017**, *43*, 405–410.

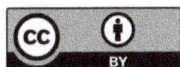

![nutrients logo]

nutrients

MDPI

Article

Stress-Reducing Function of Matcha Green Tea in Animal Experiments and Clinical Trials

Keiko Unno [1,2,*], **Daisuke Furushima** [3], **Shingo Hamamoto** [3], **Kazuaki Iguchi** [1], **Hiroshi Yamada** [3], **Akio Morita** [4], **Hideki Horie** [5] and **Yoriyuki Nakamura** [2]

[1] Department of Neurophysiology, School of Pharmaceutical Sciences, University of Shizuoka, Shizuoka 422-8526, Japan; iguchi@u-shizuoka-ken.ac.jp

[2] Tea Science Center, Graduate School of Integrated Pharmaceutical and Nutritional Sciences, University of Shizuoka, Shizuoka 422-8526, Japan; yori.naka222@u-shizuoka-ken.ac.jp

[3] Department of Drug Evaluation & Informatics, School of Pharmaceutical Sciences, University of Shizuoka, Shizuoka 422-8526, Japan; dfuru@u-shizuoka-ken.ac.jp (D.F.); m14093@u-shizuoka-ken.ac.jp (S.H.); hyamada@u-shizuoka-ken.ac.jp (H.Y.)

[4] Department of Functional Plant Physiology, Faculty of Agriculture, Shizuoka University, Shizuoka 422-8529, Japan; morita.akio@shizuoka.ac.jp

[5] Institute of Fruit Tree and Tea Science, National Agriculture and Food Research Organization, Shimada 428-8501, Japan; horie@affrc.go.jp

* Correspondence: unno@u-shizuoka-ken.ac.jp; Tel.: +81-542-645-731

Received: 14 September 2018; Accepted: 9 October 2018; Published: 10 October 2018

Abstract: Theanine, a major amino acid in green tea, exhibits a stress-reducing effect in mice and humans. Matcha, which is essentially theanine-rich powdered green tea, is abundant in caffeine. Caffeine has a strong antagonistic effect against theanine. The stress-reducing effect of matcha was examined with an animal experiment and a clinical trial. The stress-reducing effect of matcha marketed in Japan and abroad was assessed based on its composition. The stress-reducing effect of matcha in mice was evaluated as suppressed adrenal hypertrophy using territorially-based loaded stress. High contents of theanine and arginine in matcha exhibited a high stress-reducing effect. However, an effective stress-reducing outcome was only possible when the molar ratio of caffeine and epigallocatechin gallate (EGCG) to theanine and arginine was less than two. Participants ($n = 39$) consumed test-matcha, which was expected to have a stress-reducing effect, or placebo-matcha, where no effect was expected. Anxiety, a reaction to stress, was significantly lower in the test-matcha group than in the placebo group. To predict mental function of each matcha, both the quantity of theanine and the ratios of caffeine, EGCG, and arginine against theanine need to be verified.

Keywords: adrenal hypertrophy; anxiety; caffeine; catechin; green tea; matcha; salivary α-amylase activity; stress-reduction; theanine

1. Introduction

Theanine is an L-glutamate analogue and a non-protein amino acid that is particular to the tea plant (*Camellia sinensis* (L.) Kuntze) [1]. The amount of theanine, which is the most abundant amino acid in green tea leaves, depends on nitrogen supply absorbed from the roots [2]. Matcha is a fine-powdered green tea that is prepared from tea leaves protected from sunlight. When tea leaves are protected from direct sunlight, their amino acid content, especially theanine, remains high because the hydration of theanine used in the biosynthesis of catechin is lowered [3,4]. To make matcha, cultivation under shade for about three weeks is necessary before harvest [5]. Given their protection from sunlight, catechin content is lower in matcha than in other popular green teas prepared from leaves grown in sunlight [3,6]. In addition, matcha has a high content of caffeine because the buds and young leaves of

Camellia plants contain more caffeine than mature leaves [7]. The balance of these components, such as theanine, caffeine, and catechin, determines the quality of the green tea. A higher content of amino acids indicates a higher level of "umami" ingredients. Therefore, matcha is essentially the best-grade green tea, rich in theanine and caffeine, but with a low content of catechin compared with popular green tea.

Chronic psychosocial stress is associated with the development of depression, mood disorders, and various other stress-related diseases [8–10]. Addressing stress-induced alterations with dietary supplements is a potential therapeutic strategy for a healthy life. Green tea is the most popular drink in Asian countries and its consumption and that of theanine has revealed health benefits and medicinal potential for several ailments [11]. Theanine exhibits an excellent stress-reducing effect on mice and humans [12,13]. However, the effect of theanine is antagonized by caffeine and epigallocatechin gallate (EGCG), which are two major components of green tea [14–16]. In contrast, the stress-reducing effect of theanine is enhanced by arginine (Arg), which is the second most abundant amino acid in Japanese green tea [17]. Glutamate (Glu), the third most abundant amino acid in green tea, has no effect on stress in mice [17]. To enhance the stress-reducing effect of green tea, low-caffeine green tea with reduced caffeine content can be prepared from tea leaves by irrigating them with hot water at 95 °C for three minutes. Published data showed that a significant stress-reducing effect of low-caffeine green tea was observed in participants in their 20 s, 40 s–50 s, and 80 s–90 s relative to barley tea or standard green tea [18–20].

Matcha is expected to have a stress-reducing effect due to its high theanine content, although this has not been scientifically proven. Previous studies described above suggested that differences in the quantities and ratios of green tea components affect the efficiency of its stress-reducing action. Therefore, the stress-reducing effect of matcha, which contains catechins, caffeine, and amino acids whose contents were measured, was evaluated in an animal (mouse) experiment. Mice were stressed using territorial conflict between male mice [14]. The stress-reducing effect of matcha was evaluated as the suppression of adrenal hypertrophy in stressed mice because adrenal glands are sensitive to stress [14]. The relationship between suppressed adrenal hypertrophy and quantities or ratios of matcha tea components was examined. Based on these data, test-matcha with contents expected to have a stress-reducing effect, as well as placebo-matcha with contents expected to have no stress-reducing effect, were selected for a clinical trial. Participants, who were selected for a double-blind randomized controlled trial, consumed matcha (3 g) suspended in 500 mL water daily. They were fifth year college students of the University of Shizuoka, School of Pharmaceutical Sciences, Japan, who were assigned to a pharmacy practice outside the university, such as a hospital or a pharmacy. Commitment to a new environment provides a stressful condition for young students. Since anxiety is a reaction to stress, to assess the anxiety of participants, the state-trait anxiety inventory (STAI) test was administered before and on the eighth day of pharmacy practice. In addition, to assess the physiological stress response, the activity of salivary α-amylase activity (sAA), an oral cavity enzyme, was measured as a stress marker of sympathetic excitement [15]. This enzyme rapidly increases in response to physiological and psychosocial stress [21]. We examined whether test-matcha was able to reduce participants' stress. Finally, based on the quantity and ratio of components of each matcha, 76 matcha samples sold in Japan and 67 samples sold abroad were evaluated to determine whether mental function such as anxiety and stress could be expected when humans consume these forms of matcha.

2. Materials and Methods

2.1. Measurement of Tea Components by High-Performance Liquid Chromatography

The components in matcha were measured by high performance liquid chromatography (HPLC) as described previously [17]. We focused on the contents of theanine, arginine, caffeine, and EGCG. In brief, according to the method of Horie et al. [5], catechins and caffeine were measured by HPLC at 280 nm (SCL-10Avp, Shimadzu, Kyoto, Japan; Develosil packed column ODS-HG-5, 150 × 4.6 mm,

Nomura Chemical Co. Ltd., Seto, Japan). Free amino acids (Arg, alanine, aspartic acid (Asp), asparagine (Asn), glutamic acid (Glu), glutamine (Gln), γ-amino butyric acid (GABA), serine (Ser), and theanine) were measured by HPLC as described above using glycylglycine as the internal standard [22]. These amino acids were detected at an excitation wavelength of 340 nm and at an emission wavelength of 450 nm (RF-535 UV detector, Shimadzu, Kyoto, Japan). Based on these data, seven matcha samples were selected for the animal experiment.

2.2. Animal Studies

2.2.1. Animals and Stress Experiment

Male ddY mice (Slc: ddY, four weeks old) were purchased from Japan SLC Co. Ltd. (Shizuoka, Japan) and kept under conventional conditions in a temperature- and humidity-controlled environment with a 12/12 h light/dark cycle (light period, 8:00 a.m.–8:00 p.m.; temperature, 23 ± 1 °C; relative humidity, 55 ± 5%). Four-week-old mice were reared in a group of six in a cage for five days to allow them to adapt to co-habitation. Mice were fed a normal diet (CE-2; Clea Co. Ltd., Tokyo, Japan) and water *ad libitum*. All experimental protocols were approved by the University of Shizuoka Laboratory Animal Care Advisory Committee (approval no. 166197) and were in accordance with the guidelines of the U.S. National Institute of Health for the Care and Use of Laboratory Animals. To apply psychosocial stress to mice, confrontational rearing was performed in a standard polycarbonate cage that was divided into two identical subunits by a stainless-steel partition as previously described [14]. In brief, two mice were reared in a partitioned cage for one week (single rearing) to establish territorial consciousness. Then, the partition was removed to expose the mice to confrontational stress for 24 h (confrontational rearing). Adrenal glands, a critical stress-responsible organ, became significantly enlarged after confrontational rearing and peak size was reached at 24 h. The phenomenon continues for at least one week [14]. In mice under confrontational rearing, adrenal-hypertrophy, change in diurnal rhythm of corticosterone, and depression-like behavior have been observed. In addition, adrenal hypertrophy was suppressed by the intake of the antidepressant and anxiolytic drug, diazepam [14]. Since the suppression of adrenal hypertrophy is thought to be related to antidepressant and anxiolytic effects, the stress-reducing and anxiolytic effects of matcha in mice was evaluated by weighing the adrenal glands. Each cage was placed in a styrofoam box (width 30 cm, length 40 cm, height 15 cm) to avoid visual social contact between cages.

2.2.2. Ingestion of Matcha or Tea Components by Mice

The effect of matcha was examined in 15 groups of mice (4–8 mice/group, $n = 86$). Mice consumed matcha or tea components in a powder diet of CE-2 ad libitum for seven days (single rearing for six days and confrontational rearing for one day) (Scheme 1). The experimental dose was set based on the consumption in humans. Since about 2–3 g of matcha is used per cup in the tea ceremony in Japan, the intake (2–3 g/60 kg body weight) in humans corresponds to 33–50 mg/kg in mice. Based on this and considering the difference between humans and mice, the effect of matcha was examined at 0, 10, 17, 33, 50, and 100 mg/kg (body weight) doses in mice. Ingested food weight was measured using a special bait box for measurement of exact ingestion volume (Roden CAFE®, Oriental Yeast Co., Ltd., Tokyo, Japan). Mouse body weight was measured on the last day of the experiment. Seven matcha samples were used for the experiment. The stress-reducing effect was compared among matcha samples no. 1–5, at a dose of 33 mg/kg, and no. 6–7, at 50 mg/kg. Tea components used were as follows: L-theanine (Suntheanine; Taiyo Kagaku Co. Ltd., Yokkaichi, Japan), EGCG (Sunphenon EGCg, Taiyo Kagaku Co. Ltd., Yokkaichi, Japan), caffeine, and Arg (Wako Pure Chemical Co. Ltd., Osaka, Japan). The interaction of these tea components was examined on adrenal hypertrophy in stressed mice. The stress-reducing effect of tea components was compared among four groups of mice as follows: group 1 was control mice fed a powder diet; group 2 included mice fed a diet containing only theanine; group 3 included mice fed a diet containing theanine, caffeine, and EGCG; and group 4 included mice fed a diet containing theanine, caffeine, EGCG, and Arg. The concentration of theanine was 0.32 mg/kg. The molar ratio of each component was that of matcha sample no. 6, i.e., the molar ratio of theanine:caffeine:EGCG:Arg was 1:2:1:0.7. At the end of the 24 h of confrontational rearing, mice were sacrificed and adrenal glands were weighed.

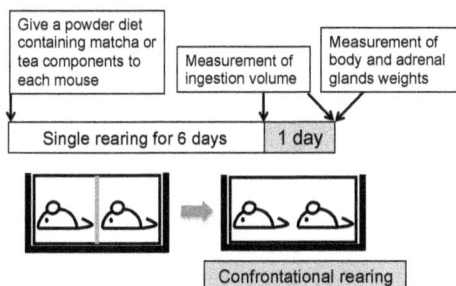

Scheme 1. Study design of the animal experiment.

2.3. Human Studies

2.3.1. Participants

Thirty-nine healthy students (23 ± 1.1 years old, 23 men and 16 women) who participated in the experiment received verbal and written information about the study. They signed an informed consent form before participating in the study. None of the participants indicated any acute or chronic diseases, regular intake of medication, or habitual smoking. Participants were instructed to drink mainly the test-matcha tea, and to not consume theanine- and caffeine-rich beverages, such as other teas, including green tea, coffee, black tea, and soda, throughout the experiment. They were also instructed not to consume caffeine-rich foods such as chocolate and candies. Participants were allowed to drink water freely, but were not permitted to consume alcohol at night to eliminate psychological effects due to alcohol intake. They were randomly divided into two groups: test-matcha ($n = 19$) and placebo-matcha ($n = 20$).

The participants were assigned to a practice outside the university, either in a hospital or at a pharmacy, for 11 weeks. Seven days of routine university life and the first eight days of the students' practice program were analyzed. The study was conducted in accordance with the Declaration of Helsinki and Ethical Guidelines for Medical and Health Research Involving Human Subjects (Public Notice of the Ministry of Education, Culture, Sports, Science, and Technology and the Ministry of Health, Labour and Welfare, 2008). This study was approved in Japan, and the study protocol, which was approved by the Ethics Committee of the University of Shizuoka (no. 28-60), was registered at the University Hospital Medical Information Network (UMIN) (registration no. UMIN26905). The study period was from April to May 2017.

2.3.2. Procedure

This study was based on a group comparison design and participants were randomly assigned to test- or placebo-matcha groups. The test- and placebo-matcha were packed 3 g each into exactly same-shaped bags. The participants did not know whether they were consuming test- or placebo-matcha. The intake of test- or placebo-matcha tea started from seven days prior to pharmacy practice and continued for eight days into the practice period, for a total of 15 days (Table 1). Since anxiety is a reaction to stress, to assess the anxiety of participants, the state-trait anxiety inventory (STAI) test (Japanese STAI Form X-1, Sankyobo, Kyoto, Japan) was administered before pharmacy

Nutrients **2018**, *10*, 1468

practice and on the eighth day of pharmacy practice. In this study, the state-anxiety of participants was compared between test- and placebo-groups.

Table 1. Experimental procedure.

Practice	University				Pharmacy	
Days	3	3–10	7		8	
Matcha intake	(−)	(−)	+		+	
sAAm	+	(−)	+		+	
STAI	(−)	(−)	(−)	+	(−)	+

sAAm: salivary α-amylase activity in the morning, STAI: state-trait anxiety inventory. That was administered before pharmacy practice and on the eighth day of pharmacy practice.

A questionnaire that included feedback on their physical condition, subjective stress, and achievement emotion was assigned for 15 days after each day's practice. The physical condition of participants was assigned an ordinal scale (5, very good; 4, good; 3, normal; 2, slightly bad; 1, bad). Subjective stress was evaluated using visual analogue scales (VAS: 0–10) from very relaxed to highly stressed. Achievement emotion was assigned an ordinal scale (5, completely; 4, better; 3, a little better; 2, a little worse; 1, much worse). Sleeping hours were also recorded. Each participant's median data for the last three days at the university and pharmacy practice were used for statistical analysis considering the influence of consecutive ingestion of matcha.

2.3.3. Measurement of sAA

To assess the physiological stress response, sAA was measured using a colorimetric system (Nipro Co., Osaka, Japan) [23]. In brief, salivary amylase hydrolyzes a substrate, 2-chloro-4-nitrophenyl-4-O-β-D-galactopyranosylmaltoside, in the presence of maltose, a competitive inhibitor. The color of a reagent strip turns from white to yellow in this reaction, and changes are quantified using a salivary amylase monitor. One unit of activity (U) per mass of enzyme is defined as the production of 1 μmol of the reduction sugar, maltose, in 1 min (NC-IUBMB, EC 3.2.1.1). Prior to sampling, participants washed their mouths with water. After saliva was collected for 30 s using a sampling tip, participants measured their own sAA immediately. Saliva was measured in the morning after waking up (sAAm). To establish a sAA baseline, participants recorded measurements every morning for three days during routine daily life at the university before intake of matcha. Next, the participants measured sAA every morning and every evening (sAAe) for seven days during routine daily life at the university, and successively for eight days during pharmacy practice (Table 1). Each participant's median sAA of the last three days at the university and pharmacy practice was used for statistical analysis considering the influence of consecutive ingestion of matcha.

2.4. Statistical Analyses

Data are expressed as the mean ± standard error of the mean (SEM). Statistical analyses were performed using Student's *t*-test and one-way analysis of variance (ANOVA) followed by Bonferroni's post-hoc test for multiple comparisons. All statistical analyses were performed in a statistical analysis program, JMP ver.13 (SAS Institute Inc., Cary, NC, USA). Differences were considered to be significant at $p < 0.05$.

3. Results

3.1. Animal Study

3.1.1. Anti-Stress Effects of Matcha in a Mouse Model of Psychosocial Stress

The relationship between the amount of matcha intake and suppression of adrenal hypertrophy was examined using matcha sample no. 1, whose theanine content represented the median of seven samples. The difference in matcha concentration did not affect food intake or body weight. The weight of adrenal glands increased to 5.0 ± 0.2 mg in mice after confrontational rearing from about 4.0 mg before confrontation. The results show that adrenal hypertrophy was significantly suppressed in mice that ingested more than 33 mg/kg of matcha (Figure 1a).

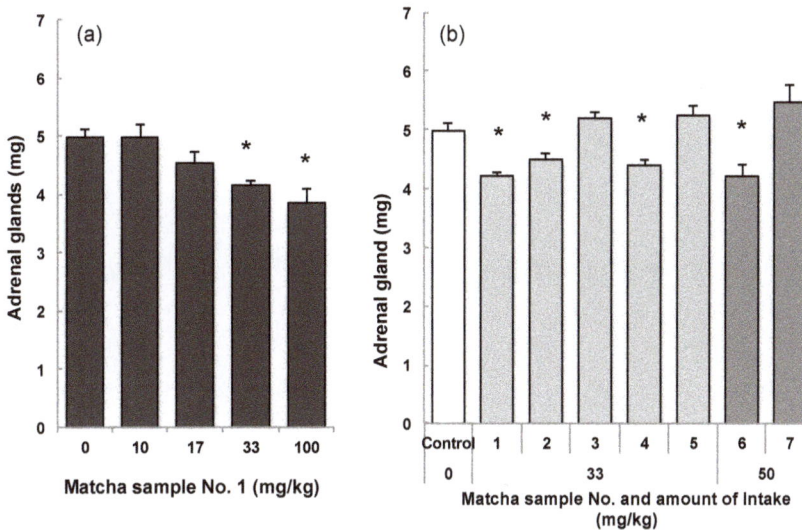

Figure 1. Suppression of adrenal hypertrophy by matcha intake in stressed mice. (**a**) Mice consumed a matcha sample (no. 1) in a powder diet for seven days (single rearing for six days and confrontational rearing for one day). Since each mouse (ca. 30 g) ingested about five grams of diet per day, the intake of matcha was set to 0, 10, 17, 33, and 100 mg/kg; (**b**) Mice were fed a diet containing matcha from no. 1 to no. 5 at a concentration of 33 mg/kg, and from no. 6 to no. 7 at a concentration of 50 mg/kg. Each bar shows the mean $\pm$ SEM ($n = 4$–8; * $p < 0.05$).

The stress-reducing effect was then compared among the seven samples of matcha. Adrenal hypertrophy was significantly suppressed in mice that consumed matcha sample nos. 1, 2, 4, and 6. Suppression of stress was not observed in mice that consumed matcha samples nos. 3, 5, or 7 (Figure 1b). The former samples had less total amino acid content than the latter batch of matcha samples (Table 2).

3.1.2. Relationship between Tea Components in Each Matcha Sample and Suppression of Adrenal Hypertrophy

We confirmed that theanine and Arg have a significant stress-reducing effect [17]. These are the most and the second most abundant amino acids in Japanese matcha. However, the third and fourth most abundant amino acids, glutamate and glutamine, had no effect. Therefore, the actual amount of theanine and arginine ingested by mice from matcha was calculated (Table 3). To suppress adrenal hypertrophy in mice, theanine is needed at 0.32 mg/kg or more [17]. This explains the lack of a stress-reducing effect in mice that ingested sample nos. 3, 5, and 7 (Table 3). The relationship between theanine intake and adrenal hypertrophy showed a dose-dependent suppression of the latter (Figure 2a, R^2 = 0.783). A similar correlation was observed for Arg (R^2 = 0.783). There was no relationship between caffeine intake and adrenal hypertrophy (Figure 2b, R^2 = 0.281).

Although the effect of theanine at 0.48 mg/kg (sample no. 1, 17 mg/kg) was slightly low, the coexistence of caffeine and EGCG may have counteracted the effect of theanine. All matcha samples contained both, equal, or higher molar amounts of caffeine and EGCG.

To examine the relationship among theanine, Arg, caffeine, and EGCG, mice ingested feed that contained each component as a molar ratio of sample no. 6 (Table 4). When the concentration of theanine was 0.32 mg/kg, adrenal hypertrophy was significantly suppressed by the ingestion of theanine (Figure 3). However, the action of theanine was antagonized by the coexistence of two-fold higher molar concentration of caffeine and an equal molar ratio of EGCG (Figure 3). In contrast, the coexistence of a 0.7 molar ratio of Arg to theanine recovered the counteraction of caffeine or EGCG (Figure 3), suggesting that Arg plays an essential role in the suppression of adrenal hypertrophy. The molar ratio of caffeine and EGCG to theanine and Arg was ≤1.8 in the effective samples, but was ≥3.6 in the non-effective samples (Table 4). These results indicate that the molar ratio of Arg, caffeine, and EGCG additionally affects theanine.

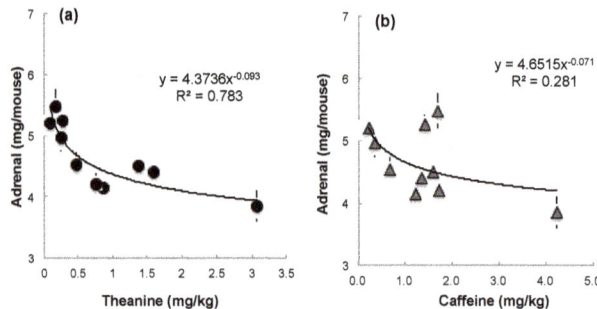

Figure 2. Correlations between adrenal hypertrophy and ingestion of matcha components in stressed mice. The amounts of (**a**) theanine and (**b**) caffeine were calculated from the matcha-containing feed that each mouse consumed, as shown in Table 3. Each point and bar shows the mean ± SEM (*n* = 4–8).

Table 2. Ingredient composition in each matcha sample.

Sample	Amino Acids (mg/g)								
No	Theanine	Arg	Glu	Asp	Asn	Ser	Gln	GABA	Total
1	28.99 ± 0.10	12.50 ± 0.04	7.52 ± 0.02	6.95 ± 0.02	2.90 ± 0.01	1.25 ± 0.00	1.08 ± 0.01	0.25 ± 0.00	61.45 ± 0.19
2	38.77 ± 0.16	18.19 ± 0.02	7.58 ± 0.05	8.47 ± 0.05	3.36 ± 0.01	1.84 ± 0.01	1.34 ± 0.01	0.22 ± 0.00	79.77 ± 0.43
3	2.48 ± 0.03	0.36 ± 0.00	0.48 ± 0.00	0.65 ± 0.01	0.09 ± 0.00	0.13 ± 0.00	0.11 ± 0.00	0.05 ± 0.00	4.35 ± 0.04
4	44.65 ± 1.73	20.39 ± 1.06	5.86 ± 0.16	7.95 ± 0.19	4.01 ± 0.12	1.74 ± 0.05	3.20 ± 0.11	0.23 ± 0.01	88.02 ± 3.41
5	7.87 ± 0.17	1.41 ± 0.06	2.64 ± 0.03	2.80 ± 0.02	0.59 ± 0.02	0.57 ± 0.03	0.51 ± 0.01	0.14 ± 0.00	16.52 ± 0.26
6	17.41 ± 0.18	12.33 ± 0.32	5.37 ± 0.04	7.60 ± 0.14	3.18 ± 0.03	1.34 ± 0.01	0.85 ± 0.01	0.13 ± 0.00	48.21 ± 0.70
7	3.91 ± 0.09	1.43 ± 0.11	2.82 ± 0.05	2.94 ± 0.06	0.82 ± 0.02	0.58 ± 0.01	0.38 ± 0.01	0.26 ± 0.01	13.15 ± 0.37

Sample	Caffeine	Catechin (mg/g)			
No	(mg/g)	EGCG	ECG	EGC	EC
1	39.95 ± 0.19	59.34 ± 0.41	12.44 ± 0.07	14.86 ± 0.06	4.26 ± 0.01
2	44.43 ± 0.47	57.20 ± 0.84	13.81 ± 0.21	9.68 ± 0.04	3.44 ± 0.02
3	5.95 ± 0.02	13.15 ± 0.08	2.20 ± 0.01	4.09 ± 0.02	0.87 ± 0.00
4	37.19 ± 0.36	48.44 ± 0.53	9.96 ± 0.15	8.40 ± 0.06	2.50 ± 0.04
5	40.35 ± 0.70	86.76 ± 1.47	06.09 ± 0.34	28.76 ± 0.38	6.48 ± 0.13
6	38.95 ± 0.55	49.15 ± 0.69	25.41 ± 0.69	9.91 ± 0.09	3.29 ± 0.03
7	37.06 ± 0.23	64.61 ± 4.30	30.54 ± 1.51	31.21 ± 0.40	6.75 ± 0.11

Data represents mean ± SEM (*n* = 2–3). ECG, epicatechin gallate; EGC, epigallocatechin; EC, epicatechin.

Table 3. Adrenal weight in mice that ingested each matcha sample, and the actual amount of each component that was ingested by mice.

Matcha	Concentration	Adrenal	Matcha Intake	Theanine	Arginine	Caffeine	EGCG
No.	(mg/kg)	(mg/Mouse)	(mg/kg)	(mg/kg)	(mg/kg)	(mg/kg)	(mg/kg)
1	10	4.97 ± 0.23	8.7 ± 2.2	0.25 ± 0.03	0.11 ± 0.01	0.35 ± 0.04	0.51 ± 0.05
1	17	4.53 ± 0.19	16.7 ± 0.4	0.48 ± 0.01	0.21 ± 0.01	0.67 ± 0.01	0.99 ± 0.02
1	33	4.15 ± 0.09	30.2 ± 1.5	0.88 ± 0.04	0.38 ± 0.02	1.21 ± 0.06	1.79 ± 0.09
1	100	3.85 ± 0.25	105.9 ± 5.0	3.07 ± 0.14	1.32 ± 0.06	4.23 ± 0.20	6.28 ± 0.30
2	33	4.50 ± 0.09	35.5 ± 0.2	1.38 ± 0.01	0.65 ± 0.00	1.58 ± 0.01	2.03 ± 0.01
3	33	5.20 ± 0.10	35.6 ± 1.1	0.09 ± 0.00	0.01 ± 0.00	0.21 ± 0.01	0.47 ± 0.01
4	33	4.40 ± 0.09	35.8 ± 0.3	1.60 ± 0.01	0.73 ± 0.01	1.33 ± 0.01	1.73 ± 0.01
5	33	5.25 ± 0.17	34.8 ± 0.6	0.27 ± 0.01	0.05 ± 0.00	1.40 ± 0.02	3.02 ± 0.05
6	50	4.21 ± 0.19	44.3 ± 1.9	0.77 ± 0.03	0.55 ± 0.02	1.73 ± 0.07	1.79 ± 0.09
7	50	5.48 ± 0.29	45.7 ± 1.7	0.18 ± 0.01	0.07 ± 0.00	1.69 ± 0.06	2.95 ± 0.11

Data represents mean $\pm$ SEM (n = 4–8).

Table 4. Molar ratios in matcha samples.

Matcha No.	Caffeine/ Theanine	EGCG/ Theanine	Arg/ Theanine	(Caffeine + EGCG) /(Theanine + Arg)
1	1.23	0.78	0.43	1.41
2	1.03	0.56	0.47	1.08
3	2.17	2.01	0.15	3.63
4	0.75	0.41	0.46	0.79
5	4.60	4.19	0.18	7.45
6	2.01	1.07	0.71	1.80
7	8.50	6.28	0.37	10.79

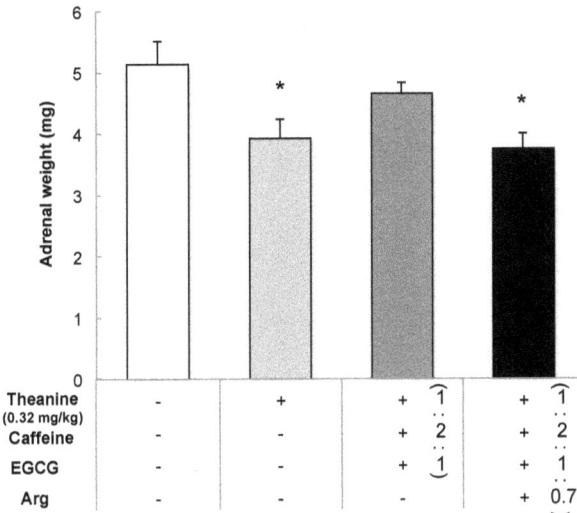

Figure 3. Interaction of tea components on adrenal hypertrophy in stressed mice. Mice consumed powder diet containing theanine, caffeine, EGCG, and Arg for seven days (single rearing for six days and confrontational rearing for one day). Control mice were fed a powder diet, CE-2. The concentration of theanine was 0.32 mg/kg. Mice ingested feed that contained each component as molar ratios of matcha sample no. 6, i.e., the molar ratio of theanine:caffeine:EGCG:Arg was 1:2:1:0.7. Each bar shows the mean $\pm$ SEM (n = 4; * $p < 0.05$).

3.2. Human Study

3.2.1. Effect of Matcha Ingestion on Stress in Students Assigned Pharmacy Practice Outside the University

Participants consumed three grams of matcha daily that were suspended in 500 mL of room-temperature water. Test-matcha was sample No. 6 and placebo-matcha was sample no. 7. These matcha samples were selected based on the mice data shown in Tables 2 and 4. Before pharmacy practice, the STAI value of those participants that consumed test-matcha was significantly lower than that of placebo-matcha ($p = 0.03$, Figure 4a). On the eighth day of pharmacy practice, the raw values and the difference between the means of these two groups was low ($p = 0.13$).

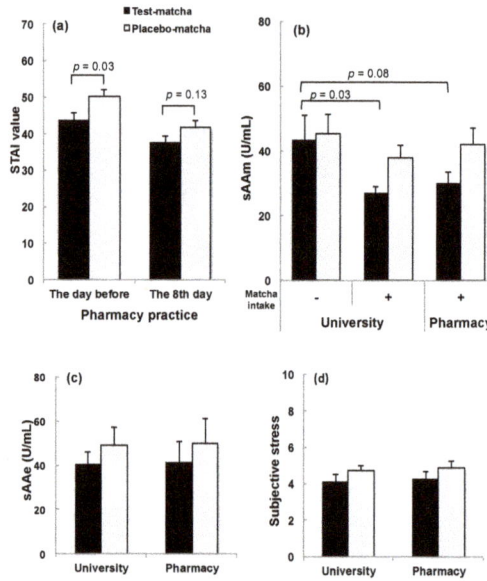

Figure 4. Effect of matcha ingestion on students during university and pharmacy practice. (**a**) The STAI test was administered before and on the eighth day of pharmacy practice. (**b**, left bars) The level of sAAm was measured in participants every morning for three days during routine daily life at the university before intake of matcha as the baseline. (**b**, middle and right bars) After the ingestion of matcha started, median sAAm of each participant for the last three days at the university and pharmacy practice was used for statistical analysis. The median of (**c**) sAAe and (**d**) subjective stress of each participant of the last three days at the university and pharmacy practice are shown. Each bar shows the mean ± SEM (test matcha, $n = 19$; placebo matcha, $n = 20$).

These data indicate that the intake of test-matcha was effective for the specific suppression of anxiety before practice outside the university. Although the basal level of sAAm before the intake of matcha was not different between the participants of the test- and placebo-matcha groups, the level at university was significantly lowered by the intake of test-matcha ($p = 0.03$, Figure 4b). Similarly, in pharmacy practice, the level of sAAm tended to be lower in the test-matcha group ($p = 0.08$, Figure 4b). In both groups, the sAA levels increased in the evening after practice (Figure 4c). The subjective stress that was recorded after practice tended to be slightly lower in the test group than in the placebo group, but it was not significantly different between both groups (Figure 4d). Nerve excitation was commonly down-regulated by the next morning [24]. Test-matcha may regulate recovery rather than suppress excitation. Differences in sex were not observed in STAI and sAA values. Other parameters such as physical condition, sleeping time, and achievement emotion were not significantly different between the two groups during pharmacy practice (Table 5).

Table 5. Effect of consumption of test- and placebo-matcha by students at university and pharmacy practice on psychosocial responses, as assess from a questionnaire.

Questionnaire Item	University			Pharmacy		
	Matcha		*p*	Matcha		*p*
	Test	Placebo	value	Test	Placebo	value
Physical condition (1–5)	3.55 ± 0.16	3.32 ± 0.13	0.30	3.44 ± 0.12	3.36 ± 0.12	0.62
Sleep time (h)	6.33 ± 0.15	6.20 ± 0.18	0.71	6.15 ± 0.17	6.40 ± 0.19	0.40
Achievement emotion (1–5)	(−)	(−)		3.49 ± 0.20	3.49 ± 0.16	0.82

3.2.2. Composition of Matcha Marketed in Japan and Overseas

The components of matcha marketed in Japan (76 samples) and overseas (67 samples) were measured (supplemental data; Tables S1 and S2). When a human takes three grams of matcha in a day, a clinical experiment showed that matcha samples that contain levels of theanine exceeding 17 mg/g might have a stress-reducing effect. As a result, 50 out of 76 samples in Japan met this condition. In contrast, of the 67 samples sold overseas, six samples met this condition (Figure 5a,b). In addition to this, the molar ratio of caffeine and EGCG to theanine and Arg might need to be lower than two. The result indicated that 32 out of 76 samples in Japan met this condition (Figure 5a). Only one sample sold overseas met the condition (Figure 5b).

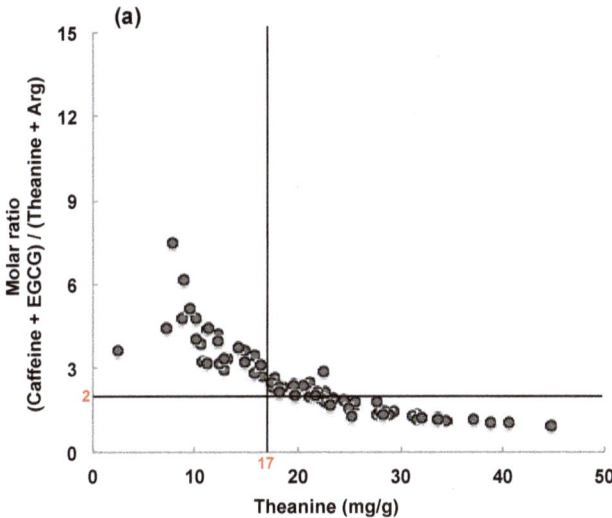

Figure 5. *Cont.*

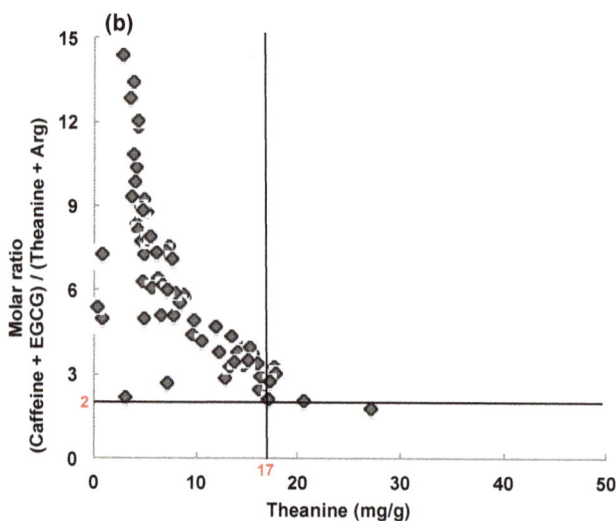

Figure 5. The amount of theanine and the molar ratio of caffeine and EGCG to theanine and Arg in (**a**) 76 samples of matcha marketed in Japan and (**b**) 67 samples of matcha marketed overseas. Based on data in humans, samples in the section, theanine > 17 mg/g, and molar ratio of caffeine and EGCG to theanine and Arg < 2 are expected to show a stress-reducing effect.

4. Discussion

Based on the quantities and ratios of matcha components, the stress-reducing effect of matcha was evaluated by mice experiments using seven kinds of matcha. These matcha samples were selected based on differences in theanine content. Since the amount of theanine in the tea leaves depends on the amount of nitrogen supply in the soil, one matcha with low theanine content was sourced from organic cultivation. The matcha sample containing high amounts of EGCG might be prepared from leaves that were not fully protected from the sunlight before harvest. Additionally, a sample with low amounts of all components was a matcha product containing additives.

Since theanine and Arg reduce stress and caffeine and EGCG antagonizes the action of theanine [16,17], we examined how these levels affect adrenal hypertrophy in stressed mice. In mice, adrenal hypertrophy was suppressed when the amount of theanine ingested was 0.32 mg/kg or more. Since the effect of theanine is cancelled by caffeine and EGCG, a molar ratio of caffeine and EGCG to theanine and Arg must be less than 3.6. Although EGC has a stress-reducing effect, EGC needed to be more than 10 times higher than EGCG [17]. As EGC was not higher than EGCG in matcha, the effect of EGC was not considered. Matcha essentially contains a high amount of caffeine, but if theanine is sufficiently high, the anti-theanine action of caffeine is counteracted. Catechin in matcha is less than in general green teas, but its increase is accompanied by a decrease in theanine. Therefore, an increase in catechin in matcha potentially increases the reduction of the stress-reducing effect of matcha.

Using test-matcha, which meets these conditions, we conducted a study in humans. Whereas the distribution of sAAm, a marker of physiological stress, was similar in the test and placebo groups before matcha was consumed, anxiety (STAI) and physiological stress (sAAm) decreased when test-matcha was consumed. The significant decrease in sAAm at university due to the intake of test-matcha may have contributed to the decrease in anxiety before pharmacy practice. Although caffeine consumption is reportedly linked to anxiety sensitivity [25,26], the caffeine content in test- and placebo-matcha were not different (Table 2). Additionally, the amount of caffeine ingested by participants was about 40 mg/day, which is about one-quarter cup of coffee, so drinking it every day would not cause a problem. Rather, in the case of matcha, the counteracting effects of caffeine and EGCG against theanine and Arg are considered to be important.

Whereas EGCG has been reported to have anxiolytic effects [27], the antagonistic effect of EGCG on theanine may be due to an increased excitatory synaptic connection by EGCG [28]. Glutamate is the main excitatory neurotransmitter and EGCG reportedly facilitates the release of glutamate [29]. Although central glutamatergic activity is crucial to cognitive function, excessive release of glutamate causes excessive excitation. The level of GABA, the main inhibitory neurotransmitter in the brain, is increased by theanine ingestion [30,31]. These data suggest that different ratios of EGCG/theanine cause a different balance of excitatory and inhibitory neurotransmitters such as glutamate and GABA.

Since the active component of matcha could be applied to evaluate the stress-reducing effect of matcha in humans, we then tried to assess the stress-reducing effect of matcha marketed in Japan and overseas. When people ingested three grams of these matcha per day, we examined whether stress-reducing effects would be expected. The results showed that, about 42% of matcha sold in Japan was expected to suppress stress versus only one of the matcha marketed overseas, because the amounts of theanine and Arg were low, and the amounts of caffeine and EGCG were high. Matcha is essentially rich in theanine and low in catechin, but not all marketed matcha satisfied this condition. This indicates that greater attention is needed to evaluate the mental function of matcha. Although the number of people drinking green tea as a health beverage is increasing in many countries, low-grade green teas with low amino acid contents are also sold as "matcha" [32]. Many matcha marketed overseas had low amino acids contents (Figure 5, Table S2). The counteracting effect of caffeine and EGCG on theanine is hardly considered. This may cause confusing results. For example, the effect of matcha tea on mood and cognitive performance has been examined [33]. The mood state measured by a Profile of Mood State (POMS) was not significantly changed by the ingestion of four grams of matcha tea. The matcha tea that those authors used contained 67 mg theanine, 280 mg EGCG, and 136 mg caffeine. Theanine content was slightly less than 17 mg/g. Although the content of Arg was not reported, the molar ratio of caffeine and EGCG against theanine was higher than two. This suggests that the result of POMS might have been different if those authors had used another matcha sample with a lower content of caffeine and EGCG. EGCG has been reported to have various beneficial functions [34]. However, when expecting mentally positive functions of matcha in anxiety, stress, and mood, the quantities of theanine and Arg must be high, and the ratios of caffeine and EGCG against theanine must be low.

5. Conclusions

We evaluated the effects of quantity and ratio of matcha components on its stress-reducing properties using an animal model of psychosocial stress. The stress-reducing effect in humans was confirmed using two kinds of matcha selected based on the animal study. In addition, we assessed the stress-reducing effect of matcha marketed in Japan and overseas. As a result, 42% of matcha samples marketed in Japan, and only one sample marketed abroad, were expected to have a stress-reducing effect. When using matcha samples to study mental function, a quality check is critical.

Supplementary Materials: The following are available online at http://www.mdpi.com/2072-6643/10/10/1468/s1, Table S1: Components of matcha marketed in Japan (mg/g), Table S2: Components of matcha marketed abroad (mg/g).

Author Contributions: K.U., H.Y., and Y.N. supervised the study. K.U. carried out the animal experiments. K.U., D.F., S.H., K.I., H.Y., and Y.N. carried out the clinical study. A.M., H.H., and Y.N. measured the tea component composition. K.U., D.F., and Y.N wrote the manuscript.

Funding: This research study was supported by a Grant-in-Aid for Scientific Research (KAKENHI 15K00828) and a grant for specifically promoted research of the University of Shizuoka.

Acknowledgments: The authors thank the participants of this study.

Conflicts of Interest: The authors declare no conflicts of interest.

References

1. Vuong, Q.V.; Bowyer, M.C.; Roach, P.D. L-Theanine: Properties, synthesis and isolation from tea. *J. Sci. Food Agric.* **2011**, *91*, 1931–1939. [CrossRef] [PubMed]
2. Ruan, J.; Haerdter, R.; Gerendás, J. Impact of nitrogen supply on carbon/nitrogen allocation: A case study on amino acids and catechins in green tea [*Camellia sinensis* (L.) O. Kuntze] plants. *Plant Biol. (Stuttg.)* **2010**, *12*, 724–734. [CrossRef] [PubMed]
3. Ikegaya, K.; Takayanagi, H.; Anan, T. Chemical composition of Matcha. *Tea Res. J. (Chagyo Kenkyu Hokoku)* **1984**, *60*, 79–81. [CrossRef]
4. Ashihara, H. Occurrence, biosynthesis and metabolism of theanine (γ-glutamyl-L-ethylamide) in plants: A comprehensive review. *Nat. Prod. Commun.* **2015**, *10*, 803–810. [PubMed]
5. Horie, H.; Ema, K.; Sumikawa, O. Chemical components of Matcha and powdered green tea. *J. Cook. Sci. Jpn. (Nippon Chourikagaku Kaishi)* **2017**, *50*, 182–188.
6. Goto, T.; Nagashima, H.; Yoshida, Y.; Kiso, M. Contents of individual tea catechins and caffeine in Japanese green tea. *Tea Res. J. (Chagyo Kenkyu Hokoku)* **1996**, *83*, 21–28. [CrossRef]
7. Ashihara, H.; Suzuki, T. Distribution and biosynthesis of caffeine in plants. *Front. Biosci.* **2004**, *9*, 1864–1876. [CrossRef] [PubMed]
8. Munakata, M. Clinical significance of stress-related increase in blood pressure: Current evidence in office and out-of-office settings. *Hypertens. Res.* **2018**. [CrossRef] [PubMed]
9. Wirtz, P.H.; von Känel, R. Psychological stress, inflammation, and coronary heart disease. *Curr. Cardiol. Rep.* **2017**, *19*, 111. [CrossRef] [PubMed]
10. Piirainen, S.; Youssef, A.; Song, C.; Kalueff, A.V.; Landreth, G.E.; Malm, T.; Tian, L. Psychosocial stress on neuroinflammation and cognitive dysfunctions in Alzheimer's disease: The emerging role for microglia? *Neurosci. Biobehav. Rev.* **2017**, *77*, 148–164. [CrossRef] [PubMed]
11. Saeed, M.; Naveed, M.; Arif, M.; Kakar, M.U.; Manzoor, R.; Abd El-Hack, M.E.; Alagawany, M.; Tiwari, R.; Khandia, R.; Munjal, A.; et al. Green tea (*Camellia sinensis*) and L-theanine: Medicinal values and beneficial applications in humans—A comprehensive review. *Biomed. Pharmacother.* **2017**, *95*, 1260–1275. [CrossRef] [PubMed]
12. Kimura, K.; Ozeki, M.; Juneja, L.R.; Ohira, H. L-Theanine reduces psychological and physiological stress responses. *Biol. Psychol.* **2007**, *74*, 39–45. [CrossRef] [PubMed]
13. Unno, K.; Fujitani, K.; Takamori, N.; Takabayashi, F.; Maeda, K.; Miyazaki, H.; Tanida, N.; Iguchi, K.; Shimoi, K.; Hoshino, M. Theanine intake improves the shortened lifespan, cognitive dysfunction and behavioural depression that are induced by chronic psychosocial stress in mice. *Free Radic. Res.* **2011**, *45*, 966–974. [CrossRef] [PubMed]
14. Unno, K.; Iguchi, K.; Tanida, N.; Fujitani, K.; Takamori, N.; Yamamoto, H.; Ishii, N.; Nagano, H.; Nagashima, T.; Hara, A.; et al. Ingestion of theanine, an amino acid in tea, suppresses psychosocial stress in mice. *Exp. Physiol.* **2013**, *98*, 290–303. [CrossRef] [PubMed]
15. Unno, K.; Tanida, H.; Ishii, N.; Yamamoto, H.; Iguchi, K.; Hoshino, M.; Takeda, A.; Ozawa, H.; Ohkubo, T.; Juneja, L.R.; et al. Anti-stress effect of theanine on students during pharmacy practice: Positive correlation among salivary α-amylase activity, trait anxiety and subjective stress. *Pharmacol. Biochem. Behav.* **2013**, *111*, 128–135. [CrossRef] [PubMed]
16. Giles, G.E.; Mahoney, C.R.; Brunyé, T.T.; Taylor, H.A.; Kanarek, R.B. Caffeine and theanine exert opposite effects on attention under emotional arousal. *Can. J. Physiol. Pharmacol.* **2017**, *95*, 93–100. [CrossRef] [PubMed]
17. Unno, K.; Hara, A.; Nakagawa, A.; Iguchi, K.; Ohshio, M.; Morita, A.; Nakamura, Y. Anti-stress effects of drinking green tea with lowered caffeine and enriched theanine, epigallocatechin and arginine on psychosocial stress induced adrenal hypertrophy in mice. *Phytomedicine* **2016**, *23*, 1365–1374. [CrossRef] [PubMed]
18. Unno, K.; Yamada, H.; Iguchi, K.; Ishida, H.; Iwao, Y.; Morita, A.; Nakamura, Y. Anti-stress effect of green tea with lowered caffeine on humans: A pilot study. *Biol. Pharm. Bull.* **2017**, *40*, 902–909. [CrossRef] [PubMed]
19. Unno, K.; Noda, S.; Kawasaki, Y.; Yamada, H.; Morita, A.; Iguchi, K.; Nakamura, Y. Ingestion of green tea with lowered caffeine improves sleep quality of the elderly via suppression of stress. *J. Clin. Biochem. Nutr.* **2017**, *61*, 210–216. [CrossRef] [PubMed]

20. Unno, K.; Noda, S.; Kawasaki, Y.; Yamada, H.; Morita, A.; Iguchi, K.; Nakamura, Y. Reduced stress and improved sleep quality caused by green tea are associated with a reduced caffeine content. *Nutrients* **2017**, *9*, 777. [CrossRef] [PubMed]

21. Van Stegeren, A.; Rohleder, N.; Everaerd, W.; Wolf, O.T. Salivary alpha amylase as marker for adrenergic activity during stress: Effect of betablockade. *Psychoneuroendocrinology* **2006**, *31*, 137–141. [CrossRef] [PubMed]

22. Goto, T.; Horie, H.; Mukai, T. Analysis of major amino acids in green tea by high-performance liquid chromatography coupled with OPA precolumn derivatization. *Tea Res. J. (Chagyo Kenkyu Hokoku)* **1993**, *77*, 29–33.

23. Yamaguchi, M.; Kanemori, T.; Kanemaru, M.; Takai, N.; Mizuno, Y.; Yoshida, H. Performance evaluation of salivary amylase activity monitor. *Biosens. Bioelectron.* **2004**, *20*, 491–497. [CrossRef] [PubMed]

24. Niethard, N.; Burgalossi, A.; Born, J. Plasticity during Sleep Is Linked to Specific Regulation of Cortical Circuit Activity. *Front. Neural Circuits* **2017**, *11*, 65. [CrossRef] [PubMed]

25. Pané-Farré, C.A.; Alius, M.G.; Modeß, C.; Methling, K.; Blumenthal, T.; Hamm, A.O. Anxiety sensitivity and expectation of arousal differentially affect the respiratory response to caffeine. *Psychopharmacology (Berl)* **2015**, *232*, 1931–1939. [CrossRef] [PubMed]

26. Vilarim, M.M.; Rocha Araujo, D.M.; Nardi, A.E. Caffeine challenge test and panic disorder: A systematic literature review. *Expert Rev. Neurother.* **2011**, *11*, 1185–1195. [CrossRef] [PubMed]

27. Dias, G.P.; Cavegn, N.; Nix, A.; do Nascimento Bevilaqua, M.C.; Stangl, D.; Zainuddin, M.S.; Nardi, A.E.; Gardino, P.F.; Thuret, S. The role of dietary polyphenols on adult hippocampal neurogenesis: Molecular mechanisms and behavioural effects on depression and anxiety. *Oxid. Med. Cell. Longev.* **2012**, *2012*, 541971. [CrossRef] [PubMed]

28. Catuara-Solarz, S.; Espinosa-Carrasco, J.; Erb, I.; Langohr, K.; Gonzalez, J.R.; Notredame, C.; Dierssen, M. Combined treatment with environmental enrichment and (−)-epigallocatechin-3-gallate ameliorates learning deficits and hippocampal alterations in a mouse model of down syndrome. *eNeuro* **2016**, *3*, e0103. [CrossRef] [PubMed]

29. Chou, C.W.; Huang, W.J.; Tien, L.T.; Wang, S.J. (-)-Epigallocatechin gallate, the most active polyphenolic catechin in green tea, presynaptically facilitates Ca^{2+}-dependent glutamate release via activation of protein kinase C in rat cerebral cortex. *Synapse* **2007**, *61*, 889–902. [CrossRef] [PubMed]

30. Inoue, K.; Miyazaki, Y.; Unno, K.; Min, J.Z.; Todoroki, K.; Toyo'oka, T. Stable isotope dilution HILIC-MS/MS method for accurate quantification of glutamic acid, glutamine, pyroglutamic acid, GABA and theanine in mouse brain tissues. *Biomed. Chromatogr.* **2016**, *30*, 55–61. [CrossRef] [PubMed]

31. Ogawa, S.; Ota, M.; Ogura, J.; Kato, K.; Kunugi, H. Effects of L-theanine on anxiety-like behavior, cerebrospinal fluid amino acid profile, and hippocampal activity in Wistar Kyoto rats. *Psychopharmacology (Berl)* **2018**, *235*, 37–45. [CrossRef] [PubMed]

32. Horie, H.; Ema, K.; Nishikawa, H.; Nakamura, Y. Comparison of the chemical components of powdered green tea sold in the US. *JARQ* **2018**, *52*, 143–147. [CrossRef]

33. Dietz, C.; Dekker, M.; Piqueras-Fiszman, B. An intervention study on the effect of matcha tea, in drink and snack bar formats, on mood and cognitive performance. *Food Res. Int.* **2017**, *99*, 72–83. [CrossRef] [PubMed]

34. Kim, H.S.; Quon, M.J.; Kim, J.A. New insights into the mechanisms of polyphenols beyond antioxidant properties; lessons from the green tea polyphenol, epigallocatechin 3-gallate. *Redox Biol.* **2014**, *2*, 187–195. [CrossRef] [PubMed]

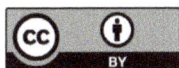

nutrients

MDPI

Article

Habitual Tea Consumption and Risk of Fracture in 0.5 Million Chinese Adults: A Prospective Cohort Study

Qian Shen [1], Canqing Yu [1], Yu Guo [2], Zheng Bian [2], Nanbo Zhu [1], Ling Yang [3], Yiping Chen [3], Guojin Luo [4], Jianguo Li [4], Yulu Qin [5], Junshi Chen [6], Zhengming Chen [3], Jun Lv [1,7,8,*], Liming Li [1] and on behalf of the China Kadoorie Biobank Collaborative Group [†]

[1] Department of Epidemiology and Biostatistics, School of Public Health, Peking University Health Science Center, Beijing 100191, China; qianshen@bjmu.edu.cn (Q.S.); yucanqing@pku.edu.cn (C.Y.); znb@pku.edu.cn (N.Z.); lmLee@vip.163.com (L.L.)

[2] Chinese Academy of Medical Sciences, Beijing 100191, China; guoyu@kscdc.net (Y.G.); bianzheng@kscdc.net (Z.B.)

[3] Clinical Trial Service Unit & Epidemiological Studies Unit (CTSU), Nuffield Department of Population Health, University of Oxford, Oxford OX1 2JD, UK; ling.yang@ndph.ox.ac.uk (L.Y.); yiping.chen@ndph.ox.ac.uk (Y.C.); zhengming.chen@ndph.ox.ac.uk (Z.C.)

[4] Pengzhou Center for Disease Control and Prevention, Pengzhou 611930, Sichuan, China; L630415@163.com (G.L.); fintear@163.com (J.L.)

[5] NCDs Prevention and Control Department, Liuzhou Center for Disease Control and Prevention, Liuzhou 545007, Guangxi, China; lzcdcmbfzk@126.com

[6] China National Center for Food Safety Risk Assessment, Beijing 100191, China; chenjunshi@cfsa.net.cn

[7] Key Laboratory of Molecular Cardiovascular Sciences (Peking University), Ministry of Education, Beijing 100191, China

[8] Peking University Institute of Environmental Medicine, Beijing 100191, China

[*] Correspondence: lvjun@bjmu.edu.cn; Tel.: +86-10-82801528 (ext. 322)

[†] The members of steering committee and collaborative group are listed in the Acknowledgements.

Received: 27 September 2018; Accepted: 23 October 2018; Published: 2 November 2018

Abstract: Background: Tea consumption may have favorable effects on risk of fracture. However, little is known about such association in Chinese adults. The aim of this study was to examine the association between tea consumption and risk of hospitalized fracture in Chinese adults. Methods: The present study included 453,625 participants from the China Kadoorie Biobank (CKB). Tea consumption was self-reported at baseline. Hospitalized fractures were ascertained through linkage with local health insurance claim databases. The results: During a median of 10.1 years of follow-up, we documented 12,130 cases of first-time any fracture hospitalizations, including 1376 cases of hip fracture. Compared with never tea consumers, daily tea consumption was associated with lower risk of any fracture (hazard ratio (HR): 0.88; 95% confidence interval (CI): 0.83, 0.93). Statistically significant reduced risk of hip fracture was shown among daily consumers who most commonly drank green tea (HR: 0.80; 95% CI: 0.65, 0.97) and those who had drunk tea for more than 30 years (HR: 0.68; 95% CI: 0.52, 0.87). Our conclusions: Habitual tea consumption was associated with moderately decreased risk of any fracture hospitalizations. Participants with decades of tea consumption and those who preferred green tea were also associated with lower risk of hip fracture.

Keywords: tea consumption; fracture; cohort study

---

1. Introduction

Bone fractures usually result from the combination of impaired bone strength and trauma from falling [1,2]. Bone fractures may lead to reduced activities, functional impairment, disability, and even increased mortality of patients [3,4]. Furthermore, bone fractures are associated with enormous economic expenditure. Hip fractures account for the majority of this burden mainly because of their severity, and requirements of medical care and hospital facilities [4,5].

Tea is among the most widely consumed beverages in the world and rich in both caffeine and polyphenols. Experimental studies demonstrated that caffeine, in a high amount, may promote differentiation of osteoclast [6,7] and increase urinary calcium [8], leading to diminished bone mineral density. Polyphenols, however, were shown to have favorable effects on bone biology [9–11]. Previous epidemiological studies have yielded inconsistent associations between tea consumption and risk of fracture. Tea consumption was associated with a decreased risk of fracture in some case-control studies [12–14], but not in others [15–17]. Most of the prospective cohort studies observed null associations between tea consumption and risk of fracture [18–22], while one study reported a positive association [23] and another reported a negative one [24]. These prospective studies were primarily conducted in Western postmenopausal women, had small sample sizes with few fracture cases, and had a relatively low consumption of tea. Even the existing meta-analyses assessing the association between tea consumption and fracture were inconsistent. Chen et al. [25], Yan et al. [26], and Guo et al. [27] reported no association between tea consumption and fracture, whereas Sheng et al. [28] reported that individuals drinking 1–4 cups of tea per day was associated with a lower risk of hip fracture. Also, the associations with various measures of tea consumption, like the amount of tea leaves added, types of tea, and duration of tea consumption, have yet to be examined. For Chinese populations, in which tea is most widely consumed, only one case-control study [14] and one cohort study [22] were performed and the results were mixed.

Thus, we aimed to prospectively examine the association between tea consumption and risk of hospitalized fracture in approximately 0.5 million Chinese adults from the China Kadoorie Biobank (CKB).

2. Materials and Methods

2.1. Study Population

Details of the CKB study design and characteristics of the study participants have been described elsewhere [29,30]. Briefly, the baseline survey took place between 2004–2008 in 10 geographically diverse areas of China (five urban and five rural areas). In each area, all nondisabled, permanent residents aged 35–74 years were invited to participate. Overall, a total of 512,891 individuals were recruited, including a few just outside the age range of 35–74 years. Each participant completed an interview-administered questionnaire and physical measurements.

After correction for errors in age and exclusion of participants with age outside of the 30–79 years, 512,715 participants were eligible for inclusion in the study. In the present analysis, participants with a history of any fracture before baseline ($n = 35,444$) were excluded. We also excluded participants with other diseases known to affect fracture risk, including a self-reported doctor diagnosis of cancer ($n = 2578$), heart disease ($n = 15,472$), or stroke ($n = 8884$) at baseline [31]. We also excluded participants who were lost to follow-up shortly after baseline ($n = 1$), and whose information on body mass index (BMI) was missing ($n = 2$). The final analysis included 453,625 participants, including 181,566 men and 272,059 women.

Ethical approval was obtained from the Ethical Review Committee of the Chinese Centre for Disease Control and Prevention, Beijing, China, and the Oxford Tropical Research Ethics Committee, University of Oxford, UK. All study participants provided written informed consent.

2.2. Assessment of Tea Consumption

At baseline survey, we asked participants "during the past 12 months, how often did you drink any tea (never, only occasionally, only at certain seasons, every month but less than weekly, or at least once a week)?" Participants who drank tea at least once a week were further asked to report: (1) days drinking in a typical week (1–2 days, 3–5 days, or almost every day), (2) cups (in 300 mL-sized) of tea consumed on days of drinking, (3) times of changing tea leaves on days of drinking, (4) amount of tea leaves (in grams) added each time, (5) types of tea most commonly consumed (green tea, oolong tea, black tea, or others), and (6) age they started drinking tea weekly. A pictorial guide was provided to demonstrate the standard sized cup and the amount of tea leaves. The total tea leaves consumed (in grams) on days of drinking was calculated as the product of the amount of tea leaves added each time and the times of changing tea leaves. Duration of tea consumption was calculated as the difference between age at baseline and age of starting drinking tea weekly. According to tea consumption frequency, participants were categorized into three groups (never, less than daily, or daily consumers). Daily consumers were further categorized into four groups according to rounded quartiles of the amount of tea consumed in grams (0.1–2.0, 2.1–3.0, 3.1–5.0, or >5.0 g per day) or in cups (1–2, 3–4, 5–6, or ≥7 cups per day).

2.3. Assessment of Outcomes

Hospitalized fracture outcomes were ascertained periodically through linkage with local health insurance (HI) claim databases. The reimbursement data of the local HI data are comprehensive and capture information on all diagnoses and treatments prescribed to patients who sought health care in a hospital. Such linkage has been achieved for about 98% of our participants, which was similar across ten survey sites. Linkage to local HI databases was renewed annually. Participants who failed to be linked to local HI databases were actively followed annually by staff to ascertain their status including hospital admission, death, and moving out of the study area. Fractures that did not require hospital admission as an in-patient were not ascertained in the present study. The date of fracture incidence was based on the admission date from the hospital inpatient discharge summaries. Trained staff who were blind to participants' baseline information coded the cause of incident cases with the 10th revision of the International Classification of Diseases (ICD-10). The present study focused on the first-time hospitalizations of interest during the follow-up. Hip fracture cases were defined with ICD-10 codes of S72.0, S72.1, and S72.2. Any fracture cases were defined with the codes of S12, S22, S32, S42, S52, S62, S72, S82, and S92. Fractures of other parts of neck (S12.8), flail chest (S22.5), scapula (S42.1), fingers (S62.5–62.7), and toes (S92.4, S92.5) as any fracture events were excluded since these fractures were less likely associated with osteoporosis [32].

2.4. Assessment of Covariates

Information on socio-demographic characteristics (age, sex, education, occupation, marital status, and household income), lifestyle (smoking, alcohol drinking, physical activity, and diet), self-reported medical history, and reproductive history (in women) was obtained from the baseline questionnaire. Daily level of physical activity was calculated by multiplying the metabolic equivalent tasks (METs) value for a particular type of physical activity by hours spent on that activity per day and summing the MET-hours for all activities. Habitual dietary intake in the past year was assessed by a qualitative food frequency questionnaire (FFQ). We conducted a reliability and validity study of the FFQ during 2015–2016. The study included 432 CKB participants who completed two FFQ (median interval: 3.3 months) and twelve 24-h dietary recalls (24-HDR). The reliability of the FFQ was assessed by comparing the frequency of food consumption from the two FFQ. Except for fresh vegetables, values of weighted kappa ranged from 0·62 to 0·90 for all food categories. As for fresh vegetables, exact agreement rate was 89.8%, and misclassification to opposite quartiles was less than 1.0%. The validity of the FFQ was evaluated by comparing the frequency of food consumption from the first FFQ and the multiple 24-HDR. Except for fresh vegetables, values of weighted kappa ranged from 0.60 to 0.90 for all food categories. As for fresh vegetables, the exact agreement rate was 89.3%, and misclassification to opposite quartiles was less than 0.3%. Height, weight, waist and hip circumferences, and blood pressure were obtained from physical measurements using standard protocol and validated instruments.

2.5. Statistical Analyses

Each participant's follow-up time was accrued from baseline survey until the admission date of the first-time fracture hospitalization, death, loss to follow up, or 31 December 2016, whichever occurred first. Stratified Cox proportional hazards models, with age as the underlying time scale, were conducted to calculate hazard ratios (HRs) and 95% confidence intervals (CIs) between tea consumption and risk of fracture. Multivariable-adjusted models were stratified jointly by 10 study areas and age at baseline in 5-year intervals, and they were adjusted for sex, education, marital status, alcohol consumption, smoking status, physical activity, frequencies of red meat, fruit, vegetable, and dairy product consumption, menopause status (only for women), BMI, waist-to-hip ratio, prevalent hypertension, and diabetes. Tests for linear trend were only conducted in daily tea consumers by assigning the median value of tea consumption (in grams or cups per day) to each of the categories as a continuous variable in regression models. Also, we examined associations between tea consumption and risk of fracture according to types of tea and duration of tea consumption. Subgroup analyses were conducted to test for interaction of tea consumption with 11 baseline factors (for example, age, region, etc.) by using likelihood ratio tests comparing models with and without a cross-product term.

We used Stata, version 15.0 (StataCorp, College Station, TX, USA), for statistical analyses. All *p* values were two-sided. Statistical significance was defined as $p < 0.05$, except that a Bonferroni corrected *p* value (0.05/11) was used in the interaction analyses since multiple testing issues might occur.

3. Results

Of 453,625 participants, the mean age was 51.4 ± 10.6 years. Overall, 26.2% of participants drank tea daily, in which 41.3% of men and 16.1% of women were daily tea consumers. Table 1 summarizes baseline characteristics of the study participants according to tea consumption. Compared with never tea consumers during the past 12 months, participants who drank tea daily were more likely to be well educated, current smokers, and daily alcohol drinkers. Daily consumers who consumed more tea leaves per day tended to start drinking tea earlier and drink more cups of tea. The majority of CKB participants most commonly consumed green tea.

During a median of 10.1 years of follow-up and 4.5 million person years at risk in total, 12,130 participants experienced their first fracture hospitalization of any type, including 1376 cases of hip fracture. After adjustment for potential confounders, compared with participants who never drank tea during the past 12 months, daily tea consumption was associated with lower risk of any fracture (Table 2). Multivariable-adjusted HR (95% CI) was 0.88 (0.83, 0.93) for daily consumers. We did not observe a statistically significant linear trend in the risk of any fracture with the grams of tea leaves consumed in daily tea consumers (*p* for trend = 0.863). The corresponding HR (95% CI) for hip fracture was 0.84 (0.71, 1.00). Also, there was no linear trend for risk of hip fracture in daily consumers (*p* for trend = 0.148). Both associations were consistent between men and women (*p* for sex interaction: 0.960 for any fracture, 0.079 for hip fracture) (Table S1). The results were similar when daily consumers were further categorized by the cups of tea consumed (Table S2).

To test the robustness of our risk estimates, we performed sensitivity analyses by additionally adjusting for occupation, household income, consumption of calcium, iron, or zinc supplements in the whole cohort; or additionally adjusting for use of oral contraceptive in women; or excluding participants who were former tea consumers from the reference group (*n* = 3809); or excluding participants whose outcomes occurred during the first two years of follow-up (any fracture *n* = 1643, hip fracture *n* = 80). Also, open fractures of the clavicle (S42.0), proximal humerus (S42.2), and proximal or shaft tibia and fibula (S82.1, S82.2, and S82.4) were less likely related with osteoporosis [32]. Given that we could not distinguish open from closed fractures of these sites, we performed sensitivity analyses by further excluding them both as any fracture events. The associations were not substantially changed (data not shown).

Table 1. Baseline characteristics of 453,625 study participants according to tea consumption.

	Never	Less than Daily	Daily (Grams/Day)			
			0.1–2.0	2.1–3.0	3.1–5.0	>5.0
No. of participants, n (%)	159,367 (35.1)	175,569 (38.7)	45,835 (10.1)	20,505 (4.5)	25,373 (5.6)	26,976 (5.9)
Age, year	52.5	49.8	52.8	52.6	52.4	51.4
Rural area, %	58.2	54.8	66.2	75.5	50.5	49.1
Married, %	89.1	91.3	92.2	92.5	93.3	93.8
Middle school and higher, %	40.6	51.6	54.9	57.4	59.3	59.8
Current smoker *, %						
Men	56.4	63.6	72.8	75.2	76.8	81.4
Women	2.3	2.7	4.3	5.3	4.8	6.9
Daily alcohol drinking, %						
Men	14.7	17.3	24.9	25.3	26.9	27.8
Women	0.6	0.9	2.3	2.9	2.6	3.9
Physical activity, MET h/day	21.2	21.9	21.0	21.4	21.2	21.5
Average weekly consumption †, day						
Red meat	3.44	3.73	3.98	3.75	4.04	4.24
Fresh vegetables	6.82	6.82	6.88	6.81	6.90	6.87
Fresh fruits	2.43	2.62	2.74	2.55	2.67	2.52
Dairy products	0.84	1.01	1.08	1.04	1.08	1.10
Body mass index, kg/m^2	23.4	23.7	23.6	23.6	23.7	23.8
Waist-to-hip ratio	0.870	0.881	0.888	0.890	0.894	0.900
Diabetes, %	5.4	5.3	5.4	5.2	5.4	5.4
Hypertension, %	32.6	33.0	34.8	35.3	36.3	36.2
Postmenopausal (in women), %	50.4	49.7	49.4	49.1	48.9	48.8
Characteristics of daily tea consumer						
Age of starting tea consumption, year	-	-	28.4	27.8	26.6	25.0
Duration of tea consumption, year	-	-	23.9	24.5	25.8	27.4
Amount of tea consumption, gram	-	-	1.7	3.1	4.1	9.5
Amount of tea consumption, cup	-	-	3.3	4.2	4.6	6.6
Green tea consumer, %	-	-	86.0	85.7	86.1	85.8

Abbreviations: MET, metabolic equivalent of task. All variables were adjusted for age and survey areas, as appropriate. * Former smoker who had stopped smoking for illness was categorized into the current smoker. † Average weekly consumption of red meat, fresh vegetables, fresh fruits, and dairy products was calculated by assigning participants to the midpoint of their consumption category.

Figure 1 presents associations of tea consumption and fracture according to types of tea and duration of tea consumption in participants who drank tea daily. The risk estimates for any fracture seemed to be similar across different types of tea or duration of tea consumption. As for hip fracture, however, daily green tea consumers had a decreased risk (RR: 0.80; 95% CI: 0.65, 0.97). Strongest risk reduction for hip fracture was observed among daily consumers who had drunk tea for more than 30 years (RR: 0.68; 95% CI: 0.52, 0.87). Risk estimates for participants who consumed tea less than daily are shown in Table S3.

Table 2. HRs (95% CIs) for associations between tea consumption (in grams/day) and risk of fracture among 453,625 participants.

Endpoints	Never	Less than Daily	Daily (Grams/Day)					p for Trend *
			All	0.1–2.0	2.1–3.0	3.1–5.0	>5.0	
Any fracture								
No. of cases	4603	4502	3025	1237	471	621	696	
No. of PYs	1,568,372	1,737,307	1164,811	446,985	200,235	249,505	268,085	
Cases/PYs (/1000)	2.93	2.59	2.60	2.77	2.35	2.49	2.60	
Model 1	1.00	0.95 (0.91, 0.99)	0.89 (0.84, 0.94)	0.90 (0.84, 0.96)	0.85 (0.77, 0.94)	0.87 (0.80, 0.95)	0.91 (0.83, 0.99)	0.952
Model 2	1.00	0.95 (0.91, 1.00)	0.88 (0.83, 0.93)	0.90 (0.84, 0.96)	0.84 (0.76, 0.93)	0.86 (0.78, 0.94)	0.89 (0.81, 0.97)	0.807
Model 3	1.00	0.95 (0.91, 1.00)	0.88 (0.83, 0.93)	0.90 (0.84, 0.97)	0.84 (0.76, 0.94)	0.86 (0.79, 0.94)	0.89 (0.81, 0.97)	0.863
Hip fracture								
No. of cases	614	420	342	162	58	67	55	
No. of PYs	1,587,266	1,754,313	1,176,665	451,421	202,121	251,979	271,144	
Cases/PYs (/1000)	0.39	0.24	0.29	0.36	0.29	0.27	0.20	
Model 1	1.00	0.86 (0.75, 0.98)	0.82 (0.70, 0.97)	0.92 (0.76, 1.13)	0.73 (0.54, 0.98)	0.81 (0.62, 1.06)	0.70 (0.52, 0.93)	0.143
Model 2	1.00	0.87 (0.76, 0.99)	0.82 (0.70, 0.97)	0.92 (0.75, 1.12)	0.74 (0.55, 0.99)	0.80 (0.61, 1.05)	0.69 (0.51, 0.92)	0.119
Model 3	1.00	0.89 (0.77, 1.01)	0.84 (0.71, 1.00)	0.94 (0.77, 1.15)	0.76 (0.56, 1.02)	0.83 (0.63, 1.09)	0.71 (0.53, 0.96)	0.148

Abbreviations: HR, hazard ratio; CI, confidence interval; PYs, person years. Model 1 was adjusted for sex (men or women); model 2 additionally included level of education (no formal school, primary school, middle school, high school, college, or university or higher), marital status (married, widowed, divorced or separated, or never married), alcohol consumption (non-drinker, former weekly drinker, weekly drinker, daily drinking <15, 15–29, 30–59, or ≥60 g of pure alcohol), smoking status (never smoker, former smoker who had stopped smoking for reasons other than illness, current smoker, or former smoker who had stopped smoking for illness consuming 1–14, 15–24, or ≥25 cigarettes or equivalent per day), physical activity (MET h/day), frequencies of red meat, fruits, vegetables, and dairy products intake (daily, 4–6 days/week, 1–3 days/week, monthly, or rarely or never); model 3 additionally included BMI (kg/m²), waist-to-hip ratio, prevalent hypertension (presence or absence), and prevalent diabetes (presence or absence). * Tests for linear trend were only conducted in daily consumers by assigning the median value of tea consumption (in grams/day) to each of the categories as a continuous variable in regression models.

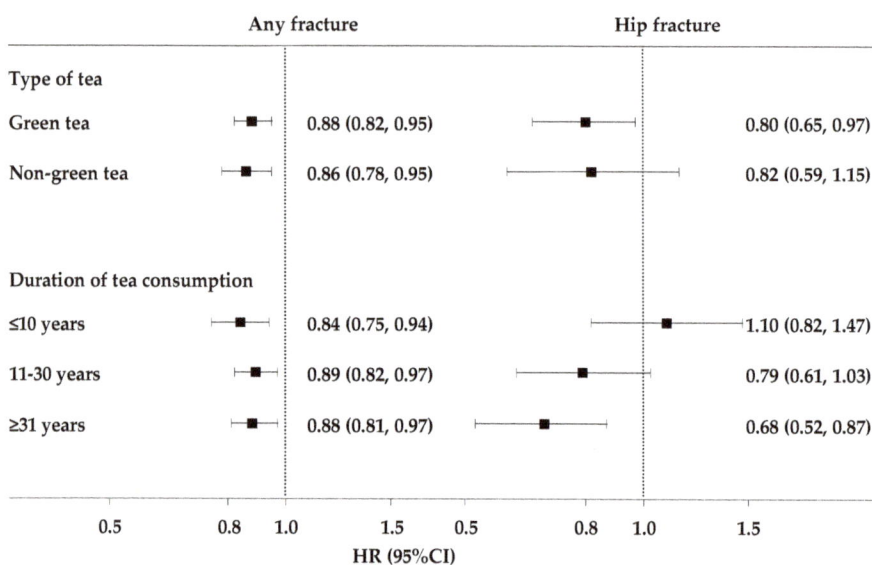

Figure 1. Subgroup analyses of associations between tea consumption and risk of fracture according to types of tea and duration of tea consumption in daily consumers. Hazard ratios are for comparison of daily tea consumers with participants who never consumed tea during the past 12 months. Risk estimates for participants who consumed tea less than daily are shown in Table S3. Solid squares represent point estimates, and horizontal lines represent 95% confidence intervals.

Further analyses were conducted according to prespecified baseline subgroups. Although statistically significant interaction with age was observed for incident any fracture (p values for interaction <0.001), the HRs were similar across different age subgroups. (Table S4). Associations between tea consumption and hip fracture were generally consistent across all subgroups (all p values for interaction >0.05/11).

4. Discussion

In this large prospective cohort study of Chinese adults, compared to participants who never drank tea during the past 12 months, daily tea consumers were associated with a 12% decreased risk of any fracture hospitalizations. Also, there was a suggestive association of a 16% lower risk of hip fracture hospitalizations among those who drank tea daily; such risk reduction became obvious among green tea consumers (18%) and prolonged tea consumers (32%). The associations were consistent in both men and women.

Existing prospective studies have yielded inconclusive results on the relationship between tea consumption and risk of fracture. Prospective studies conducted in Western women found no associations of tea consumption with the risks of hip fracture [18–20,24], forearm/wrist fracture [18,20], fracture other than hip and forearm/wrist [20], osteoporosis fracture [21], or any fracture [19]. However, these studies were primarily performed decades ago. Their confidence intervals of estimates tended to be wide due to small sample size and a limited number of outcomes, leading to less powerful results. The Singapore Chinese Health study with 16 years of follow-up and 2502 hip fracture cases also did not find associations between daily consumption of any tea and hip fracture (RR: 0.95; 95% CI: 0.85, 1.06) [22]. A cohort study of 1188 Australia women aged >75 years and 10-year follow-up showed that consumption of ≥3 cups of black tea per day was associated with a decreased risk of osteoporotic fracture that required hospitalization (RR: 0.70; 95% CI: 0.50, 0.96) compared with reference group of ≤1 cup per week [24]. Conversely, another study based on the Framingham cohort examined the association of caffeine consumption from both coffee and tea with hip fracture risk, with 135 cases occurred during 12 years of follow-up [23]. Its findings showed that consumption of ≥2.5 units of caffeine per day, an equivalent of 5 cups of tea, was associated with an increased risk of hip fracture. However, the results should be interpreted cautiously since researchers did not consider tea and coffee separately.

In the current analysis of 10-year follow-up data of Chinese adults, we observed that daily tea consumption was associated with a reduction in risk of any fracture in both men and women. Despite the apparently smaller number of hip fracture cases, a reduced risk of hip fracture was also shown among participants with decades of tea consumption and those who were used to drinking green tea. The findings that tea consumption was associated with lower fracture risk are biologically reasonable based on previous experimental evidence. Tea polyphenols could enhance osteoblastogenesis, suppress osteoclastogenesis, increase bone formation, and inhibit bone resorption through antioxidant or anti-inflammatory pathways, which result in greater bone strength [9–11]. However, in the present study, the fracture risk associated with daily tea consumption did not follow any linear trend with the amount of tea leaves added, which may correspond to the amount of both polyphenols and caffeine in the tea. Adverse effects of increased caffeine on bone health may counterbalance the beneficial effect of tea polyphenols [8]. But at least we did not observe that stronger tea consumption, averaged about 9.5 g/day of tea leaves, increased the risk of fracture. Our findings also do not preclude the possibility that tea consumption exerts positive effects on attention and alertness throughout the day [33,34], reducing the risk of severe injury. Further studies are needed to verify our findings.

To the best of our knowledge, this is by far the largest prospective cohort study among a wide age range of Chinese adults investigating the association between habitual tea consumption and the risk of fracture. The strengths of our study included prospective study design, large study population, the inclusion of both men and women and a geographically spread Chinese population living in urban and rural areas, and available information on a broad range of covariates. We measured tea consumption in grams of tea leaves which may better reflect the intake of active ingredients and also collected detailed information on types of tea and duration of tea consumption. With the electronic linkage to local HI databases, we are able to obtain data on hospitalized fractures comprehensively, which could be difficult to be captured with the linkage to local disease and death registries or by face-to-face interviews.

Inevitably, there are some limitations in our study. First, there was measurement error in tea consumption since it was self-reported. However, misclassification in this prospective study should be non-differential and attenuate the associations to be null. Second, tea consumption was measured only once at baseline. However, tea consumers in our cohort usually had drunk tea for decades. Third, we could only ascertain fractures that required hospitalization. Underreporting of hospitalized fractures might exist, and other fractures that were not serious enough to lead to hospitalization were not captured in our study. Fourth, our analyses have adjusted for a range of potential confounders, but residual confounding may remain. For instance, coffee consumption, which was not collected at baseline survey, may be a confounder given that coffee may influence the risk of fracture [35]. However, the prevalence of coffee consumption is likely to be relatively low in our population. A re-survey involving about 5% of randomly chosen surviving participants was conducted during 2008, in which less than 2% of participants consumed coffee at least once a week. Thus the potential confounding from coffee consumption, if any, might be trivial. Fifth, we did not further analyze the effects of black tea, oolong tea or other types of tea on the risk of fracture separately since fewer participants consumed other types tea than green tea in our population. Sixth, we didn't have data on bone mineral density at baseline survey, thus we couldn't identify whether tea consumption reduced the risk of fracture through improving bone health.

5. Conclusions

In summary, this large prospective cohort of Chinese adults provided evidence that habitual tea consumption was associated with moderately decreased risk of any fracture hospitalizations in both men and women. Participants with decades of tea consumption and those who preferred green tea were also at lower risk of hip fracture. Given the observational nature of our study, causality cannot be established. Further randomized trials studies are needed to elucidate whether tea consumption has the potential to reduce the risk of fracture hospitalizations through improving bone health directly or improving attention and alertness, or if it is merely a marker of other dietary and lifestyle factors.

Supplementary Materials: The following are available online at http://www.mdpi.com/2072-6643/10/11/1633/s1, Table S1: Sex-specific HRs (95% CIs) for associations between tea consumption (in grams/day) and risk of fracture among 453,625 participants, Table S2: HRs (95% CIs) for associations of tea consumption (in cups/day) and risk of fracture among 453,625 participants, Table S3: Subgroup analyses of associations between tea consumption and risk of fracture according to types of tea and duration of tea consumption, Table S4: Subgroup analyses of associations between tea consumption and risk of fracture according to potential baseline risk factors.

Author Contributions: J.L. and L.L. conceived and designed the study. L.L., Z.C., and J.C., as the members of CKB steering committee, designed and supervised the conduct of the whole study, obtained funding, and together with Y.G., Z.B., C.Y., L.Y., Y.C., G.L., J.L., and Y.Q. acquired the data. Q.S. and N.Z. analyzed the data. Q.S. drafted the manuscript. J.L. and L.L. contributed to the interpretation of the results and critical revision of the manuscript for important intellectual content and approved the final version of the manuscript. All authors reviewed and approved the final manuscript. J.L. and L.L. are the guarantors.

Funding: This work was supported by grants (2016YFC0900500, 2016YFC0900501, 2016YFC0900504) from the National Key R&D Program of China. The CKB baseline survey and the first re-survey were supported by a grant from the Kadoorie Charitable Foundation in Hong Kong. The long-term follow-up is supported by grants from the UK Wellcome Trust (202922/Z/16/Z, 088158/Z/09/Z, 104085/Z/14/Z), National Natural Science Foundation of China (81390540, 81390541, 81390544), and Chinese Ministry of Science and Technology (2011BAI09B01). The funders had no role in the study design, data collection, data analysis and interpretation, writing of the report, or the decision to submit the article for publication.

Acknowledgments: The most important acknowledgment is to the participants in the study and the members of the survey teams in each of the 10 regional centers, as well as to the project development and management teams based at Beijing, Oxford and the 10 regional centers.

Conflicts of Interest: The authors declare no conflict of interest.

References

1. Kannus, P.; Uusi-Rasi, K.; Palvanen, M.; Parkkari, J. Non-pharmacological means to prevent fractures among older adults. *Ann. Med.* **2005**, *37*, 303–310. [CrossRef] [PubMed]
2. Jarvinen, T.L.; Sievanen, H.; Khan, K.M.; Heinonen, A.; Kannus, P. Shifting the focus in fracture prevention from osteoporosis to falls. *BMJ* **2008**, *336*, 124–126. [CrossRef] [PubMed]
3. Kannus, P.; Niemi, S.; Parkkari, J.; Palvanen, M.; Heinonen, A.; Sievanen, H.; Jarvinen, T.; Khan, K.; Jarvinen, M. Why is the age-standardized incidence of low-trauma fractures rising in many elderly populations? *J. Bone Miner. Res.* **2002**, *17*, 1363–1367. [CrossRef] [PubMed]
4. Cummings, S.R.; Melton, L.J. Epidemiology and outcomes of osteoporotic fractures. *Lancet* **2002**, *359*, 1761–1767. [CrossRef]
5. Kanis, J.A.; Oden, A.; McCloskey, E.V.; Johansson, H.; Wahl, D.A.; Cooper, C.; IOF Working Group on Epidemiology and Quality of Life. A systematic review of hip fracture incidence and probability of fracture worldwide. *Osteoporos. Int.* **2012**, *23*, 2239–2256. [CrossRef] [PubMed]
6. Liu, S.H.; Chen, C.; Yang, R.S.; Yen, Y.P.; Yang, Y.T.; Tsai, C. Caffeine enhances osteoclast differentiation from bone marrow hematopoietic cells and reduces bone mineral density in growing rats. *J. Orthop. Res.* **2011**, *29*, 954–960. [CrossRef] [PubMed]
7. Shankar, V.S.; Pazianas, M.; Huang, C.L.; Simon, B.; Adebanjo, O.A.; Zaidi, M. Caffeine modulates Ca^{2+} receptor activation in isolated rat osteoclasts and induces intracellular Ca^{2+} release. *Am. J. Physiol.* **1995**, *268*, F447–F454. [CrossRef] [PubMed]
8. Nash, L.A.; Ward, W.E. Tea and bone health: Findings from human studies, potential mechanisms, and identification of knowledge gaps. *Crit. Rev. Food Sci. Nutr.* **2017**, *57*, 1603–1617. [CrossRef] [PubMed]

9. Yun, J.H.; Kim, C.S.; Cho, K.S.; Chai, J.K.; Kim, C.K.; Choi, S.H. (-)-Epigallocatechin gallate induces apoptosis, via caspase activation, in osteoclasts differentiated from RAW 264.7 cells. *J. Periodont. Res.* **2007**, *42*, 212–218. [CrossRef] [PubMed]

10. Oka, Y.; Iwai, S.; Amano, H.; Irie, Y.; Yatomi, K.; Ryu, K.; Yamada, S.; Inagaki, K.; Oguchi, K. Tea polyphenols inhibit rat osteoclast formation and differentiation. *J. Pharmacol. Sci.* **2012**, *118*, 55–64. [CrossRef] [PubMed]

11. Shen, C.L.; Chyu, M.C.; Wang, J.S. Tea and bone health: Steps forward in translational nutrition. *Am. J. Clin. Nutr.* **2013**, *98*, 1694S–1699S. [CrossRef] [PubMed]

12. Johnell, O.; Gullberg, B.; Kanis, J.A.; Allander, E.; Elffors, L.; Dequeker, J.; Dilsen, G.; Gennari, C.; Lopes Vaz, A.; Lyritis, G.; et al. Risk factors for hip fracture in European women: The MEDOS Study. Mediterranean Osteoporosis Study. *J. Bone Miner. Res.* **1995**, *10*, 1802–1815. [CrossRef] [PubMed]

13. Kanis, J.; Johnell, O.; Gullberg, B.; Allander, E.; Elffors, L.; Ranstam, J.; Dequeker, J.; Dilsen, G.; Gennari, C.; Vaz, A.L.; et al. Risk factors for hip fracture in men from southern Europe: The MEDOS study. Mediterranean Osteoporosis Study. *Osteoporos. Int.* **1999**, *9*, 45–54. [CrossRef] [PubMed]

14. Xie, H.L.; Ouyang, W.F.; Wu, B.H.; Tu, S.L.; Xue, W.Q.; Fan, F.; Chen, Y.M. A case-control study regarding tea consumption and risk of hip fractures in middle-aged and elderly Chinese. *Zhonghua Liu Xing Bing Xue Za Zhi* **2013**, *34*, 385–388. [PubMed]

15. Kreiger, N.; Gross, A.; Hunter, G. Dietary factors and fracture in postmenopausal women: A case-control study. *Int. J. Epidemiol.* **1992**, *21*, 953–958. [CrossRef] [PubMed]

16. Nieves, J.W.; Grisso, J.A.; Kelsey, J.L. A case-control study of hip fracture: Evaluation of selected dietary variables and teenage physical activity. *Osteoporos. Int.* **1992**, *2*, 122–127. [CrossRef] [PubMed]

17. Suzuki, T.; Yoshida, H.; Hashimoto, T.; Yoshimura, N.; Fujiwara, S.; Fukunaga, M.; Nakamura, T.; Yoh, K.; Inoue, T.; Hosoi, T.; et al. Case-control study of risk factors for hip fractures in the Japanese elderly by a Mediterranean Osteoporosis Study (MEDOS) questionnaire. *Bone* **1997**, *21*, 461–467. [CrossRef]

18. Hernandez-Avila, M.; Colditz, G.A.; Stampfer, M.J.; Rosner, B.; Speizer, F.E.; Willett, W.C. Caffeine, moderate alcohol intake, and risk of fractures of the hip and forearm in middle-aged women. *Am. J. Clin. Nutr.* **1991**, *54*, 157–163. [CrossRef] [PubMed]

19. Hansen, S.A.; Folsom, A.R.; Kushi, L.H.; Sellers, T.A. Association of fractures with caffeine and alcohol in postmenopausal women: The Iowa Women's Health Study. *Public Health Nutr.* **2000**, *3*, 253–261. [CrossRef] [PubMed]

20. Chen, Z.; Pettinger, M.B.; Ritenbaugh, C.; LaCroix, A.Z.; Robbins, J.; Caan, B.J.; Barad, D.H.; Hakim, I.A. Habitual tea consumption and risk of osteoporosis: A prospective study in the women's health initiative observational cohort. *Am. J. Epidemiol.* **2003**, *158*, 772–781. [CrossRef] [PubMed]

21. Hallstrom, H.; Wolk, A.; Glynn, A.; Michaelsson, K. Coffee, tea and caffeine consumption in relation to osteoporotic fracture risk in a cohort of Swedish women. *Osteoporos. Int.* **2006**, *17*, 1055–1064. [CrossRef] [PubMed]

22. Dai, Z.; Jin, A.; Soh, A.Z.; Ang, L.W.; Yuan, J.M.; Koh, W.P. Coffee and tea drinking in relation to risk of hip fracture in the Singapore Chinese Health Study. *Bone* **2018**, *112*, 51–57. [CrossRef] [PubMed]

23. Kiel, D.P.; Felson, D.T.; Hannan, M.T.; Anderson, J.J.; Wilson, P.W. Caffeine and the risk of hip fracture: The Framingham Study. *Am. J. Epidemiol.* **1990**, *132*, 675–684. [CrossRef] [PubMed]

24. Myers, G.; Prince, R.L.; Kerr, D.A.; Devine, A.; Woodman, R.J.; Lewis, J.R.; Hodgson, J.M. Tea and flavonoid intake predict osteoporotic fracture risk in elderly Australian women: A prospective study. *Am. J. Clin. Nutr.* **2015**, *102*, 958–965. [CrossRef] [PubMed]

25. Chen, B.; Shi, H.-F.; Wu, S.-C. Tea consumption didn't modify the risk of fracture: A dose–response meta-analysis of observational studies. *Diagn. Pathol.* **2014**, *9*, 44. [CrossRef] [PubMed]

26. Yan, A.; Zhang, H.-H.; Wang, S.-Q.; Zhao, Y. Does tea consumption correlate to risk of fracture? A meta-analysis. *Int. J. Clin. Exp. Med.* **2015**, *8*, 8347–8357. [PubMed]

27. Guo, M.; Qu, H.; Xu, L.; Shi, D.-Z. Tea consumption may decrease the risk of osteoporosis: An updated meta-analysis of observational studies. *Nutr. Res.* **2017**, *42*, 1–10. [CrossRef] [PubMed]

28. Sheng, J.; Qu, X.; Zhang, X.; Zhai, Z.; Li, H.; Liu, X.; Li, H.; Liu, G.; Zhu, Z.; Hao, Y.; et al. Coffee, tea, and the risk of hip fracture: A meta-analysis. *Osteoporos. Int.* **2014**, *25*, 141–150. [CrossRef] [PubMed]

29. Chen, Z.; Lee, L.; Chen, J.; Collins, R.; Wu, F.; Guo, Y.; Linksted, P.; Peto, R. Cohort profile: The Kadoorie Study of Chronic Disease in China (KSCDC). *Int. J. Epidemiol.* **2005**, *34*, 1243–1249. [CrossRef] [PubMed]

30. Chen, Z.; Chen, J.; Collins, R.; Guo, Y.; Peto, R.; Wu, F.; Li, L.; China Kadoorie Biobank collaborative, g. China Kadoorie Biobank of 0.5 million people: Survey methods, baseline characteristics and long-term follow-up. *Int. J. Epidemiol.* **2011**, *40*, 1652–1666. [CrossRef] [PubMed]

31. Janghorbani, M.; Feskanich, D.; Willett, W.C.; Hu, F. Prospective study of diabetes and risk of hip fracture: The Nurses' Health Study. *Diabetes Care* **2006**, *29*, 1573–1578. [CrossRef] [PubMed]

32. Warriner, A.H.; Patkar, N.M.; Curtis, J.R.; Delzell, E.; Gary, L.; Kilgore, M.; Saag, K. Which fractures are most attributable to osteoporosis? *J. Clin. Epidemiol.* **2011**, *64*, 46–53. [CrossRef] [PubMed]

33. Einother, S.J.; Martens, V.E. Acute effects of tea consumption on attention and mood. *Am. J. Clin. Nutr.* **2013**, *98*, 1700S–1708S. [CrossRef] [PubMed]

34. De Bruin, E.A.; Rowson, M.J.; Van Buren, L.; Rycroft, J.A.; Owen, G.N. Black tea improves attention and self-reported alertness. *Appetite* **2011**, *56*, 235–240. [CrossRef] [PubMed]

35. Lee, D.R.; Lee, J.; Rota, M.; Lee, J.; Ahn, H.S.; Park, S.M.; Shin, D. Coffee consumption and risk of fractures: A systematic review and dose-response meta-analysis. *Bone* **2014**, *63*, 20–28. [CrossRef] [PubMed]

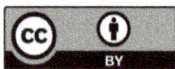

nutrients

Article

Targeting the DNA Repair Endonuclease ERCC1-XPF with Green Tea Polyphenol Epigallocatechin-3-Gallate (EGCG) and Its Prodrug to Enhance Cisplatin Efficacy in Human Cancer Cells

Joshua R. Heyza [1,†], Sanjeevani Arora [2,†,‡], Hao Zhang [1], Kayla L. Conner [1], Wen Lei [1], Ashley M. Floyd [1], Rahul R. Deshmukh [3,§], Jeffrey Sarver [4], Christopher J. Trabbic [5], Paul Erhardt [5], Tak-Hang Chan [6,7], Q. Ping Dou [8] and Steve M. Patrick [1,*]

[1] Department of Oncology, Karmanos Cancer Institute, Wayne State University, Detroit, MI 48201, USA; jrheyza@med.wayne.edu (J.R.H.); hzhang1@hfhs.org (H.Z.); connerk@karmanos.org (K.L.C.); leiwen314@gmail.com (W.L.); floyda@karmanos.org (A.M.F.)
[2] Department of Cancer Biology, University of Toledo Health Science Campus, Toledo, OH 43614, USA; sanjeevani.arora@fccc.edu
[3] Department of Pathology, Wayne State University School of Medicine, Detroit, MI 48201, USA; rdeshmukh@lecom.edu
[4] Department of Pharmacology and Experimental Therapeutics, University of Toledo College of Pharmacy and Pharmaceutical Sciences, Toledo, OH 43614, USA; jeffrey.sarver@utoledo.edu
[5] Center for Drug Design and Development, Department of Medicinal and Biological Chemistry, University of Toledo College of Pharmacy and Pharmaceutical Sciences, Toledo, OH 43614, USA; christrabbic51@gmail.com (C.J.T.); paul.erhardt@utoledo.edu (P.E.)
[6] State Key Laboratory of Chemical Biology and Drug Discovery, Department of Applied Biology and Chemical Technology, The Hong Kong Polytechnic University, Hong Kong, China; tak-hang.chan@mcgill.ca
[7] Department of Chemistry, McGill University, Montreal, QC H3A 0B8, Canada
[8] Departments of Oncology, Pharmacology, and Pathology, Karmanos Cancer Institute, Wayne State University, Detroit, MI 48201, USA; doup@karmanos.org
* Correspondence: patricks@karmanos.org; Tel.: +1-313-576-8313
† These authors contributed equally.
‡ Current Address: Cancer Prevention and Control Program, Fox Chase Cancer Center, Lewis Katz School of Medicine, Philadelphia, PA 19111, USA.
§ Current Address: School of Pharmacy, Lake Erie College of Osteopathic Medicine, Bradenton, FL 34211, USA.

Received: 8 October 2018; Accepted: 29 October 2018; Published: 3 November 2018

Abstract: The $5'$-$3'$ structure-specific endonuclease ERCC1/XPF (Excision Repair Cross-Complementation Group 1/Xeroderma Pigmentosum group F) plays critical roles in the repair of cisplatin-induced DNA damage. As such, it has been identified as a potential pharmacological target for enhancing clinical response to platinum-based chemotherapy. The goal of this study was to follow up on our previous identification of the compound NSC143099 as a potent inhibitor of ERCC1/XPF activity by performing an in silico screen to identify structural analogues that could inhibit ERCC1/XPF activity in vitro and in vivo. Using a fluorescence-based DNA-endonuclease incision assay, we identified the green tea polyphenol (-)-epigallocatechin-3-gallate (EGCG) as a potent inhibitor of ERCC1/XPF activity with an IC_{50} (half maximal inhibitory concentration) in the nanomolar range in biochemical assays. Using DNA repair assays and clonogenic survival assays, we show that EGCG can inhibit DNA repair and enhance cisplatin sensitivity in human cancer cells. Finally, we show that a prodrug of EGCG, Pro-EGCG (EGCG octaacetate), can enhance response to platinum-based chemotherapy in vivo. Together these data support a novel target of EGCG in cancer cells, namely ERCC1/XPF. Our studies also corroborate previous observations that EGCG enhances sensitivity to cisplatin in multiple cancer types. Thus, EGCG or its prodrug makes an ideal candidate for further pharmacological development with the goal of enhancing cisplatin response in human tumors.

Keywords: ERCC1/XPF; cisplatin; DNA repair; chemoresistance; green tea polyphenols

---

1. Introduction

The use of agents that induce interstrand crosslinks (ICLs), notably the platinum-based analogues, remains a mainstay of cancer treatment and they are used to treat a variety of cancer types including lung, ovarian, and head and neck cancers. Platinum-based drugs induce DNA damage by forming a variety of DNA lesions including ICLs, intrastrand crosslinks, and monoadducts. While platinum-based chemotherapy is often initially effective, resistance to these drugs usually occurs. Resistance to platinums has been attributed to several mechanisms including decreased drug accumulation, loss of mismatch and base excision repair, increased translesion synthesis as well as increased DNA repair [1]. Extensive work devoted to understanding mechanisms of resistance to these therapies has led to the identification of novel drug targets for enhancing therapeutic response and overcoming chemoresistance, including targeting the 5′-3′ structure-specific endonuclease ERCC1/XPF (Excision Repair Cross-Complementation Group 1/Xeroderma Pigmentosum Group F) [2,3]. ERCC1/XPF is a critical complex involved in the repair of DNA ICLs with essential functions in both replication-independent and -dependent ICL repair pathways [4,5]. As such, it is well-established that ERCC1 expression is altered in several tumor types, including lung, head and neck, and ovarian cancers, suggesting its potential use as a drug target or biomarker for response to platinum-based chemotherapy. Indeed, this possibility has been thoroughly investigated in preclinical and clinical studies. Clinical data have shown that low ERCC1 expression is associated with increased overall survival in response to chemotherapy [6]. Further data showed that low ERCC1 expression was associated with a positive response to platinum-based chemotherapy in non-small cell lung cancer patients [7]. Some mixed results have now hampered further clinical development of ERCC1 as a first-in-class platinum biomarker, most notably in a prospective international, randomized Phase III clinical trial where there was an absence of clinical benefit for patients with low ERCC1 receiving a platinum agent [8]. However, these mixed results have been largely attributed to problems pertaining to accurate detection of functional ERCC1/XPF (e.g., antibody specificity and splice variant expression), rather than its usefulness as a potential biomarker for response to platinum-based chemotherapy [9]. Clear evidence from extensive data from biochemical, in vitro, and in vivo approaches suggests critical roles for the complex in repair of platinum-induced DNA damage, suggesting the inhibition of ERCC1/XPF as a potential means of sensitizing tumors to platinum-based chemotherapy.

ERCC1/XPF plays key roles in nucleotide excision repair, ICL repair, and homologous recombination. In the response to DNA-ICLs, ERCC1/XPF plays a key role in incising 5′ to the DNA lesion resulting in the unhooking of the interstrand crosslink from the DNA helix [5]. In both replication-independent and -dependent pathways, ERCC1/XPF-mediated incision appears to be a generally required step for at least a subset of ICLs. In replication-dependent repair of interstrand crosslinks, however, several groups have also postulated that ERCC1/XPF nuclease activity is also essential at a second step downstream from initial unhooking likely during homologous recombination [10]. In line with critical roles for ERCC1/XPF in ICL repair, we have previously shown that siRNA knockdown of ERCC1/XPF could enhance sensitivity of lung cancer cells to cisplatin [3]. Additionally, this sensitivity was induced as a result of decreased DNA repair of interstrand and intrastrand crosslinks.

Several recent developments have been made in identifying small molecular inhibitors of ERCC1/XPF activity. The Melton and Saxty groups have published several papers identifying several classes of molecules capable of inhibiting ERCC1/XPF activity, including catechols, 3-hydroxypyridones, N-hydroxyimides, and hydroxypyrimidones, with micromolar potency in in vitro assays [11–13]. In one of these studies, Compound 13 inhibited DNA repair in vitro, and led to increased γH2AX foci formation in human cells, suggesting inhibition of ERCC1/XPF in vitro [12] (Figure 1A). In another study, Compound AS5-4 disrupted ERCC1/XPF activity and enhanced cisplatin sensitivity in a melanoma cell line [13] (Figure 1A). Inhibitors of the ERCC1/XPF interaction have also been identified [13]. An in silico screen identified the compound E-X PPI2 which could disrupt the ERCC1/XPF interaction, disrupt DNA repair mediated by ERCC1/XPF, and sensitize a melanoma cell line to cisplatin [13]. In addition to these studies, we previously performed a high-throughput screen using the NCI-DTP (National Cancer Institute Developmental Therapeutics Program) diversity set and identified the compounds NSC16168 (Figure 1A) and NSC143099, which were potent and selective inhibitors of ERCC1/XPF activity both in biochemical assays as well as in lung cancer cell lines [14]. Furthermore, the compound NSC16168 was also capable of significantly enhancing tumor response to platinum-based chemotherapy in vivo [14].

In this study, we expanded upon our previous identification of the lead compound NSC143099 as an ERCC1/XPF inhibitor by performing an in silico analysis to identify molecules with structural similarities to NSC143099 that may have activity against ERCC1/XPF both in vitro and in vivo. This preliminary screen and subsequent testing identified the green tea polyphenol epigallocatechin-3-gallate (EGCG), which has approximately 90% structural similarity to the partial structure of NSC143099, as a potent, partially reversible inhibitor of ERCC1/XPF activity in vitro. Interestingly, a number of previous studies have identified EGCG as a compound capable of enhancing cisplatin sensitivity in cancer cells and in xenograft models, but the mechanism of this interaction was not established [15–17]. In addition, EGCG has been shown to pharmacologically inhibit 20S proteasome activity [18,19]. However, we are the first to identify the DNA endonuclease ERCC1/XPF as a pharmacological target of EGCG, helping to further explain previous observations in regard to EGCG and enhanced cisplatin sensitization. Further characterization of this compound shows it is capable of inhibiting ICL repair in vitro leading to enhanced sensitivity to cisplatin in lung cancer cell lines. Finally, we show that the inhibition of ERCC1/XPF by the EGCGprodrug, Pro-EGCG (EGCG octaacetate), could significantly enhance response to cisplatin in tumor xenografts in vivo by increasing tumor cell death and decreasing proliferation. Together, these data suggest EGCG or its prodrug may be a suitable candidate for further preclinical development as an agent capable of enhancing platinum sensitivity in tumors and overcoming drug resistance.

2. Materials and Methods

2.1. Cell Lines and Cell Culture

H1299 and H460 non-small cell lung cancer cell lines used in this study were cultured in RPMI-1640 medium (Dharmacon, Lafayette, CO, USA) supplemented with 10% Fetal Bovine Serum (Atlanta Biologicals, Flowery Branch, GA, USA) and 1% penicillin/streptomycin (Dharmacon, Lafayette). Cells were grown at 37 °C in 5% CO_2. Cell lines were authenticated by the Biobanking and Correlative Sciences Core Facility at the Karmanos Cancer Institute.

2.2. In Vitro ERCC1/XPF Fluorescence Incision Assay

The in vitro ERCC1/XPF fluorescence incision assay was utilized to assess the ability of small molecules to inhibit ERCC1/XPF-mediated incision of a forked DNA substrate and was performed as previously described [14]. Purified ERCC1/XPF and XPG (Xeroderma Pigmentosum Group G) was utilized for these experiments and the purification protocol is described in [14]. The DNA substrate is described in Arora et al. [14]. Briefly, the forked DNA substrate was designed to have a 14-base dsDNA region flanked by a 12-base non-complementary ssDNA region mimicking the ssDNA:dsDNA preferred substrate for ERCC1/XPF cleavage. One strand contained a site-specific fluorescein (F) modification (5′-GCCAGCGCTCGGAT (AminoC6dT) (FLSN) TTTTTTTTTTT-3′), whereas the complementary strand contained a site-specific DABCYL quencher (Q) (5′-TTTTTTTTTTT (AminoC6dT) (Dabcyl) ATCCGAGCGCTGGC-3′) directly opposed to the fluorescein modification. An uncleaved substrate thus would not release a fluorescent signal when excited at 485 nm due to the quenching activity of the DABCYL. On the other hand, ERCC1/XPF-mediated cleavage of the forked substrate would lead to the release of the fluorescein-labeled DNA into the solution and would result in an increased fluorescent signal when measuring emission at 525 nm. The substrate was also designed with a HhaI restriction enzyme cut site in the DNA duplex, which served as a positive control for these experiments. The reactions for this experiment consisted of 10 nM DNA annealed DNA duplex, 7.5 nM ERCC1/XPF or 7.5 nM XPG in buffer (50 mM Tris-HCl pH 8.0, 2 mM MgCl$_2$, 0.1 mM bovine serum albumin, 0.5 mM β-mercaptoethanol) or HhaI (20 U/mL) (New England Biolabs, Ipswich, MA, USA) and increasing concentrations of each compound prepared in DMSO. Reactions were incubated at 37 °C for 30 min after which samples were excited with a 485 nm laser and emission at 525 nm was measured using a Spectramax M5 plate reader (Molecular Devices, -San Jose, CA, USA). Data were plotted as percent fluorescence (% incision) relative to wells containing no compound.

2.3. Rapid Dilution Assay

Rapid dilution assays were utilized to determine the irreversible or reversible binding of the EGCG and (-)-gallocatechin gallate compounds to ERCC1/XPF. These experiments were performed as described in Liu et al. [20]. In a 10 μL reaction, the concentration of ERCC1/XPF enzyme was added at 100-fold higher than normal concentrations used in the fluorescence incision assay (7.5 nM) and then mixed with 10× the IC$_{90}$ concentration of either EGCG, (-)-gallocatechin gallate, or diluent control (90:10, v/v DMSO:glycerol) and incubated at 37 °C for 30 min. After incubation, 2 μL of the drug-enzyme solution was diluted in 198 μL consisting of reaction buffer and the fluorescent DNA forked substrate in a 96-well plate. The reaction was monitored and the fluorescence was measured at various time points over 60 min. Data from the experiment were represented as the increase in fluorescence over time indicating the amount of activity of ERCC1/XPF on the DNA substrate.

2.4. Modified Alkaline Comet Assay

Modified alkaline comet assays were utilized to assess interstrand crosslink repair and were performed essentially as previously described [21,22]. H460 cells were treated with 15 M EGCG or (-)-gallocatechin gallate for two hours and then cisplatin was added to the media using the IC90 concentration for the cell line used for an additional two hours. After treatment, cells were washed with PBS and complete media was added (24 h and 48 h samples) or immediately processed for analysis at 0 h post-treatment. Prior to cell harvesting but after the experimental treatment, cells were treated with 100 μM hydrogen peroxide (H$_2$O$_2$) for 15 min to induce DNA double strand breaks. Following treatment with hydrogen peroxide, cells were trypsinized, pelleted, resuspended, and counted. Approximately 10,000 cells were embedded in 1% low melting point agarose and added onto slides pre-coated with a layer of 1% normal melting point agarose and allowed to solidify. A top layer of 0.5% low melting point agarose was then added and allowed to solidify. Following solidification, slides were incubated for 1 h at 4 °C in the absence of light in lysis buffer (2.5 M NaCl, 10 mM Tris, 100 mM EDTA, 1% Triton X-100, pH 10). Slides were removed from the lysis buffer and excess buffer was removed. Slides were then placed in an electrophoresis tank containing 4 °C alkaline electrophoresis buffer (300 mM NaOH, 1 mM EDTA, pH > 13), incubated for 20 min followed by electrophoresis for 30 min at 0.7 V/cm, 300 mA. Slides were removed and placed for 10 min in neutralizing buffer (0.4 M Tris-HCl, pH 7.5). Slides were stained with SYBR green (Trevigen, Gaithersburg, MD, USA) and images were taken using a Nikon epifluorescence microscope at 20 magnification. For analysis, DNA tails for at least 50 cells were measured for each slide using Komet Assay Software 5.5F (Kinetic Imaging, Liverpool, UK). Data were analyzed and quantified as in Arora et al. [14].

2.5. Clonogenic Survival Assays

Approximately 300–400 cells were seeded in triplicate in 60 mm dishes and allowed to attach for ~24 h. For treatments with EGCG or Pro-EGCG alone, the following day cells were titrated with the indicated concentrations of each drug for 4 h in serum-free medium followed by replacement with complete medium. For colony assays combining EGCG or Pro-EGCG with cisplatin, cells were pre-treated for 2 h and then cisplatin was added for 2 h (total treatment time with EGCG or Pro-EGCG was 4 h). After treatment, serum-free medium was replaced with complete medium. Cells were allowed to grow for approximately seven days after which plates were washed with PBS, fixed in 95% methanol, and stained in 20% ethanol containing 0.2% crystal violet dye. Colonies with >50 cells were counted using a light microscope, and percent colony survival was measured relative to the control for each group and normalized to 100%.

2.6. Chemicals

Cisplatin was purchased from Sigma-Aldrich (St. Louis, MO, USA) and prepared fresh prior to each experiment by making a 1 mM stock solution in PBS. (-)-epigallocatechin-3-gallate (EGCG) and (-)-gallocatechin gallate were purchased from Sigma-Aldrich and were prepared in dimethyl sulfoxide. Pro-EGCG was prepared as we previously described, and a 50 mM solution was prepared in DMSO for in vitro studies [23].

2.7. In Vivo Studies

For the study, 20 female athymic nude mice (five mice per group) were purchased from Taconic Biosciences (Rensselaer, NY, USA) and were maintained in accordance with protocols approved by the Wayne State University Institutional Laboratory Animal Care and Use Committee. The mice were allowed to acclimate for 1 week. Approximately 2.5×10^6 H460 cells were suspended in 100 L RPMI media containing no fetal bovine serum or penicillin/streptomycin. Cells were injected subcutaneously into the right flank of each mouse. Tumor volume was measured by caliper measurements every day starting on day 3. Tumor volume was defined as (width^2 × length/2). Weight of the mice was also measured regularly starting on the day of inoculation and through the experimental end-point. At three days post-inoculation, the mice were treated with vehicle or Pro-EGCG at 60 mg/kg by intraperitoneal IP injection. Pro-EGCG was prepared in DMSO and cremophor/ethanol (60:20:20 $v/v/v$). Once tumors reached a volume of ~100 mm^3, cisplatin or vehicle treatment began. The mice were treated with 4 mg/kg pharmaceutical grade, sterile cisplatin three times weekly by IP injection. Drugs were prepared fresh daily. The mice were sacrificed once tumors reached ~1000 mm^3 or at day 24, and the tumors were collected for further analysis of apoptosis and cell proliferation by immunohistochemistry.

2.8. Immunohistochemistry

Immunohistochemistry was performed by the Biobanking and Correlative Sciences Core at the Karmanos Cancer Institute (KCI). Subcutaneous tumors harvested from the mice were fixed in 10% formalin and were paraffin-embedded. Five μm slices were hematoxylin- and eosin-stained. Slides were stained using the Terminal nucleotidyl transferase-mediated nick end labeling assay (TUNEL) using an in situ apoptosis detection kit. Tissues were also probed for Ki67 and PCNA using standardized protocols optimized by the KCI Biobanking and Correlative Sciences Core. Images were taken at a magnification of 20. Images were quantified using ImageJ software and plotted as percent of stained area.

2.9. Statistical Analysis

The mouse xenograft study had five mice per treatment group, each bearing one tumor. Tumor volumes were log-transformed to meet the normality assumption, and growth curves were compared using a linear-mixed effects model with mice-specific effect as a random variable. P values were adjusted using Bonferroni correction. For the clonogenic survival assays, dose-response curve IC_{50} values for EGCG or Pro-EGCG in combination with cisplatin met distributional assumptions. Statistical comparisons were performed by two-sided unpaired t-test followed by Holm's post-hoc analysis. Data analyses were completed using R version 3.5.0. and RStudio: Integrated Development for R (version 1.1.447, RStudio Inc.; Boston, MA, USA).

3. Results

3.1. Hits from an in Silico Screen to Identify Structural Analogues of NSC143099 with Activity Against ERCC1/XPF Activity

We previously identified the compound NSC143099 in a high-throughput screen using the NCI-DTP diversity set, as a potent, selective inhibitor of ERCC1/XPF activity both biochemically and in vitro (Figure 1C) [14]. To expand upon the initial characterization of this compound, we performed an in silico screen to identify other structurally similar compounds that may also be capable of inhibiting ERCC1/XPF activity. A search for compounds having 80% or higher structural similarity to NSC143099 was conducted for all commercially available compounds listed in the Chemical Abstract Service (CAS) database using the online SciFinder® search tool (CAS, Columbus, OH, USA), whereas a locally available compound library established in the University of Toledo Center for Drug Design and Development (approximately 1000 compounds synthesized or purchased for multiple projects) was searched using ChemBioFinder Ultra (v14.0, Cambridge Soft Corp, Perkin Elmer Inc., Waltham, MA, USA). No hits were identified at this level of similarity from either source for the full NSC143099 molecule. However, a similarity search using just half of the molecule (the three-ring partial structure repeated in the upper and lower sections of the molecule) did identify six molecules available commercially or in the local compound library with a similarity of greater than 85% [24]. All six of these agents were surveyed in our frontline screening assay. From the screen, we identified three compounds with nanomolar potency against ERCC1/XPF activity in an in vitro, fluorescence-based ERCC1/XPF DNA-incision assay. The ERCC1/XPF incision assay consists of a forked DNA substrate sharing a 14-base complementary region followed by a 12-base non-complementary region (Figure 1B). The substrate contains both a fluorophore and quencher directly opposed to one another such that if a nuclease cleaves the substrate, the fluorophore will be released into solution and release a fluorescent signal when excited at 485 nm. This Y-shaped forked DNA structure represents an optimal substrate for ERCC1/XPF cleavage as shown in Arora et al. [14]. Additionally, the DNA substrate has a HhaI restriction enzyme cleavage site allowing for the use of HhaI as a positive control as well as assessing indiscriminate inhibition of compounds against an unrelated DNA endonuclease. Finally, because of the forked nature of the DNA substrate, it also serves as a prime substrate for cleavage by XPG, allowing us to evaluate off-target inhibition of a related DNA endonuclease. All three identified compounds share structural similarities to NSC143099 (Figure 1C). Myricetin, (-)-epigallocatechin-3-gallate (EGCG), and (-)-gallocatechin gallate (GCG) all inhibited ERCC1/XPF activity in vitro (IC_{50}s ranging from ~40–150 nM) (Figure 1C). Myricetin is known to have multiple targets in mammalian cells, including the DNA endonuclease, Ape1, (25), so we did not further assess myricetin's ERCC1/XPF inhibitory activity. Notably, EGCG and GCG had potent inhibitory activity against ERCC1/XPF-mediated DNA incision, while having no activity against HhaI or XPG (Figure 1D).

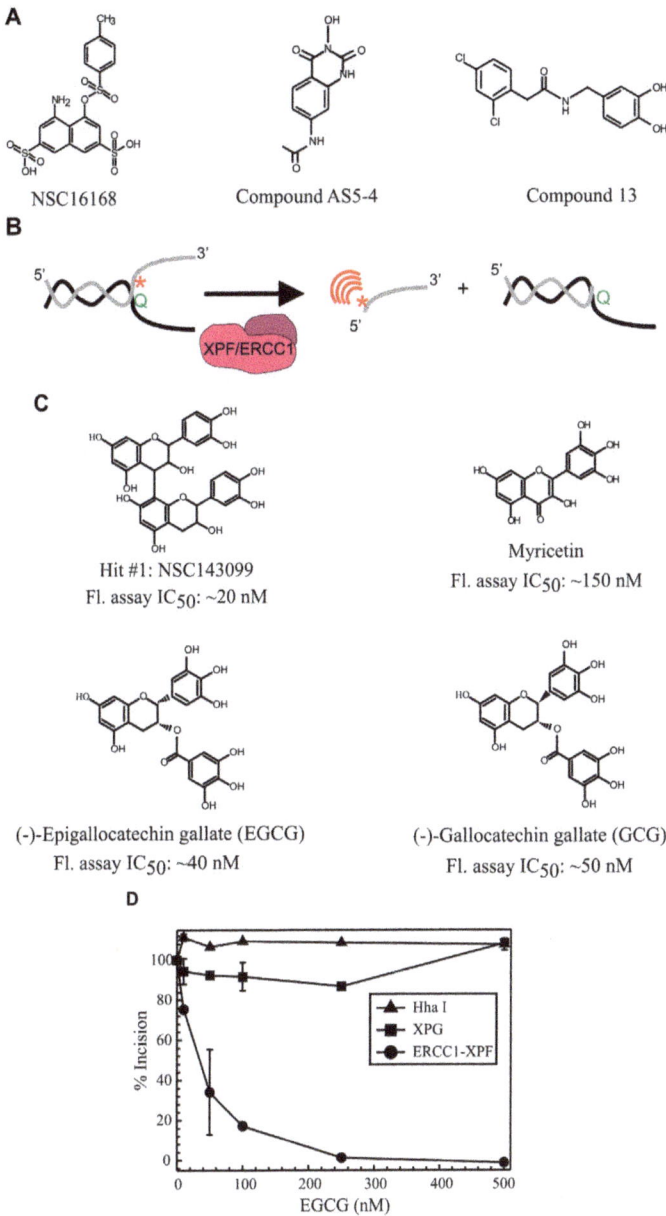

Figure 1. (**A**) Structures of ERCC1/XPF (Excision Repair Cross-Complementation Group 1/Xeroderma Pigmentosum Group F) inhibitors identified in previous studies. The structure of NSC16168 is undergoing further investigation. (**B**) Model of the DNA substrate and product produced by ERCC1/XPF cleavage in the fluorescent–DNA-incision assay. * represents fluorescein and Q represents DABCYL quencher. (**C**) Structure of NSC143099 and the three identified hits from the in silico screen along with their IC_{50}s in the DNA-incision assay. (**D**) Plotted results of EGCG-mediated inhibition of ERCC1/XPF in the DNA-incision assay. Results show selectivity for ERCC1/XPF as EGCG did not inhibit HhaI- or XPG-mediated incision of the DNA substrate. EGCG: (-)-epigallocatechin-3-gallate; IC_{50}: half maximal inhibitory concentration.

3.2. EGCG Is a Partially Reversible ERCC1/XPF Inhibitor Capable of Blocking Interstrand Crosslink Repair In Vitro

After identifying EGCG and GCG as structurally similar compounds to NSC143099 with inhibitory activity against ERCC1/XPF, we assessed the reversibility of the inhibition in vitro using a rapid dilution assay. The rapid dilution assay allowed us to assess whether the inhibition of ERCC1/XPF by EGCG or GCG was reversible in nature. The initial reaction consisted of 100ERCC1/XPF enzyme and the IC_{90} concentration of either compound determined in the ERCC1/XPF incision assay followed by a 30 min incubation at 37 °C to allow for compound binding to the enzyme. Following this initial incubation, the reaction was diluted 100-fold into a solution containing buffer and the fluorescent DNA substrate. Fluorescence was monitored over time to assess whether the enzyme recovered incision capability or if this activity was continually inhibited after dilution. As a positive control, adding ERCC1/XPF to the DNA substrate increased the fluorescent signal over time (Figure 2A). It appears that GCG is a nearly completely reversible inhibitor of ERCC1/XPF activity, as dilution of the enzyme/drug solution led to an increased fluorescent signal over time very similar to the addition of ERCC1/XPF alone to the reaction (Figure 2A). On the other hand, the rapid dilution of EGCG/enzyme solution led to a slight increase in fluorescent signal over time, suggesting that this inhibitory activity of the compound may be partially, but incompletely reversible with slow kinetics of reversibility (Figure 2A). EGCG and GCG are diastereomers, namely, they have identical structures but differ in their stereochemistries. EGCG, the most abundant polyphenol in green tea extract, has the 2S, 3S configurations with the two groups cis- to each other, whereas (-)-GCG has the 2R, 3S configuration with the two groups trans- to each other (Figure 1B). These data may indicate that the stereochemistry of the benzenetriol group at the 2-position may influence the reversibility of the inhibition of ERCC1/XPF activity by these natural compounds.

Next, we assessed the ability of EGCG and GCG to inhibit repair of cisplatin-induced interstrand crosslinks in human cancer cells via a modified alkaline comet assay. Because ERCC1/XPF endonuclease activity is critical for repair of DNA interstrand crosslinks, we chose to assess the ability of these compounds to inhibit repair of these DNA lesions. Furthermore, the modified alkaline comet assay is an established method to indirectly monitor interstrand crosslink repair over time in cells. H460 lung cancer cells were treated with 15 µM EGCG or GCG for 2 h, after which an IC_{90} concentration of cisplatin was added for an additional 2 h followed by drug removal and replacement with complete medium. Just following the experimental treatment and time-course, cells were treated with 100 µM H_2O_2 to induce random DNA double strand breaks, a critical component of the assay to be able to distinguish ICL containing from repaired DNA segments during denaturing electrophoresis. Immediately after initial treatment, single cell electrophoresis and staining of the DNA was performed and the level of interstrand crosslinking was determined and normalized to 100% interstrand crosslinks remaining for each treatment group (Figure 2B,C). Then, 24 h post-treatment, we observed a decrease in the amount of ICLs remaining as evident by the increased tail length over time, as observed in the comet assay images which were indicative of increased ICL repair over time (Figure 2B,C). Persistence of ICLs in this assay resulted in a maintenance of shorter tail length as the crosslink retarded the DNA mobility. This trend continued into the 48 h time point (Figure 2B,C). On the other hand, treatment with EGCG or GCG led to decreased repair of DNA ICLs over time which was observed starting at the 24 h time point and continuing into the 48 h time point (Figure 2B,C). Together these data indicate that EGCG is a potentially partially reversible inhibitor of ERCC1/XPF and GCG is a reversible inhibitor of ERCC1/XPF activity; however, both compounds are capable of inhibiting ICL DNA repair in vitro.

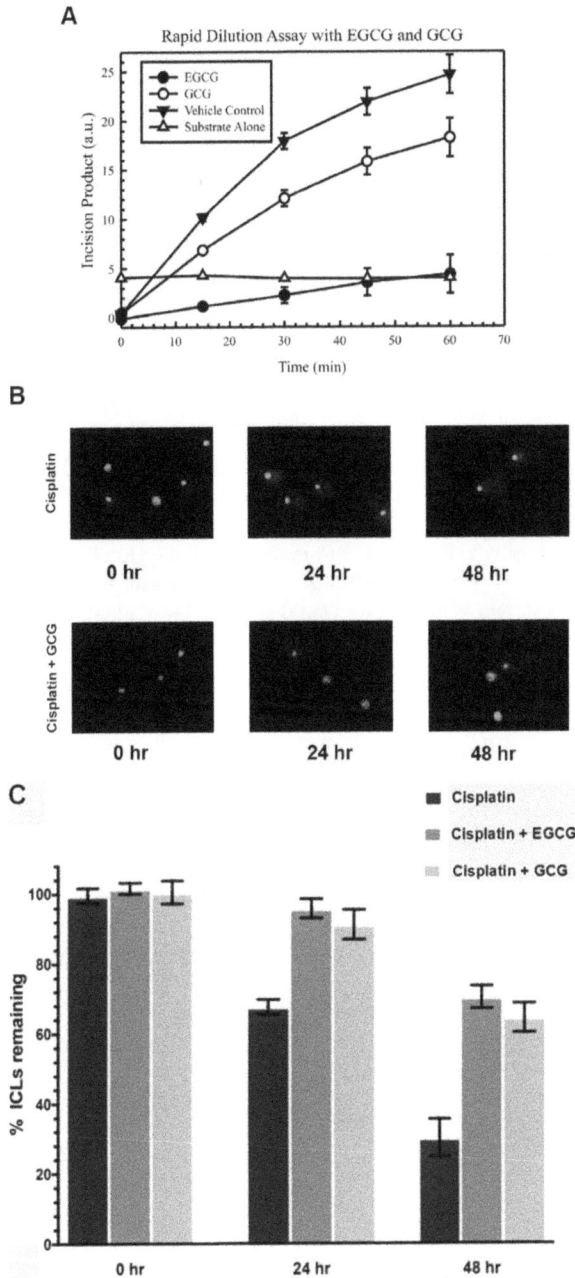

Figure 2. (**A**) Results from the rapid dilution assay showing GCG is a reversible inhibitor of ERCC1/XPF and EGCG is either partially reversible with slow kinetics or is irreversible. Data represented as average ± standard deviation. (**B**) Representative images of modified alkaline comet assay results for cisplatin and cisplatin + GCG in H460 cells. (**C**) Quantified data from the modified alkaline comet assay resulted in H460 cells showing inhibition of interstrand crosslink repair in cells treated with cisplatin + EGCG or cisplatin + GCG. GCG: (-)-gallocatechin gallate.

3.3. EGCG and Pro-EGCG Enhance Cisplatin Sensitivity in Lung Cancer Cell Lines In Vitro

After observing that EGCG and GCG could inhibit repair of ICLs in human cancer cells, we assessed the sensitivity of H460 lung cancer cells to EGCG in vitro either alone or in combination with cisplatin. For these studies, we also utilized a prodrug of EGCG, known as Pro-EGCG, which is the octaacetate of EGCG, which was first described by Lam et al. [23]. EGCG is known to have poor oral bioavailability and is subject to extensive rapid metabolic transformations [25,26]. Pro-EGCG differs from EGCG in having the reactive hydroxyl groups of EGCG converted by acetylation to peracetate-protecting groups (Figure 3A). These acetate groups are hydrolyzed back to the hydroxy groups upon entering cells of plasma due to esterases present within the cells or plasma thereby regenerating EGCG [27]. Thus, in the absence of esterases or in biochemical assays with purified protein, pro-EGCG has no inhibitory effect on ERCC1/XPF activity (Figure 3A) but showed inhibitory activity on clonogenic formation in H460 colony survival assays comparable to EGCG (Figure 3B). These inhibitory effects on colony formation are likely due to other targets of EGCG, including the proteasome [19]. This is supported by the observation that Pro-EGCG titration in H1299 wild-type and ERCC1 knockout cells led to similar inhibition of clonogenicity, indicating that the sensitivity of cells to EGCG and Pro-EGCG as a single agent is likely due to additional molecular targets (Figure 3C) [14]. It is important to note that a major genetic difference between H460 and H1299 cells is p53 status where H460 cells are p53 wild-type and H1299 cells are p53 null. We cannot exclude the possibility that p53 status may impact the sensitivity of cell lines or tumors to inhibition of ERCC1/XPF activity. However, the addition of a single ~IC_{50} dose of cisplatin in H460 cells enhanced sensitivity to EGCG and Pro-EGCG >10-fold, consistent with what we would expect if ERCC1/XPF were inhibited (Figure 3D).

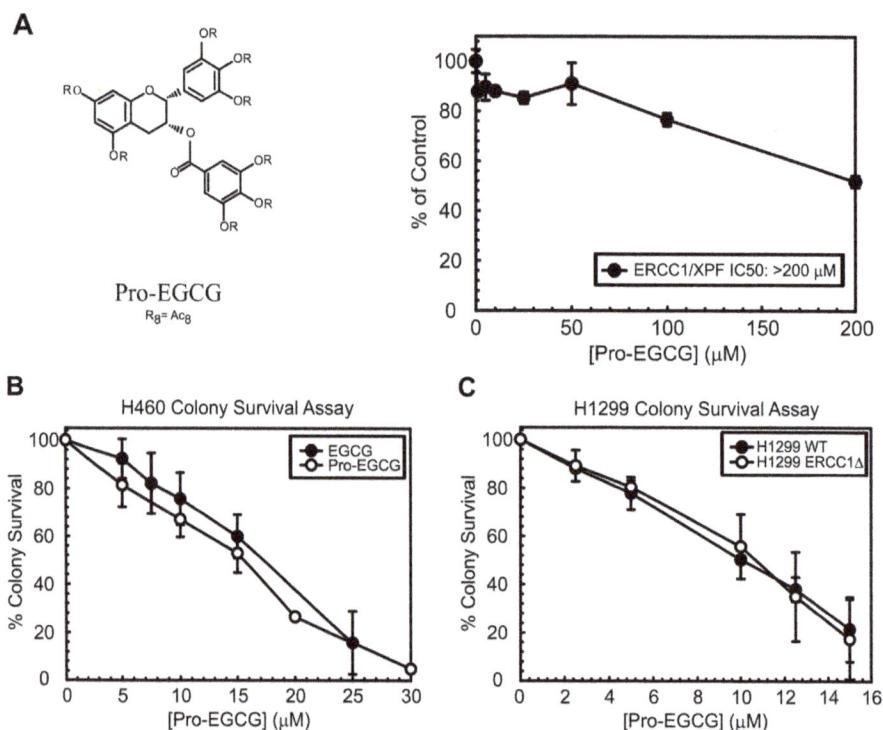

Figure 3. *Cont.*

D

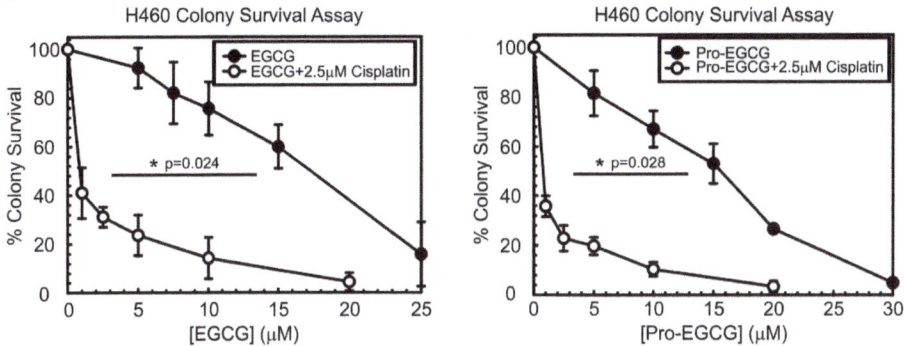

Figure 3. (**A**) Structure (Left) and activity (Right) of Pro-EGCG, the EGCG prodrug containing acetylated hydroxyl groups which are cleaved by esterases upon entry into the cell, in the DNA-incision assay. Data represented as average ± standard deviation. (**B**) Titration of EGCG and Pro-EGCG in H460 cells showing the both reduce clonogenicity to approximately the same extent. (**C**). Inhibition of clonogenicity by Pro-EGCG as a single agent appears to be independent of its targeting of ERCC1/XPF as shown by titration in H1299 wild-type and ERCC1 knockout cells. (**D**) H460 cells treated with increasing concentrations of EGCG (Left) or Pro-EGCG (Right) ± a single IC$_{50}$ dose of cisplatin. All clonogenic assay data represented as average of experimental repeats ± standard deviation. Dose-response curves were compared by two-sided unpaired *t*-test followed by Holm's post-hoc analysis.

3.4. Pro-EGCG Enhances Cisplatin Response In Vivo

Next, we evaluated the effect of combining Pro-EGCG with cisplatin in the treatment of H460 lung cancer xenografts. For this study, 20 female athymic nude mice (five mice per group) were inoculated subcutaneously with H460 lung cancer cells and tumors were allowed to grow. Pro-EGCG was administered daily beginning on day 3 by IP injection at 60 mg/kg. The route of administration and doses used for Pro-EGCG were similar to what we have utilized in previous studies [27]. Cisplatin treatment began once tumors reached ~100 mm^3 and the mice were treated three times weekly with cisplatin at 4 mg/kg by IP injection. Tumor volume was measured daily by caliper measurements and plotted over time. Once tumors reached a volume of ~1000 mm^3, the mice were sacrificed and the tumors were harvested for further analysis. Control, untreated tumors grew rapidly and all mice were sacrificed by day 19 of the experiment (Figure 4A). The addition of 60 mg/kg Pro-EGCG had some inhibitory effects on tumor growth with all mice being sacrificed by day 21. Cisplatin alone also had inhibitory effects on its own, but the combination of cisplatin and Pro-EGCG greatly enhanced these effects, with mice in the dual-treatment group having barely palpable tumors at the experimental endpoint (day 24) (Figure 4A). These inhibitory effects on tumor growth can be observed in tumors harvested from mice where at day 19 the combination-treatment group had tumors approximately the same size as the cisplatin-treated group, but by day 24, the differences in tumor size were quite dramatically different with the combination-treatment group bearing much smaller tumors than the cisplatin-treated group (Figure 4B).

A

B

Tumor size Days 19 and 24 post implantation

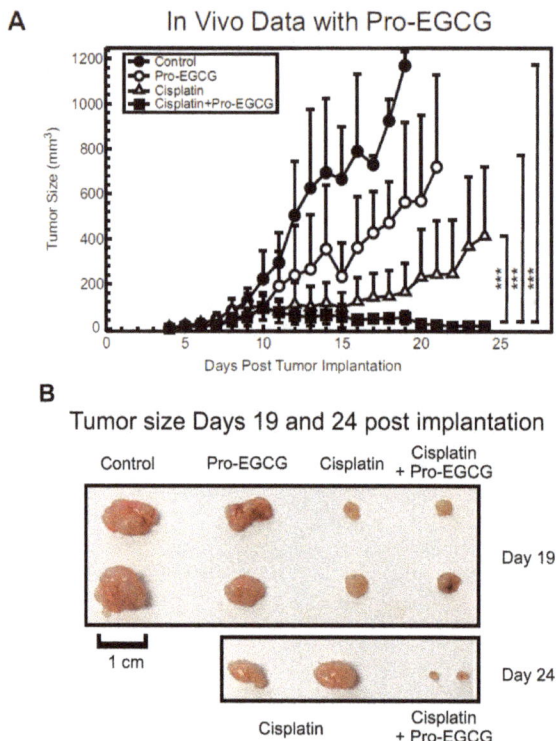

Figure 4. (**A**) Plot representing tumor growth of untreated, cisplatin-treated, Pro-EGCG-treated, or combination-treated mice. Data represented as tumor size (mm^3) over time. (**B**) Images of tumors harvested from sacrificed mice at day 19 and day 24. Growth curves were compared using a linear-mixed effects model with mice-specific effect as a random variable. *P* values were adjusted using Bonferroni correction. *** $p < 0.001$.

3.5. Enhanced Cisplatin Response in Tumors Treated with Pro-EGCG Is Associated with Increased Apoptotic Markers and Decreased Cellular Proliferation

Tumors harvested from the mice were further processed for immunohistochemical analysis. Tissue slices were analyzed for the presence of Ki67 and PCNA to evaluate markers of cellular proliferation. In addition, TUNEL staining was performed to detect cells undergoing cell death. While the Pro-EGCG- and cisplatin-treated tumors had reduced Ki67 and PCNA staining, this effect was exacerbated in combination-treated tumors, especially in terms of Ki67 staining (Figure 5). This would be indicative of reduced tumor cell proliferation in the combination-treated group. In the context of tumor cell death, we observed the opposite effect. Pro-EGCG-treated tumors had very little increase in TUNEL staining compared to untreated, control tumors (Figure 5). This staining was increased in cisplatin-treated mice as we would expect with a cytotoxic, DNA damaging agent. However, in the combination-treated group, the increase in TUNEL staining was quite dramatic compared to the Pro-EGCG- and cisplatin-treated tumors, suggesting the combination treatment concurrently decreases the amount of cellular proliferation in the tumors and dramatically increases tumor cell death (Figure 5).

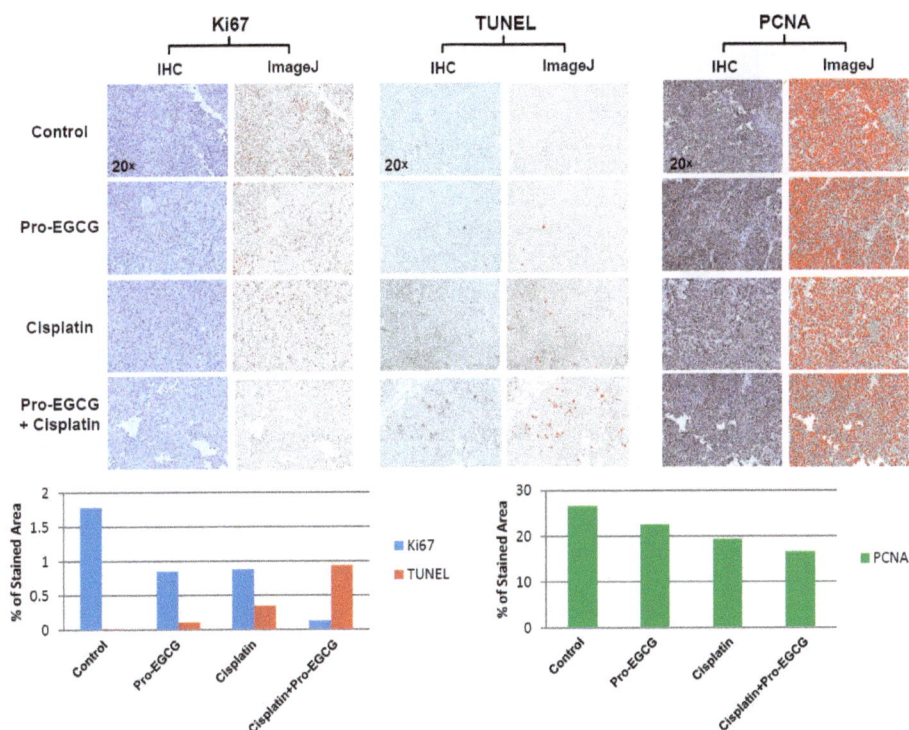

Figure 5. Raw images, ImageJ-processed images (**Top**), and quantification of immunohistochemical analysis of Ki67, TUNEL, and PCNA staining in tumors harvested from sacrificed mice (**Bottom**). Data showing increased TUNEL staining, decreased Ki67 staining, and decreased PCNA staining in the cisplatin+Pro-EGCG-treated tumors compared to other groups.

4. Discussion

Despite recent advances in cancer treatment such as using PD-1 and PD-L1 related therapies, platinum-based chemotherapy remains a mainstay option for a variety of tumor types either as first- or second-line therapy. Due to the prevalence of acquired or intrinsic resistance to platinum-based chemotherapy, it remains a valuable effort to identify factors that, when inhibited, can sensitize tumor cells to cisplatin. We previously have shown that ERCC1/XPF knockdown can sensitize ovarian and lung cancer cell lines to cisplatin [3]. Additionally, our group previously identified the compound NSC16168 as a potent inhibitor of ERCC1/XPF that can sensitive tumors to cisplatin [14]. The wide interest in ERCC1/XPF expression as a predictive biomarker for response to platinum-based chemotherapy also lends credence to the possibility of using inhibitors of this enzyme complex to enhance therapeutic response.

In our previous work, we performed a high-throughput screen and identified the compound NSC143099 as a potent inhibitor of ERCC1/XPF activity in vitro in both biochemical and cell-based assays [14]. In this work, we performed an in silico screen to identify other agents with structural similarity to NSC143099 that could have the potential for inhibiting ERCC1/XPF activity. From this screen, we identified three hits with nanomolar potency against ERCC1/XPF activity in a fluorescence-based DNA-incision assay: myricetin, EGCG, and GCG (Figure 1A). These compounds had substantial similarities and all shared a similar flavonoid structure. Myricetin was capable of inhibiting ERCC1/XPF activity with an IC_{50} of ~150 nM in our DNA-incision assay. However, myricetin has also been shown to inhibit a variety of other enzymes, including MEK1, PI3Kγ, and the

DNA endonuclease Ape1, among others [28–30]. Due to the known targeting of this compound to Ape1, we did not move further with this compound in this study.

EGCG as an anti-cancer agent has been thoroughly investigated in multiple studies and in multiple cancer types, including in breast, colorectal, gastric, ovarian, and lung cancers [31]. It has been established that EGCG has multiple cellular targets including work from the Dou lab, characterizing EGCG's inhibitory effects on the proteasome [27]. In line with these observations, treatment with EGCG or Pro-EGCG alone reduced clonogenicity in vitro in multiple lung cancer cell lines (Figure 3B). Additionally, these effects appear to be independent of any toxicity induced by inhibition of ERCC1/XPF as the sensitivity of H1299 wild-type and ERCC1 knockout cells were identical to each other (Figure 3C). Additionally, EGCG was described to have enhancing effects for cisplatin sensitivity both in vitro and in vivo. The studies assessing the cisplatin-sensitizing effects of EGCG implicated a number of different pathways and events as critical for this sensitization, including demethylation of gene promoters, increased expression of the copper transporter, CTR1, and enhancing autophagic flux [15–17]. In this work, we identified another target of EGCG, ERCC1/XPF, which has important implications for understanding the mechanism of the EGCG-mediated sensitization of tumors to cisplatin and for improving current cancer treatment strategies.

The EGCG compound had no activity against XPG or HhaI, suggesting its inhibition is largely specific to ERCC1/XPF (Figure 1B). Next, we showed that GCG, differing from EGCG only in the relative stereochemistry of the substitutions in the 2- and 3-positions, is a reversible inhibitor of ERCC1/XPF activity in a rapid dilution assay (Figure 2B). Conversely, EGCG is either partially reversible with slow kinetics or is an irreversible inhibitor of ERCC1/XPF activity (Figure 2A). This was similar to what we observed with another compound we identified from our original screen, NSC16168 [14]. While there were differences in the reversibility of this inhibition in biochemical assays, both EGCG and GCG could inhibit repair of cisplatin-induced interstrand crosslinks in vitro (Figure 2B,C). Not only did these compounds inhibit ERCC1/XPF activity in vitro, but this inhibition enhanced sensitivity to cisplatin in lung cancer cell lines (Figure 3). Due to the poor bioavailability and the facile metabolic transformations of EGCG, we also utilized a prodrug form of EGCG for our studies. Previous study showed that Pro-EGCG was converted intracellularly into EGCG, presumably by cellular esterases. Furthermore, Pro-EGCG was better absorbed into the cells, giving higher accumulation of EGCG by at least 2.4-fold than when the cells were treated with similar levels of EGCG [23,27]. In our DNA-incision assay, as expected, we observed that Pro-EGCG has no inhibitory effect on the purified ERCC1/XPF protein (Figure 3A). However, both EGCG and Pro-EGCG can sensitize lung cancer cells to an IC_{50} dose of cisplatin in clonogenic assays indicating these cell line models have sufficient esterase activity to convert the Pro-EGCG to active EGCG (Figure 3B).

Furthermore, after observing that EGCG could inhibit ERCC1/XPF and, along with Pro-EGCG, could sensitize lung cancer cells to cisplatin in vitro, we assessed the effects of combination treatment with cisplatin and Pro-EGCG in vivo. While Pro-EGCG and cisplatin had modest inhibitory effects on tumor growth as single agents, the combination treatment group had substantially smaller tumors at the day 24 endpoint (Figure 4A,B). The tumors in the combination treatment group were barely palpable at the experimental endpoint. Further analysis of these tumors by immunohistochemistry revealed that this sensitization was associated with the decreased presence of markers of cell growth and DNA replication and a dramatic increase in TUNEL staining indicative of cell death (Figure 5). Together these data suggest that EGCG and Pro-EGCG are potent inhibitors of ERCC1/XPF activity both in vitro and in vivo and that they are capable of sensitizing tumors to cisplatin therapy. In conclusion, we have identified the NSC143099 structural analogue, EGCG, as a potent inhibitor of ERCC1/XPF endonuclease activity capable of decreasing DNA repair in vitro and Pro-EGCG in enhancing cisplatin sensitivity in vivo. These data provide evidence that the green tea polyphenol, EGCG, and its prodrug could represent a potential structure for further pharmacological development in efforts to target the ERCC1/XPF endonuclease to enhance platinum-based chemotherapeutic response.

5. Conclusions

The data presented in this paper shows results from an in silico screen to identify structurally similar compounds to our lead compound NSC143099 that are capable of inhibiting ERCC1/XPF activity. The screen identified the green tea polyphenol, (-)-epigallocatechin gallate (EGCG), as a compound capable of inhibiting ERCC1/XPF activity in biochemical assays and blocking intrastrand crosslink repair in vitro. Furthermore, treatment of cells with EGCG or the prodrug form of EGCG, Pro-EGCG) was capable of sensitizing lung cancers to the chemotherapeutic agent, cisplatin. Additionally, Pro-EGCG treatment could enhance cisplatin efficacy in vivo. This increase in sensitization to cisplatin and Pro-EGCG combination treatment was correlated with decreased immunohistochemical staining of markers of cellular proliferation and increased staining for the apoptotic marker, TUNEL. Together these data suggest EGCG and its prodrug Pro-EGCG can target ERCC1/XPF activity and enhance cisplatin efficacy in vitro and in vivo.

Author Contributions: Conceptualization, Q.P.D. and S.M.P.; Data curation, J.R.H., S.A., H.Z., W.L. and A.M.F.; Formal analysis, J.R.H., S.A., H.Z., K.L.C., W.L., A.M.F. and J.S.; Funding acquisition, Q.P.D. and S.M.P.; Investigation, S.A.; Methodology, R.R.D.; Project administration, S.M.P.; Resources, C.J.T., P.E., T-H.C., Q.P.D. and S.M.P.; Supervision, S.M.P.; Writing—original draft, J.R.H.; Writing—review and editing, J.R.H., S.A., K.L.C., R.R.D., J.S., C.J.T., P.E., T-H.C., Q.P.D. and S.M.P.

Funding: This study was supported by grants from the American Cancer Society (RSG-06-163-01) and the National Institutes of Health (GM088249) both awarded to S.M.P, the National Cancer Institute T32 CA009035 and DOD CA171000 (W81XWH-18-1-0148) both awarded to S.A.; the National Cancer Institute NRSA T32CA009531 to J.R.H. and K.L.C.; the Wayne State University Thomas C. Rumble Fellowship to R.R.D.; the National Cancer Institute-National Institutes of Health to Q.P.D. (1R01CA120009; 1R01CA120009-04S1), and from the Natural Sciences and Engineering Research Council (NSERC) of Canada to T.H.C. as well as a Karmanos internal pilot fund for SMP and QPD.

Acknowledgments: We would like to thank Pershang Farshi for her assistance in the initial phase of the animal study and members of the Patrick lab for critical reading of the manuscript. We also wish to thank the Karmanos Cancer Institute KCI Biobanking and Correlative Sciences Core for assistance with the TUNEL and immunohistochemistry assays.

Conflicts of Interest: T.H.C. and Q.P.D. are inventors of patents on pro-EGCG; the other authors declare no conflict of interest. The funders had no role in the design of the study; in the collection, analyses, or interpretation of data; in the writing of the manuscript; or in the decision to publish the results.

References

1. Kelland, L. The resurgence of platinum-based cancer chemotherapy. *Nat. Rev. Cancer* **2007**, *7*, 573–584. [CrossRef] [PubMed]

2. McNeil, E.M.; Melton, D.W. DNA repair endonuclease ERCC1-XPF as a novel therapeutic target to overcome chemoresistance in cancer therapy. *Nucleic Acids Res.* **2012**, *40*, 9990–10004. [CrossRef] [PubMed]

3. Arora, S.; Kothandapani, A.; Tillison, K.; Kalman-Maltese, V.; Patrick, S.M. Downregulation of XPF-ERCC1 enhances cisplatin efficacy in cancer cells. *DNA Repair* **2010**, *9*, 745–753. [CrossRef] [PubMed]

4. Muniandy, P.A.; Liu, J.; Majumdar, A.; Liu, S.T.; Seidman, M.M. DNA interstrand crosslink repair in mammalian cells: Step by step. *Crit. Rev. Biochem. Mol. Biol.* **2010**, *45*, 23–49. [CrossRef] [PubMed]

5. Zhang, J.; Walter, J.C. Mechanism and regulation of incisions during DNA interstrand cross-link repair. *DNA Repair* **2014**, *19*, 135–142. [CrossRef] [PubMed]

6. Lord, R.V.; Brabender, J.; Gandara, D.; Alberola, V.; Camps, C.; Domine, M.; Cardenal, F.; Sanchez, J.M.; Gumerlock, P.H.; Taron, M.; et al. Low ERCC1 expression correlates with prolonged survival after cisplatin plus gemcitabine chemotherapy in non-small cell lung cancer. *Clin. Cancer Res.* **2002**, *8*, 2286–2291. [PubMed]

7. Olaussen, K.A.; Dunant, A.; Fouret, P.; Brambilla, E.; Andre, F.; Haddad, V.; Taranchon, E.; Filipits, M.; Pirker, R.; Popper, H.H.; et al. DNA repair by ERCC1 in non-small-cell lung cancer and cisplatin-based adjuvant chemotherapy. *N. Engl. J. Med.* **2006**, *355*, 983–991. [CrossRef] [PubMed]

8. Bepler, G.; Williams, C.; Schell, M.J.; Chen, W.; Zheng, Z.; Simon, G.; Gadgeel, S.; Zhao, X.; Schreiber, F.; Brahmer, J.; et al. Randomized international phase III trial of ERCC1 and RRM1 expression-based chemotherapy versus gemcitabine/carboplatin in advanced non-small-cell lung cancer. *J. Clin. Oncol. Off. J. Am. Soc. Clin. Oncol.* **2013**, *31*, 2404–2412. [CrossRef] [PubMed]

9. Friboulet, L.; Olaussen, K.A.; Pignon, J.P.; Shepherd, F.A.; Tsao, M.S.; Graziano, S.; Kratzke, R.; Douillard, J.Y.; Seymour, L.; Pirker, R.; et al. ERCC1 isoform expression and DNA repair in non-small-cell lung cancer. *N. Engl. J. Med.* **2013**, *368*, 1101–1110. [CrossRef] [PubMed]

10. Rahn, J.J.; Adair, G.M.; Nairn, R.S. Multiple roles of ERCC1-XPF in mammalian interstrand crosslink repair. *Environ. Mol. Mutagen.* **2010**, *51*, 567–581. [CrossRef] [PubMed]

11. Chapman, T.M.; Wallace, C.; Gillen, K.J.; Bakrania, P.; Khurana, P.; Coombs, P.J.; Fox, S.; Bureau, E.A.; Brownlees, J.; Melton, D.W.; et al. N-Hydroxyimides and hydroxypyrimidinones as inhibitors of the DNA repair complex ERCC1-XPF. *Bioorg. Med. Chem. Lett.* **2015**, *25*, 4104–4108. [CrossRef] [PubMed]

12. Chapman, T.M.; Gillen, K.J.; Wallace, C.; Lee, M.T.; Bakrania, P.; Khurana, P.; Coombs, P.J.; Stennett, L.; Fox, S.; Bureau, E.A.; et al. Catechols and 3-hydroxypyridones as inhibitors of the DNA repair complex ERCC1-XPF. *Bioorg. Med. Chem. Lett.* **2015**, *25*, 4097–4103. [CrossRef] [PubMed]

13. McNeil, E.M.; Astell, K.R.; Ritchie, A.M.; Shave, S.; Houston, D.R.; Bakrania, P.; Jones, H.M.; Khurana, P.; Wallace, C.; Chapman, T.; et al. Inhibition of the ERCC1-XPF structure-specific endonuclease to overcome cancer chemoresistance. *DNA Repair* **2015**, *31*, 19–28. [CrossRef] [PubMed]

14. Arora, S.; Heyza, J.; Zhang, H.; Kalman-Maltese, V.; Tillison, K.; Floyd, A.M.; Chalfin, E.M.; Bepler, G.; Patrick, S.M. Identification of small molecule inhibitors of ERCC1-XPF that inhibit DNA repair and potentiate cisplatin efficacy in cancer cells. *Oncotarget* **2016**, *7*, 75104–75117. [CrossRef] [PubMed]

15. Hu, F.; Wei, F.; Wang, Y.; Wu, B.; Fang, Y.; Xiong, B. EGCG synergizes the therapeutic effect of cisplatin and oxaliplatin through autophagic pathway in human colorectal cancer cells. *J. Pharmacol. Sci.* **2015**, *128*, 27–34. [CrossRef] [PubMed]

16. Wang, X.; Jiang, P.; Wang, P.; Yang, C.S.; Wang, X.; Feng, Q. EGCG enhances cisplatin sensitivity by regulating expression of the copper and cisplatin influx transporter ctr1 in ovary cancer. *PLoS ONE* **2015**, *10*, e0125402. [CrossRef]

17. Yuan, C.H.; Horng, C.T.; Lee, C.F.; Chiang, N.N.; Tsai, F.J.; Lu, C.C.; Chiang, J.H.; Hsu, Y.M.; Yang, J.S.; Chen, F.A. Epigallocatechin gallate sensitizes cisplatin-resistant oral cancer CAR cell apoptosis and autophagy through stimulating AKT/STAT3 pathway and suppressing multidrug resistance 1 signaling. *Environ. Toxicol.* **2017**, *32*, 845–855. [CrossRef] [PubMed]

18. Yang, H.; Landis-Piwowar, K.; Chan, T.H.; Dou, Q.P. Green tea polyphenols as proteasome inhibitors: Implication in chemoprevention. *Curr. Cancer Drug Targets* **2011**, *11*, 296–306. [CrossRef] [PubMed]

19. Nam, S.; Smith, D.M.; Dou, Q.P. Ester bond-containing tea polyphenols potently inhibit proteasome activity in vitro and in vivo. *J. Biol. Chem.* **2001**, *276*, 13322–13330. [CrossRef] [PubMed]

20. Liu, T.; Toriyabe, Y.; Kazak, M.; Berkman, C.E. Pseudoirreversible inhibition of prostate-specific membrane antigen by phosphoramidate peptidomimetics. *Biochemistry* **2008**, *47*, 12658–12660. [CrossRef] [PubMed]

21. Sawant, A.; Floyd, A.M.; Dangeti, M.; Lei, W.; Sobol, R.W.; Patrick, S.M. Differential role of base excision repair proteins in mediating cisplatin cytotoxicity. *DNA Repair* **2017**, *51*, 46–59. [CrossRef] [PubMed]

22. Kothandapani, A.; Sawant, A.; Dangeti, V.S.; Sobol, R.W.; Patrick, S.M. Epistatic role of base excision repair and mismatch repair pathways in mediating cisplatin cytotoxicity. *Nucleic Acids Res.* **2013**, *41*, 7332–7343. [CrossRef] [PubMed]

23. Lam, W.H.; Kazi, A.; Kuhn, D.J.; Chow, L.M.; Chan, A.S.; Dou, Q.P.; Chan, T.H. A potential prodrug for a green tea polyphenol proteasome inhibitor: Evaluation of the peracetate ester of (-)-epigallocatechin gallate [(-)-EGCG]. *Bioorg. Med. Chem.* **2004**, *12*, 5587–5593. [CrossRef] [PubMed]

24. Bajusz, D.; Racz, A.; Heberger, K. Why is Tanimoto index an appropriate choice for fingerprint-based similarity calculations? *J. Cheminform.* **2015**, *7*, 20. [CrossRef] [PubMed]

25. Lambert, J.D.; Yang, C.S. Cancer chemopreventive activity and bioavailability of tea and tea polyphenols. *Mutat. Res.* **2003**, *523*, 201–208. [CrossRef]

26. Kida, K.; Suzuki, M.; Matsumoto, N.; Nanjo, F.; Hara, Y. Identification of biliary metabolites of (-)-epigallocatechin gallate in rats. *J. Agric. Food Chem.* **2000**, *48*, 4151–4155. [CrossRef] [PubMed]

27. Landis-Piwowar, K.R.; Huo, C.; Chen, D.; Milacic, V.; Shi, G.; Chan, T.H.; Dou, Q.P. A novel prodrug of the green tea polyphenol (-)-epigallocatechin-3-gallate as a potential anticancer agent. *Cancer Res.* **2007**, *67*, 4303–4310. [CrossRef] [PubMed]

28. Simeonov, A.; Kulkarni, A.; Dorjsuren, D.; Jadhav, A.; Shen, M.; McNeill, D.R.; Austin, C.P.; Wilson, D.M. Identification and characterization of inhibitors of human apurinic/apyrimidinic endonuclease APE1. *PLoS ONE* **2009**, *4*, e5740. [CrossRef] [PubMed]

29. Lee, K.W.; Kang, N.J.; Rogozin, E.A.; Kim, H.G.; Cho, Y.Y.; Bode, A.M.; Lee, H.J.; Surh, Y.J.; Bowden, G.T.; Dong, Z. Myricetin is a novel natural inhibitor of neoplastic cell transformation and MEK1. *Carcinogenesis* **2007**, *28*, 1918–1927. [CrossRef] [PubMed]
30. Walker, E.H.; Pacold, M.E.; Perisic, O.; Stephens, L.; Hawkins, P.T.; Wymann, M.P.; Williams, R.L. Structural determinants of phosphoinositide 3-kinase inhibition by wortmannin, LY294002, quercetin, myricetin, and staurosporine. *Mol. Cell* **2000**, *6*, 909–919. [CrossRef]
31. Chen, D.; Wan, S.B.; Yang, H.; Yuan, J.; Chan, T.H.; Dou, Q.P. EGCG, green tea polyphenols and their synthetic analogs and prodrugs for human cancer prevention and treatment. *Adv. Clin. Chem.* **2011**, *53*, 155–177. [PubMed]

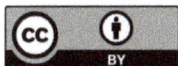

nutrients

MDPI

Review

Health Benefits of Bioactive Compounds from the Genus *Ilex*, a Source of Traditional Caffeinated Beverages

Ren-You Gan [†], Dan Zhang [†], Min Wang and Harold Corke *

Department of Food Science & Technology, School of Agriculture and Biology, Shanghai Jiao Tong University, Shanghai 200240, China; renyougan@sjtu.edu.cn (R.-Y.G.); zhang.dan@sjtu.edu.cn (D.Z.); wangmin799@outlook.com (M.W.)
* Correspondence: hcorke@sjtu.edu.cn or hcorke@yahoo.com; Tel.: +86-21-3420-6880
† These authors equally contributed to this paper.

Received: 10 October 2018; Accepted: 1 November 2018; Published: 5 November 2018

Abstract: Tea and coffee are caffeinated beverages commonly consumed around the world in daily life. Tea from *Camellia sinensis* is widely available and is a good source of caffeine and other bioactive compounds (e.g., polyphenols and carotenoids). Other tea-like beverages, such as those from the genus *Ilex*, the large-leaved Kudingcha (*Ilex latifolia* Thunb and *Ilex kudingcha* C.J. Tseng), Yerba Mate (*Ilex paraguariensis* A. St.-Hil), Yaupon Holly (*Ilex vomitoria*), and Guayusa (*Ilex guayusa* Loes) are also traditional drinks, with lesser overall usage, but have attracted much recent attention and have been subjected to further study. This review summarizes the distribution, composition, and health benefits of caffeinated beverages from the genus *Ilex*. Plants of this genus mainly contain polyphenols and alkaloids, and show diverse health benefits, which, as well as supporting their further popularization as beverages, may also lead to potential applications in the pharmaceutical or nutraceutical industries.

Keywords: kudingcha; yerba mate; yaupon holly; guayusa; caffeine; polyphenols

1. Introduction

Caffeine (1,3,7-trimethylxanthine) is a member of a group of compounds known as purine alkaloids [1], occurs naturally in plants used to make beverages such as coffee and tea, and is added in the formulation of many soft drinks. Caffeine is a well-known central nervous system stimulant in humans. Tea from *Camellia sinensis* is the most popular non-alcoholic caffeine-containing beverage, and has a long consumption history all over the world. Major chemical constituents in tea are polyphenols, proteins, enzymes, caffeine, carbohydrates, and inorganics, which provide health beneficial properties [1,2]. However, caffeinated tea-like beverages with somewhat comparable chemical characteristics are also obtained from plants of the genus *Ilex*, mainly the large-leaved Kudingcha, Yerba Mate, Yaupon tea, and Guayusa tea, which have been well studied in recent years. The genus *Ilex*, comprising some 600 species, is widely distributed across most non-tropical parts of the world. The best-known species in Western literature is the European or English Holly, *I. aquifolium* L., with its characteristic red drupes (berries) and leaves widely used in Christmas decorations.

Kudingcha has a long consumption history in China and its commercial products are commonly found in the market. The large-leaved Kudingcha, including *Ilex latifolia* Thunb and *Ilex kudingcha* C.J. Tseng, have been reported to show significant medicinal or bioactive properties such as antioxidant, anti-inflammatory, anti-obesity, anti-cancer, modulation of gut microbiota, and antiproliferative effects [3–10]. In addition, Yerba Mate produced from leaves of the tree *Ilex paraguariensis* is a widely consumed beverage in South American countries such as Argentina, Brazil, Chile, Paraguay, and Uruguay, and the average annual consumption reaches around 3 kg to 10 kg per person.

Yerba Mate tea has developed into a main alternative to coffee and black tea since it is characterized as having various health benefits, such as antimicrobial, antioxidant, anti-obesity, anti-diabetic, and cardiovascular protective effects [11–18]. Moreover, in the southeastern part of the United States, Yaupon tea (Yaupon Holly, *Ilex vomitoria*) is prepared as a healthy beverage by Native Americans [19]. The polyphenolics extracted from Yaupon Holly are free of catechin, and exhibit antioxidant, anti-inflammatory, and chemo-preventive effects [19–21]. Compared to green tea, processing and packaging have less effect on the degradation of polyphenolics in Yaupon Holly, indicating an advantage for commercial products of Yaupon tea. Guayusa tea, commercially known as Runa tea, is natively grown in the Amazon and has long been consumed by Amazonian indigenous tribes [22,23]. *Ilex guayusa* tea contains high levels of phenolic compounds, a good dietary resource with cellular antioxidant and anti-inflammatory properties [23,24].

Therefore, in order to provide a better understanding of *Ilex*-based caffeinated beverages, the relevant literature from the last ten years was searched in Web of Science. The geographical distributions of different *Ilex* species are summarized, followed by a discussion of their main bioactive compounds, and finally we highlight the potential health benefits and related molecular mechanisms. Since many *Ilex* species are already commonly consumed in the world, the information in this review will help to provide a scientific structure to explain the health benefits of *Ilex*-based beverages, which may encourage further development by the *Ilex* tea industry and lead to new products for the public.

2. Distribution

Plants of the genus *Ilex* are distributed widely in various parts of the world (Table 1). Large-leaved Kudingcha, an infusion made from evergreen trees of two species (*I. kudingcha* C.J. Tseng and *I. latifolia* Thunb.), is a popular bitter-tasting infused tea found in China and other Southeastern Asian countries (e.g., Singapore, Malaysia, and Vietnam) [3,25]. Yerba Mate tea, from a native South American holly shrub, is mainly produced and consumed in South America [26,27]. A study from Marcelo et al. reported that Yerba Mate could possibly be identified as to country of origin in South America by elemental concentration and chemometrics [28]. Leaves of Yaupon Holly (*Ilex vomitoria*), from an evergreen and caffeine-containing shrub native to the southeastern United States, was used to make a healthy beverage by Amerindians and later European colonists [19,29]. Guayusa is made from leaves of an evergreen tree native to South America and is grown in the Amazon. Guayusa has recently gained more attention [22,23].

Table 1. Distribution of the most commonly consumed species of the genus *Ilex*.

Common Name	Species	Distribution	References
Large-leaved Kudingcha	*I. kudingcha* C.J. Tseng	China: Guangxi; Guangdong; Hainan	[3,25,30]
	I. latifolia Thunb.	China: Zhejiang; Jiangsu; Fujian; Anhui; Hainan	[3,6,7,10]
Yerba Mate	*Ilex paraguariensis* A. St.-Hil	South America: Argentina; Brazil; Paraguay; Uruguay	[26,27,31–33]
Yaupon Holly	*Ilex vomitoria*	Southeastern United States	[19,21,29,34]
Guayusa	*Ilex guayusa* Loes	South America: Argentina, Southern of Brazil, Paraguay and Uruguay	[22,24,35,36]

3. Bioactive Compounds

Ilex genus plants are generally known to be rich in a wide variety of bioactive compounds, mainly polyphenols and alkaloids, which play an essential role in their health benefits.

3.1. Polyphenols

3.1.1. Polyphenols in Large-Leaved Kudingcha

Structurally, polyphenols are a class of compounds composed of benzene rings bonded to one or more hydroxyl groups. In previous published studies, different methods have been applied to determine the phenolic composition in Kudingcha. For example, the use of tyrosinase biosensor, Folin-Ciocalteu assay, high performance liquid chromatography (HPLC), HPLC-nuclear magnetic resonance (NMR), ultra-high performance liquid chromatography (UHPLC), UHPLC-diode array detector-linear ion trap-Orbitrap (UHPLC-DAD-LTQ-Orbitrap), liquid chromatography-photodiode array detector-atmospheric pressure chemical ionization-mass spectrometry (LC-PDA–APCI-MS), and the quantitative analysis of multiple components with a single marker (QAMS) methods were reported [3,24,25,30,37]. Using these methods, polyphenols can be identified and quantified effectively.

The total polyphenolic content (TPC) in *I. latifolia* was 188 mg gallic acid equivalent (GAE) per g dry plant material using the Folin–Ciocalteu method [10]. Caffeoylquinic acids (Figure 1) and their derivatives are the main polyphenols in Kudingcha. Compounds such as ethyl caffeate, 3,4-di-O-caffeoylquinic acid methyl ester, 3,5-di-O-caffeoylquinic acid methyl ester, and chlorogenic acid were identified in *I. latifolia* [38]. Chlorogenic acid (CGA), the ester of caffeic acid and quinic acid, is known for its biological functionality. The CGA derivatives 3-O-caffeoylquinic acid, 5-O-caffeoylquinic acid, 3,5-O-dicaffeoylquinic acid, and 4,5-O-dicaffeoylquinic acid have been identified as major compounds in methanol and ether acetate extracts of *I. kudingcha* [39]. This was confirmed by Che et al., who detected a total of 68 CGA candidates belonging to 12 categories [40]. Our previous study also reported that isomers of mono- and di-caffeoylquinic acids were the predominant compounds from Kudingcha genotypes of two *Ilex* species, and the average amount of major CGAs from these Kudingcha of different origins was 97 mg/g [25]. Furthermore, 18 active components including polyphenols, such as hydroxycasein, protocatechuic acid, rutin, neochlorogenic acid, chlorogenic acid, cryptochlorogenic acid, caffeic acid, and isochlorogenic acid, were first determined in *I. kudingcha* by the QAMS method, which was efficiently applied for simultaneous determination of different phenolic compounds [30]. Moreover, three caffeoylquinic acids, including neochlorogenic, chlorogenic, and cryptochlorogenic acids, and three dicaffeoylquinic acids, were identified as the main constituents in *I. kudingcha* [37].

3.1.2. Polyphenols in Yerba Mate

Polyphenols have been extracted from different parts of Yerba Mate, such as the whole plant, leaves, and stems. Of these, the highest level of phenolic compounds was found in the leaf extract [15]. From chromatographic analyses, the TPC was determined as about 51 mg/g dry mass (DM) in *I. paraguariensis* [41]. Moreover, determination of the TPC in Yerba Mate was performed by the Folin-Ciocalteu method, where 111 samples from the Parana State in Brazil were characterized [18]. Additionally, 46 different polyphenols from four commercial Yerba Mate products have been quantified, with hydroxycinnamic acid derivatives and flavonols accounting for 90% and 10% of the polyphenols present. Of these, 3-caffeoylquinic (26.8% to 28.8%), 5-caffeoylquinic (21.1% to 22.4%), 4-caffeoylquinic (12.6% to 14.2%), and 3,5-dicaffeoylquinic acids (9.5% to 11.3%) along with rutin (7.1% to 7.8%) were found to be the predominant polyphenolic compounds. In conclusion, *I. paraguariensis* was shown to be a good source of polyphenols [18,27]. Moreover, the content of lutein in aqueous extracts of Yerba Mate varied in different commercial samples, giving further prospects for a role in risk reduction for certain diseases [42].

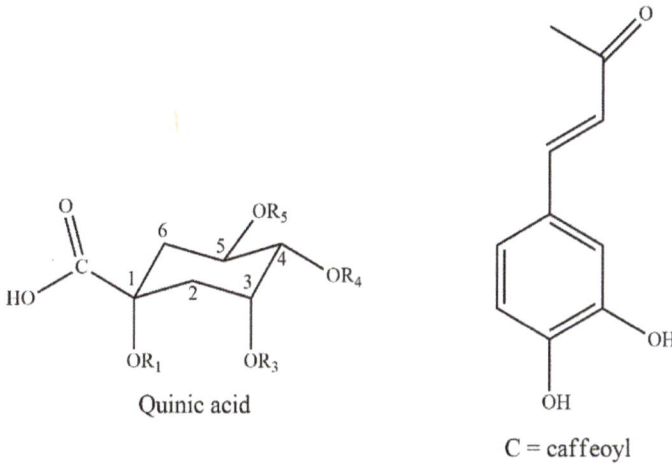

Figure 1. The chemical structures of caffeoylquinic acids.

Caffeoylquinic acids	R1	R3	R4	R5
3-O-caffeoylquinic acid	H	C	H	H
4-O-caffeoylquinic acid	H	H	C	H
5-O-caffeoylquinic acid	H	H	H	C
3,5-di-O-caffeoylquinic acid	H	C	H	C
4,5-di-O-caffeoylquinic acid	H	H	C	C

3.1.3. Polyphenols in Yaupon Holly

Recently, limited research has been carried out on Yaupon Holly (*I. vomitoria*). In infusions, eight polyphenolic compounds were identified including mono-caffeoylquinic acids, di-caffeoylquinic acids, and two flavonol glycosides (quercetin 3-rutinosides and kaempferol 3-rutinoside), where the mono- and di-caffeoylquinic acids comprised 70% of the total polyphenolics [20]. Kim and Talcott also determined the composition of diverse polyphenolic compounds in tea infusion of Yaupon Holly, and found that 3-O-caffeoylquinic acid (chlorogenic acid), quercetin 3-rutinoside (rutin), 5-O-caffeoylquinic acid (neochlorogenic acid), and 4-O-caffeoylquinic acid (cryptochlorogenic acid) were the main phenolic compounds, with 423, 392, 318, and 125 mg/L rutin equivalents, respectively [21].

3.1.4. Polyphenols in Guayusa

I. guayusa teas showed high polyphenolic content totaling between 54 and 67 mg GAE/g DM, and phenolic mono- and di-caffeoylquinic acid derivatives were the major compounds determined by mass spectrometry [23]. Moreover, determination of TPC by the Slinkard and Singleton method showed a very different content in green leaves and in processed Guayusa [22]. For green leaves, TPC was about 55 mg/g DM, with hydroxycinnamic acid derivatives as the major constituents. The levels of 5-O-CQA (chlorogenic acid), 3,5-Dicaffeoylquinic acid (isochlorogenic acid), and 3-O-CQA (neochlorogenic acid) were 24, 16, and 8 mg/g DM, respectively. Processing methods such as blanching and fermentation are important factors affecting the TPC in Guayusa [22]. Kapp et al. reported that catechin, epicatechin, epicatechin gallate, epigallocatechin, and epigallocatechin gallate (EGCG) were found in *I. guayusa* leaves [36]. Other research showed that the major constituents of phenolics were hydroxycinnamic acid, and chlorogenic acid was the main phenolic compound found in both young and old leaves of Guayusa [24].

Overall, caffeoylquinic acids and their derivatives are the main phenolic compounds in the genus *Ilex*, which are summarized in Table 2.

Table 2. Main phenolic compounds in the genus *Ilex*.

Tea Name	Species	Main Polyphenols	Reference
Large-leaved Kudingcha	*Ilex kudingcha* C. J. Tseng	Neochlorogenic acid Chlorogenic acid Cryptochlorogenic acid	[30,37]
		Protocatechuic acid Caffeic acid Isochlorogenic acid Rutin	[37]
		Caffeic acid derivatives	[3]
	I. latifolia	Ethyl caffeate 3,4-di-*O*-caffeoylquinic acid methyl ester 3,5-di-*O*-caffeoylquinic acid methyl ester Chlorogenic acid	[5]
Yerba Mate	*Ilex paraguariensis* A. St.-Hil	Hydroxycinnamic acid derivatives Flavonols 3-caffeoylquinic acid 5-caffeoylquinic acid 4-caffeoylquinic acid 3, 5-dicaffeoylquinic acid Rutin	[18]
Yaupon holly	*I. vomitoria*	Rutin	[20,21]
		Chlorogenic acid Neochlorogenic acid Cryptochlorogenic acid	[21]
Guayusa	*I. guayusa*	Chlorogenic acid	[22,24]
		Isochlorogenic acid Neochlorogenic acid	[22]

3.2. Alkaloids

3.2.1. Alkaloids in Large-Leaved Kudingcha

Alkaloids are a class of naturally occurring compounds that mostly contain basic nitrogen atoms, showing a wide range of physiological and pharmacological effects. Methylxanthines, mainly caffeine and theobromine (Figure 2), are the main alkaloids in large-leaved kudingcha. However, alkaloid content is relatively low. It was reported that the content of total methylxanthines was around 7% to 9%, of which caffeine accounted for 3% to 6%, while theobromines made up only 0.1% [1].

3.2.2. Alkaloids in Yerba Mate

Methylxanthines are alkaloids naturally present in Yerba Mate, mainly comprising caffeine and theobromine [18,27,31]. It was reported that near infrared spectroscopy analysis could be applied to predict the total methylxanthine content in Yerba Mate. The total amount of methylxanthine in 25 samples of Yerba Mate ranged from 3.69 to 12.7 mg/g, with concentrations of caffeine and theobromine as 0.001 to 10.1 and 0.02 to 5.03 mg/g, respectively [31]. To quantify theobromine and caffeine in *I. paraguariensis* extracts, quality by design (QbD) models and UHPLC were optimized and applied, and indicated good future potential for application of this methodology [32]. In another study of samples of Yerba Mate methylxanthines were quantified by HPLC–DAD, with caffeine consistently higher in content than theobromine. Overall, Yerba Mate, with the total methylxanthines ranging from 8.2 to 10.2 mg/g, can be regarded as a moderate source of these purine alkaloids [18].

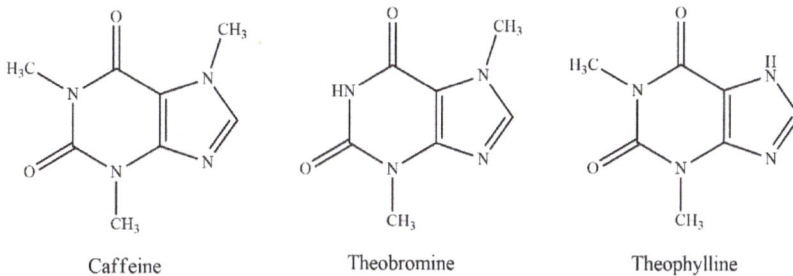

Caffeine Theobromine Theophylline

Figure 2. The chemical structures of main alkaloids in the genus *Ilex*.

3.2.3. Alkaloids in Yaupon Holly

To identify residues of caffeinated beverages, three xanthines theobromine, theophylline, and caffeine (Figure 2) are commonly used as standards. It was found that Yaupon beverages contained all three, but their concentrations were significantly different between wild and domesticated types [34]. Moreover, the caffeine content in dioecious Yaupon Holly was 0% to 1.91% of dry weight, with the level strongly affected by nitrogen fertilizer but not by gender [19,29]. In another study, caffeine was undetectable by HPLC in Yaupon Holly leaves [43].

3.2.4. Alkaloids in Guayusa

The tea of *I. guayusa*, prepared by steeping leaves in boiling water, is consumed by Amazonian families and has a high caffeine content [23]. Kapp et al. found that the extract of Guayusa contained several secondary metabolites, such as caffeine and theobromine, at 36 and 0.3 mg/mL, respectively [36]. Extracts from *I. guayusa* have also been shown to contain caffeine [23].

4. Health Benefits

Some of the physiological effects of caffeinated beverages from *Ilex* are potentially beneficial for human health (Figure 3). Here, we further discuss the actions and related mechanisms of these potential benefits from different *Ilex* species.

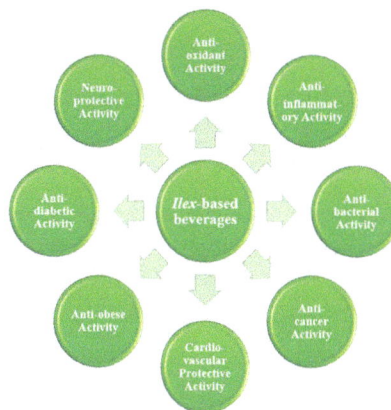

Figure 3. The health benefits of caffeinated beverages from the genus *Ilex*.

4.1. Antioxidant Activity

Consumption of herbal teas prepared from *I. paraguariensis*, *I. vomitoria*, *I. kudingcha*, and *I. guayusa* have been reported to exhibit high reducing power, 2,2-diphenyl-1-picrylhydrazyl (DPPH) scavenging and lipid peroxidation inhibition activities, thus relieving oxidative damage [44]. Based on the in vitro ferric-reducing antioxidant power (FRAP) assay, one extracted alkaloid constituent from *I. latifolia* had high reducing power [5]. Our previous study also found that the methanol extracts of six Kudingcha genotypes of the genus *Ilex* had relatively high in vitro antioxidant activity based on different antioxidant assays [25]. *I. guayusa* tea aqueous extracts (1 g/mL) prepared by conventional means protected 70% to 80% Caco-2 cells from oxidative damage [23], and prevented lipid peroxidation and DNA oxidative damage induced by ultraviolet radiation [45]. Similar antioxidant ability was also found in vivo and in human studies. Pereira et al. found that giving a gavage of Mate tea (20 mg/kg BW/day) to female Wistar rats minimized oxidative stress induced by hormonal changes during perimenopause [46]. Moreover, the impaired endogenous antioxidant defense system in the host could also be recovered by these widely consumed non-alcoholic beverages. As reported, the long-term ingestion of Mate tea (1 L/day) contributed to the increase in ferric-reducing antioxidant potential in dyslipidemic subjects [44], as well as the increased glutathione (GSH) concentration and decreased serum lipid hydroperoxides (LOOH) levels in type 2 diabetic mellitus (T2DM) subjects [47]. In addition, the acute consumption of freeze concentrated Yerba Mate infusion (100 mL) also enhanced the activities of antioxidant enzymes in healthy individuals, including catalase (CAT, 28.7%), superoxide dismutase (SOD, 21.3%), and glutathione peroxidase (GPx, 9.6%) in blood samples [48].

It is widely accepted that the counteraction on oxidative stress is mainly attributable to the existing phenolic compounds, especially chlorogenic acids (like mono- and dicaffeoylquinic acids) as well as flavonols [49,50], since in vitro antioxidant capacity has been confirmed to be positively correlated with their concentrations [13,51]. In order to better retain the contents and stability of health-beneficial antioxidants in *Ilex* teas, more attention should be paid to the adjustment of industrial processing methods and the improvement of packaging methods [22,52].

4.2. Anti-Inflammatory Activity

The inflammatory response is usually accompanied by the activation of macrophages, neutrophils, and various released inflammatory cytokines, such as tumor necrosis factor-α (TNF-α), interleukin (IL)-1β, -6, and -12, triggering histological damage to specific tissues. Reduction of the exudate concentration, reestablishment of the balance between pro- and anti-inflammatory cytokines (IL-4 and -10), and suppression of the pro-inflammatory enzyme activity are considered to be major therapeutic targets in inflammation treatment.

High anti-inflammatory effects were observed in RAW 264.7 cells treated with *I. latifolia* ethanol extract (50 µg/mL), coupled with reduced nitric oxide (NO) production, which could dilate small blood vessels and increase the infiltration of pro-inflammatory mediators [5,10]. Similarly, a 10% to 30% NO inhibition rate was also reported in *I. guayusa* aqueous extracts (1 g/mL) treatment [23]. In addition, several animal experiments also reported the anti-inflammatory effects of these tea-like beverages. For instance, *I. kudingcha* C. J. Tseng methanol extracts (KME) administration upregulated the mRNA expression of inducible nitric oxide synthase (iNOS) and reduced the formation of pro-inflammatory factors like TNF-α, IL-1β, and IL-6 in dextran sulfate sodium (DSS)-induced ulcerative colitis (UC) mice [53]. Besides, *I. paraguariensis* has been reported to show anti-inflammatory effects in various animal models, such as pleurisy in mice [54], cigarette smoke-induced acute lung inflammation in mice [55], obesity-related inflammation in rats [56,57], azoxymethane-induced inflammation in a rat colon [58], and acute edema in a mouse model [59] at concentrations ranging from 150 mg/kg to 250 mg/kg. The anti-inflammatory mechanism of Yerba Mate was reported to inhibit the NF-κB signaling pathway through restraining the phosphorylation of upstream IκB-α and GSK-3β, leading to blocking downstream iNOS and cyclooxygenase-2 (COX-2) expression, and the secretion of inflammatory cytokines [56,58]. However, the anti-inflammatory effects observed in several animal models have not been reported in human studies. Preliminary evidence has shown that Yerba Mate consumption (3 g Yerba Mate diluted in 200 mL water once a day for sixty days) did not alter the inflammatory parameters like high-sensitivity C-reactive protein (hs-CRP), fibrinogen, and HDL-C levels in 92 HIV/AIDS-positive individuals. The discrepancy between basic research and clinical cases could be due to the amount of beverage offered, the concentration of bioactive compounds in Mate tea, and the metabolic conditions of specific populations [60].

4.3. Antibacterial Activity

Compared to tea from *Camellia sinensis*, research on the antibacterial properties of Yerba Mate is relatively limited [27]. The antibacterial effects of Yerba Mate have been reported for *Escherichia (E.) coli, Salmonella typhimurium, Listeria monocytogenes, Staphylococcus (S.) aureus*, and even methicillin-resistant *S. aureus* (MRSA), with the antibacterial concentration ranging from 40 µg/mL to 7.4 mg/mL, and the inhibitory effects seemingly better on gram-positive bacteria than gram-negative bacteria [61]. Commonly, higher concentrations are required when applied to food systems due to the interaction of antibacterial substances with food components like proteins and lipids. Burris et al. found that the concentration of lyophilized aqueous extract of Yerba Mate in apple juice (40 mg/mL) was eight-fold higher than that in a medium (5 mg/mL) for equivalent bacterial inactivation [62]. A similar conclusion was also reached for ground beef, where the anti-MRSA concentration of Mate tea increased dose-dependently with increase of fat content [63].

Although the composition of Yerba Mate extract is relatively clear, conflicting results are shown with regards to the identification of bioactive compounds responsible for antimicrobial activity. Apart from the generally believed phenolic compounds [64], 3,4-dihydroxybenzaldehyde could significantly inhibit MRSA growth even at the lowest concentration of 100 µg/mL [65]. Besides, macromolecules like protein, occupying about 26% of Yerba Mate, might be responsible for the antibacterial activity since dialyzed aqueous extracts have also shown inhibitory effects on *E. coli* and *S. aureus* [62]. The antibacterial mechanism has been much less investigated, and it was pointed out that the tea extract of *I. paraguariensis* had a destructive effect on the central carbon metabolism and energy production pathways, as well as cell membrane integrity [66]. Overall, it is still unclear whether the ingredients that have important antibacterial properties are completely identified and whether they have synergistic or additive antibacterial effects.

4.4. Lipid-Reducing Activity

Several in vitro, in vivo, and human studies have reported the lipid-lowering benefits of the extract of *I. paraguariensis*. The inhibited accumulation of triglycerides in HepG2 cells and attenuated blood lipid levels were demonstrated in *I. latifolia* aqueous extracts [7,67]. Besides, N-butanolic fraction (n-BFIP), a standardized fraction rich in phenolic compounds derived from Yerba Mate was also shown to reduce triglycerides (TG) and low-density lipoprotein cholesterol (LDL-C) in high-fat-diet induced (HFD) rats by 30% and 26%, respectively [68]. This was consistent with the conclusion that polyphenols and methylxanthines in Yerba Mate showed higher lipid-reducing activity than saponins [69]. In addition, the lipid-reducing effect of Yerba Mate extract was proven to be effective not only in animal models, such as hyperlipidemic hamster model [70], rats [68], and rabbits [69], but also in humans. Dyslipidemic and normolipidemic subjects supplemented with 50 g (330 mL infusion and 3 times/day) Yerba Mate had about 10% reduction in lipid parameters (LDL-C and TG) [71,72]. In addition, it was reported that heavy drinkers of *I. paraguariensis* beverage (>1 L/day) had lower total cholesterol, LDL-C, and fasting glucose, but interestingly, their body weight was higher, compared with moderate drinkers [73]. This low-lipids high-body-weight paradox observed in the population of heavy drinkers of *I. paraguariensis* beverages could be due to the induced hypoglycemia and compensatory higher intake of refined carbohydrates, since their consumption of carbohydrates was higher than moderate drinkers [73].

For the lipid-reducing molecular mechanism, triterpenoid saponins (200 mg/kg/day) derived from *I. latifolia* was reported to lower lipids by the inhibition of sterol regulatory element-binding proteins (SREBPs) via enhancing AMP-activated protein kinase (AMPK) phosphorylation in a non-alcoholic fatty liver disease mouse model [74,75]. In addition, Yerba Mate aqueous extract was reported to improve plasma lipid profile both in vitro (3T3-L1 cells model) and in vivo (mice model), probably by inhibiting adipogenesis via downregulating the expression of adipogenesis related genes (Creb-1 and C/EBPα) [76].

4.5. Regulation of Gut Microbiota

More recently, growing attention has been paid to the effect of tea beverages on gut microbiota. Enhanced probiotic colonization was observed in a broiler chicken model fed with ground Yerba Mate leaf supplement (0.55% inclusion rate) [77]. Moreover, *Ilex kudingcha* extract (400 mg/kg) was demonstrated to change the diet-disrupted gut microbiota composition to normal state and increase their diversity in HFD-fed mice [78]. It was reported that polyphenols from *I. latifolia* played a critical role in establishing the structure of gut microbiota, since dietary polyphenols, especially dicaffeoylquinic acids (diCQAs), exhibited low bioavailability in the upper digestive tract, and reached the colon with an intact form and interacted with the colonic microbiota, contributing to the amelioration of the intestinal flora [79]. In addition, Xie et al. reported that diCQAs from Kudingcha enhanced the diversity of intestinal microbiota in vitro and promoted the generation of short-chain fatty acids (SCFAs) through gut microbiota, which in turn provided nutrients and energy for the optimization of gut microbial profile [9]. Therefore, the interaction between tea consumption and intestinal microbes can further improve the microbial colonization and promote human health.

4.6. Anti-Cancer Activity

Although epidemiological studies have reported a correlation between Mate tea consumption and esophageal cancer, it is most likely due to confounding factors, such as high consumption temperature rather than the carcinogenic constituents present [80,81], since any beverages with temperature above 65 °C are "likely carcinogenic to humans" [82]. In fact, the cytotoxic action against diverse cancer cells, such as breast cancer, oral cancer, nasopharyngeal carcinoma, and colon adenocarcinoma cells, was reported in Yaupon Holly leaves [20], Kudingcha extracts [5], and Yerba Mate extracts [83,84], which were tested with concentrations ranging from 10 µg/mL to 1000 µg/mL, and could not only inhibit the viability and proliferation of cancer cells, but also prevent metastasis and promote apoptosis of cancer cells. The presence of characteristic ingredients, mainly chlorogenic acid derivatives, may be responsible for the anti-cancer effects of *Ilex* Kudingcha [39].

Several studies also elucidated the anti-cancer molecular mechanisms. It was reported that caffeoylquinic acids in *Ilex* tea extracts were able to activate the pro-apoptotic factors caspase-3 and caspase-9 in TCA8113 cancer cells, and caspase-8 and caspase-3 in HT-29 human colon cancer cells, accompanied with the decreased expression of the inflammatory mediator NF-κB, which regulates cell proliferation, anti-apoptosis, and cell metastasis [6,85]. Overall, induction of cancer cell apoptosis and suppression of chronic inflammation could be two main mechanisms of the anti-cancer activity of *Ilex* tea.

4.7. Cardiovascular Protective Activity

Research on cardiovascular protection is limited, and only reported for *I. paraguariensis* and *I. kudingcha*. Kudingcha extract showed ameliorative effects on blood vessel contractility and blood flow in both rats and rabbits [3]. Kudingcha polysaccharides were also reported to have a protective effect against vascular dysfunction in high fructose-fed mice [86]. Yerba Mate consumption had great potential for reducing intermediate factors for cardiovascular diseases in both animal and human interventional studies [87]. In addition, improved blood viscosity and microcirculation were observed in 142 subjects supplemented with Yerba Mate tea (5 g/day) [88]. Moreover, reduced cardiovascular diseases were observed in 95 postmenopausal women consuming more than 1 L/day of mate infusion [89]. Thus, *Ilex* tea has great potential to be used as a preventive or therapeutic ingredient against cardiovascular diseases.

4.8. Anti-Obesity Activity

In recent years, reports have shown that caffeinated beverages from the genus *Ilex*, including Yerba Mate and Kudingcha, can reduce body weight and have great potential to be developed into anti-obesity drugs [78]. *I. latifolia* (0.33% aqueous extract was added to the HFD) showed protective effects against HFD-induced body weight gain in mice, accompanied by decreased adipocyte lipid accumulation and suppressed expression of lipogenic genes in the liver [90]. Furthermore, adipocyte size, adipocyte differentiation, and fat accumulation were also suppressed in obese rats after treatment with *I. paraguariensis* aqueous solution [91–94]. In addition to direct impact on adipogenesis, the anti-obesity effects of Mate extract were correlated with decreased appetite [95]. Hussein et al. found that chronic administration of Yerba Mate (50 mg/kg) induced elevated levels of the satiety markers glucagon-like peptide 1 (GLP-1) and leptin in high-fat diet-fed mice, leading to appetite-suppression and reduced food intake, thus decreasing body weight (BW) and body mass index [96].

Besides, the anti-obesity activity of Yerba Mate beverages has been validated in clinical trials. A randomized double-blind trial conducted by Kim et al. showed that body fat mass was significantly reduced in obese subjects supplemented with oral Yerba Mate capsules (3 g/day) for twelve weeks [97]. In addition, acute intake of Yerba Mate was confirmed to augment energy expenditure in healthy people [98], and it was interesting that a higher increase in energy expenditure could be induced by ingesting Yerba Mate at cold temperatures (e.g., 3 °C) rather than hot temperatures (e.g., 55 °C), without exerting negative impacts on the cardiovascular system [99]. Thus Yerba Mate appears to have great potential to be developed into an anti-obesity functional food.

4.9. Anti-Diabetic Activity

Increasing in vitro and in vivo studies support *I. latifolia* as an effective way to control postprandial hyperglycemia. Kudingcha aqueous extracts (6 mg/mL) could decrease 36% and 50% of the Na^+-dependent and Na^+-independent glucose absorption by Caco-2 cells in vitro, respectively [100]. In addition, blood glucose levels in the epinephrine hyperglycemia rat models also returned to normal levels under treatment with 5 or 10 g/kg Kudingcha extracts [3]. This result was in agreement with another in vivo study that oral administration of Yerba Mate (100 mg/kg) aqueous extract for seven weeks decreased blood glucose levels and improved insulin sensitivity in Tsumura Suzuki obese diabetic (TSOD) mice, thus reducing the risk of hyperglycemia [97]. The caffeoylquinic acid (CQA) derivatives derived from *I. latifolia* were further confirmed to play an important role in producing these effects, by means of binding to α-glucosidase via stable hydrogen bonding and hydrophobic interaction, thus reducing blood sugar levels [8]. In addition, clinical trials demonstrated the possibility of *I. paraguariensis* beverages for the prevention of diabetes complication, since long-term *I. paraguariensis* consumption (1 L/day, sixty days) improved glycemic profile and pre-diabetes related conditions (oxidative stress and dyslipidemia) in T2DM and pre-diabetic individuals [47]. Therefore, the consumption of herbal teas prepared from *Ilex* species is likely to be beneficial for the treatment of diabetes.

4.10. Neuroprotective Activity

The caffeinated beverages from the genus *Ilex* also show neuroprotective activity [101]. For instance, the exposure of cortical neurons to *I. latifolia* (1–100 μg/mL) was reported to inhibit neuronal death induced by glutamate, hypoxia, and amyloid β protein (Aβ) through suppressing the pathway of apoptosis [102,103]. Additionally, in vivo experiments also demonstrated that *I. latifolia* supplement (25 to 200 mg/kg) significantly inhibited Aβ (25–35)-induced memory impairment in mice and ischemia-induced neurological deficits in rats in a dose-dependent manner [103,104]. Clinical results further revealed its potential to inhibit the development of Parkinson's disease [105].

4.11. Other Health Benefits

In addition to the health benefits mentioned above, Yerba Mate was also reported to improve bone mineral density in postmenopausal women and accelerated the healing of the alveolar socket in rats after tooth extraction [106,107]

5. Conclusions

In conclusion, this review summarized the distribution and chemical composition of the caffeinated beverages from the genus *Ilex*, including the large-leaved Kudingcha, Yerba Mate, Yaupon Holly, and Guayusa, along with their potential health benefits, including antioxidant, anti-inflammatory, antibacterial, lipid-reducing, regulation of gut microbiota, anti-cancer, cardiovascular protective, anti-obesity, anti-diabetic, neuroprotection, etc. However, the genus *Ilex* contains about 600 species, most of which still lack detailed investigation. In the future, intensive bioprospecting of the whole range of genetic resources is sure to reveal interesting and useful new compounds and new sources of high levels of known compounds. In addition, further research should aim at designing controlled clinical trials to investigate the effects of long-term consumption of well-characterized *Ilex*-based beverages on human health.

Author Contributions: Conceptualization, R.-Y.G. and H.C.; writing—original draft preparation, D.Z. and M.W.; writing—review and editing, R.-Y.G. and H.C.; supervision, H.C.; funding acquisition, R.-Y.G. and H.C.

Funding: This study was supported by the National Key R&D Program of China (2017YFC1600100), the Shanghai Pujiang Talent Plan (No. 18PJ1404600), the Shanghai Basic and Key Program (No. 18JC1410800), and the Shanghai Agricultural Science and Technology Key Program (18391900600).

Conflicts of Interest: The authors declare no conflict of interest.

References

1. Mohanpuria, P.; Kumar, V.; Yadav, S.K. Tea caffeine: Metabolism, functions, and reduction strategies. *Food Sci. Biotechnol.* **2010**, *19*, 275–287. [CrossRef]
2. Zhang, C.; Suen, C.L.C.; Yang, C.; Quek, S.Y. Antioxidant capacity and major polyphenol composition of teas as affected by geographical location, plantation elevation and leaf grade. *Food Chem.* **2018**, *244*, 109–119. [CrossRef] [PubMed]
3. Li, L.; Xu, L.J.; Ma, G.Z.; Dong, Y.M.; Peng, Y.; Xiao, P.G. The large-leaved kudingcha (*Ilex latifolia* thunb and *Ilex kudingcha* C.J. Tseng): A traditional Chinese tea with plentiful secondary metabolites and potential biological activities. *J. Nat. Med.* **2013**, *67*, 425–437. [CrossRef] [PubMed]
4. Fan, J.L.; Wu, Z.W.; Zhao, T.H.; Sun, Y.; Ye, H.; Xu, R.J.; Zeng, X.X. Characterization, antioxidant and hepatoprotective activities of polysaccharides from *Ilex latifolia* Thunb. *Carbohyd. Polym.* **2014**, *101*, 990–997. [CrossRef] [PubMed]
5. Hu, T.; He, X.W.; Jiang, J.G. Functional analyses on antioxidant, anti-inflammatory, and antiproliferative effects of extracts and compounds from *Ilex latifolia* thunb., a Chinese bitter tea. *J. Agric. Food Chem.* **2014**, *62*, 8608–8615. [CrossRef] [PubMed]
6. Zhu, K.; Li, G.; Sun, P.; Wang, R.; Qian, Y.; Zhao, X. In vitro and in vivo anti-cancer activities of kuding tea (*Ilex kudingcha* C.J. Tseng) against oral cancer. *Exp. Ther. Med.* **2014**, *7*, 709–715. [CrossRef] [PubMed]
7. Wang, C.Q.; Li, M.M.; Zhang, W.; Wang, L.; Fan, C.L.; Feng, R.B.; Zhang, X.Q.; Ye, W.C. Four new triterpenes and triterpene glycosides from the leaves of *Ilex latifolia* and their inhibitory activity on triglyceride accumulation. *Fitoterapia* **2015**, *106*, 141–146. [CrossRef] [PubMed]
8. Xu, D.; Wang, Q.; Zhang, W.; Hu, B.; Zhou, L.; Zeng, X.; Sun, Y. Inhibitory activities of caffeoylquinic acid derivatives from *Ilex kudingcha* C.J. Tseng on α-glucosidase from *Saccharomyces cerevisiae*. *J. Agric. Food Chem.* **2015**, *63*, 3694–3703. [CrossRef] [PubMed]

9. Xie, M.; Chen, G.; Wan, P.; Dai, Z.; Hu, B.; Chen, L.; Ou, S.; Zeng, X.; Sun, Y. Modulating effects of dicaffeoylquinic acids from *Ilex kudingcha* on intestinal microecology in vitro. *J. Agric. Food Chem.* **2017**, *65*, 10185–10196. [CrossRef] [PubMed]

10. Zhang, T.-T.; Hu, T.; Jiang, J.-G.; Zhao, J.-W.; Zhu, W. Antioxidant and anti-inflammatory effects of polyphenols extracted from *Ilex latifolia* thunb. *RSC Adv.* **2018**, *8*, 7134–7141. [CrossRef]

11. Burris, K.P.; Davidson, P.M.; Stewart, C.N., Jr.; Zivanovic, S.; Harte, F.M. Aqueous extracts of yerba mate (*Ilex paraguariensis*) as a natural antimicrobial against *Escherichia coli* O157:H7 in a microbiological medium and pH 6.0 apple juice. *J. Food Prot.* **2012**, *75*, 753–757. [CrossRef] [PubMed]

12. Bassani, D.C.; Nunes, D.S.; Granato, D. Optimization of phenolics and flavonoids extraction conditions and antioxidant activity of roasted yerba-mate leaves (*Ilex paraguariensis* a. St.-Hil., aquifoliaceae) using response surface methodology. *An. Acad. Bras. Cienc.* **2014**, *86*, 923–933. [CrossRef]

13. Molin, R.F.; Dartora, N.; Borges, A.C.P.; Gonçalves, I.L.; Di Luccio, M.; Valduga, A.T. Total phenolic contents and antioxidant activity in oxidized leaves of mate (*Ilex paraguariensis* St. Hil). *Braz. Arch. Biol. Technol.* **2014**, *57*, 997–1003. [CrossRef]

14. Boado, L.S.; Fretes, R.M.; Brumovsky, L.A. Bioavailability and antioxidant effect of the *Ilex paraguariensis* polyphenols. *Nutr. Food Sci.* **2015**, *45*, 326–335. [CrossRef]

15. Souza, A.H.P.; Correa, R.C.G.; Barros, L.; Calhelha, R.C.; Santos-Buelga, C.; Peralta, R.M.; Bracht, A.; Matsushita, M.; Ferreira, I.C.F.R. Phytochemicals and bioactive properties of *Ilex paraguariensis*: An *in-vitro* comparative study between the whole plant, leaves and stems. *Food Res. Int.* **2015**, *78*, 286–294. [CrossRef] [PubMed]

16. Colpo, A.C.; de Lima, M.E.; Maya-Lopez, M.; Rosa, H.; Marquez-Curiel, C.; Galvan-Arzate, S.; Santamaria, A.; Folmer, V. Compounds from *Ilex paraguariensis* extracts have antioxidant effects in the brains of rats subjected to chronic immobilization stress. *Appl. Physiol. Nutr. Metab.* **2017**, *42*, 1172–1178. [CrossRef] [PubMed]

17. Konieczynski, P.; Viapiana, A.; Wesolowski, M. Comparison of infusions from black and green teas (*Camellia sinensis* l. Kuntze) and erva-mate (*Ilex paraguariensis* a. St.-Hil.) based on the content of essential elements, secondary metabolites, and antioxidant activity. *Food Anal. Method* **2017**, *10*, 3063–3070. [CrossRef]

18. Mateos, R.; Baeza, G.; Sarria, B.; Bravo, L. Improved LC-MSn characterization of hydroxycinnamic acid derivatives and flavonols in different commercial mate (*Ilex paraguariensis*) brands. Quantification of polyphenols, methylxanthines, and antioxidant activity. *Food Chem.* **2018**, *241*, 232–241. [CrossRef] [PubMed]

19. Palumbo, M.J.; Talcott, S.T.; Putz, F.E. *Ilex vomitoria* ait. (yaupon): A native north American source of a caffeinated and antioxidant-rich tea. *Econ. Bot.* **2009**, *63*, 130–137. [CrossRef]

20. Noratto, G.D.; Kim, Y.; Talcott, S.T.; Mertens-Talcott, S.U. Flavonol-rich fractions of yaupon holly leaves (*Ilex vomitoria*, aquifoliaceae) induce microRNA-146a and have anti-inflammatory and chemopreventive effects in intestinal myofribroblast CCD-18Co cells. *Fitoterapia* **2011**, *82*, 557–569. [CrossRef] [PubMed]

21. Kim, Y.; Talcott, S.T. Tea creaming in nonfermented teas from *Camellia sinensis* and *Ilex vomitoria*. *J. Agric. Food Chem.* **2012**, *60*, 11793–11799. [CrossRef] [PubMed]

22. Garcia-Ruiz, A.; Baenas, N.; Benitez-Gonzalez, A.M.; Stinco, C.M.; Melendez-Martinez, A.J.; Moreno, D.A.; Ruales, J. Guayusa (*Ilex guayusa* L.) new tea: Phenolic and carotenoid composition and antioxidant capacity. *J. Sci. Food Agric.* **2017**, *97*, 3929–3936. [CrossRef] [PubMed]

23. Pardau, M.D.; Pereira, A.S.P.; Apostolides, Z.; Serem, J.C.; Bester, M.J. Antioxidant and anti-inflammatory properties of *Ilex guayusa* tea preparations: A comparison to *Camellia sinensis* teas. *Food Funct.* **2017**, *8*, 4601–4610. [CrossRef] [PubMed]

24. Villacis-Chiriboga, J.; Garcia-Ruiz, A.; Baenas, N.; Moreno, D.A.; Melendez-Martinez, A.J.; Stinco, C.M.; Jerves-Andrade, L.; Leon-Tamariz, F.; Ortiz-Ulloa, J.; Ruales, J. Changes in phytochemical composition, bioactivity and in vitro digestibility of guayusa leaves (*Ilex guayusa* loes.) in different ripening stages. *J. Sci. Food Agric.* **2018**, *98*, 1927–1934. [CrossRef] [PubMed]

25. Zhu, F.; Cai, Y.Z.; Sun, M.; Ke, J.X.; Lu, D.Y.; Corke, H. Comparison of major phenolic constituents and in vitro antioxidant activity of diverse kudingcha genotypes from *Ilex kudingcha*, *Ilex cornuta*, and *Ligustrum robustum*. *J. Agric. Food Chem.* **2009**, *57*, 6082–6089. [CrossRef] [PubMed]

26. Heck, C.I.; De Mejia, E.G. Yerba mate tea (*Ilex paraguariensis*): A comprehensive review on chemistry, health implications, and technological considerations. *J. Food Sci.* **2007**, *72*, R138–R151. [CrossRef] [PubMed]

27. Burris, K.P.; Harte, F.M.; Davidson, P.M.; Stewart, C.N.; Zivanovic, S. Composition and bioactive properties of yerba mate (*Ilex paraguariensis* a. St.-Hil.): A review. *Chil. J. Agric. Res.* **2012**, *72*, 268–274. [CrossRef]

28. Marcelo, M.C.A.; Martins, C.A.; Pozebon, D.; Dressler, V.L.; Ferrao, M.F. Classification of yerba mate (*Ilex paraguariensis*) according to the country of origin based on element concentrations. *Microchem. J.* **2014**, *117*, 164–171. [CrossRef]

29. Palumbo, M.J.; Putz, F.E.; Talcott, S.T. Nitrogen fertilizer and gender effects on the secondary metabolism of yaupon, a caffeine-containing north American holly. *Oecologia* **2007**, *151*, 1–9. [CrossRef] [PubMed]

30. Yi, H.; Zhou, J.; Shang, X.Y.; Zhao, Z.X.; Peng, Q.; Zhu, M.J.; Zhu, C.C.; Lin, C.Z.; Liu, Q.D.; Liao, Q.F.; et al. Multi-component analysis of *Ilex kudingcha* C. J. Tseng by a single marker quantification method and chemometric discrimination of HPLC fingerprints. *Molecules* **2018**, *23*, 854. [CrossRef] [PubMed]

31. Mazur, L.; Peralta-Zamora, P.G.; Demczuk, B.; Ribani, R.H. Application of multivariate calibration and NIR spectroscopy for the quantification of methylxanthines in yerba mate (*Ilex paraguariensis*). *J. Food Compos. Anal.* **2014**, *35*, 55–60. [CrossRef]

32. Pinto, R.M.C.; Lemes, B.M.; Zielinski, A.A.F.; Klein, T.; de Paula, F.; Kist, A.; Marques, A.S.F.; Nogueira, A.; Demiate, I.M.; Beltrame, F.L. Detection and quantification of phytochemical markers of *Ilex paraguariensis* by liquid chromatography. *Quim. Nova* **2015**, *38*, 1219–1225. [CrossRef]

33. Mateos, R.; Baeza, G.; Martinez-Lopez, S.; Sarria, B.; Bravo, L. LC-MSn characterization of saponins in mate (*Ilex paraguariens*, St. Hil) and their quantification by HPLC-DAD. *J. Food Compos. Anal.* **2017**, *63*, 164–170. [CrossRef]

34. King, A.; Powis, T.G.; Cheong, K.F.; Gaikwad, N.W. Cautionary tales on the identification of caffeinated beverages in north America. *J. Archaeol. Sci.* **2017**, *85*, 30–40. [CrossRef]

35. Duenas, J.F.; Jarrett, C.; Cummins, I.; Logan-Hines, E. Amazonian guayusa (*Ilex guayusa* Loes.): A historical and ethnobotanical overview. *Econ. Bot.* **2016**, *70*, 85–91. [CrossRef]

36. Kapp, R.W.; Mendes, O.; Roy, S.; McQuate, R.S.; Kraska, R. General and genetic toxicology of guayusa concentrate (*Ilex guayusa*). *Int. J. Toxicol.* **2016**, *35*, 222–242. [CrossRef] [PubMed]

37. Zhou, J.; Yi, H.; Zhao, Z.X.; Shang, X.Y.; Zhu, M.J.; Kuang, G.J.; Zhu, C.C.; Zhang, L. Simultaneous qualitative and quantitative evaluation of *Ilex kudingcha* C.J. Tseng by using UPLC and UHPLC-QTOE-MS/MS. *J. Pharm. Biomed.* **2018**, *155*, 15–26. [CrossRef] [PubMed]

38. Hu, T.; He, X.W.; Jiang, J.G.; Xu, X.L. Efficacy evaluation of a Chinese bitter tea (*Ilex latifolia* thunb.) via analyses of its main components. *Food Funct.* **2014**, *5*, 876–881. [CrossRef] [PubMed]

39. Zhong, T.; Piao, L.H.; Kim, H.J.; Liu, X.D.; Jiang, S.N.; Liu, G.M. Chlorogenic acid-enriched extract of *Ilex kudingcha* C.J. Tseng inhibits angiogenesis in zebrafish. *J. Med. Food* **2017**, *20*, 1160–1167. [CrossRef] [PubMed]

40. Che, Y.Y.; Wang, Z.B.; Zhu, Z.Y.; Ma, Y.Y.; Zhang, Y.Q.; Gu, W.; Zhang, J.Y.; Rao, G.X. Simultaneous qualitation and quantitation of chlorogenic acids in kuding tea using ultra-high-performance liquid chromatography-diode array detection coupled with linear ion trap-orbitrap mass spectrometer. *Molecules* **2016**, *21*, 1728. [CrossRef] [PubMed]

41. Zwyrzykowska, A.; Kupczynski, R.; Jarosz, B.; Szumny, A.; Kucharska, A.Z. Qualitative and quantitative analysis of polyphenolic compounds in *Ilex* sp. *Open Chem.* **2015**, *13*, 1303–1312. [CrossRef]

42. da Silveira, T.F.F.; Meinhart, A.D.; Coutinho, J.P.; de Souza, T.C.L.; Cunha, E.C.E.; de Moraes, M.R.; Godoy, H.T. Content of lutein in aqueous extracts of yerba mate (*Ilex paraguariensis* St. Hil). *Food Res. Int.* **2016**, *82*, 165–171. [CrossRef]

43. Kim, Y.; Welt, B.A.; Talcott, S.T. The impact of packaging materials on the antioxidant phytochemical stability of aqueous infusions of green tea (*Camellia sinensis*) and yaupon holly (*Ilex vomitoria*) during cold storage. *J. Agric. Food Chem.* **2011**, *59*, 4676–4683. [CrossRef] [PubMed]

44. Boaventura, B.C.; Di Pietro, P.F.; Stefanuto, A.; Klein, G.A.; de Morais, E.C.; de Andrade, F.; Wazlawik, E.; da Silva, E.L. Association of mate tea (*Ilex paraguariensis*) intake and dietary intervention and effects on oxidative stress biomarkers of dyslipidemic subjects. *Nutrition* **2012**, *28*, 657–664. [CrossRef] [PubMed]

45. Barg, M.; Rezin, G.T.; Leffa, D.D.; Balbinot, F.; Gomes, L.M.; Carvalho-Silva, M.; Vuolo, F.; Petronilho, F.; Dal-Pizzol, F.; Streck, E.L.; et al. Evaluation of the protective effect of *Ilex paraguariensis* and *Camellia sinensis* extracts on the prevention of oxidative damage caused by ultraviolet radiation. *Environ. Toxicol. Pharmacol.* **2014**, *37*, 195–201. [CrossRef] [PubMed]

46. Pereira, A.A.F.; Tirapeli, K.G.; Chaves-Neto, A.H.; da Silva Brasilino, M.; da Rocha, C.Q.; Bello-Klein, A.; Llesuy, S.F.; Dornelles, R.C.M.; Nakamune, A. *Ilex paraguariensis* supplementation may be an effective nutritional approach to modulate oxidative stress during perimenopause. *Exp. Gerontol.* **2017**, *90*, 14–18. [CrossRef] [PubMed]

47. Boaventura, B.C.B.; Di Pietro, P.F.; Klein, G.A.; Stefanuto, A.; de Morais, E.C.; de Andrade, F.; Wazlawik, E.; da Silva, E.L. Antioxidant potential of mate tea (*Ilex paraguariensis*) in type 2 diabetic mellitus and pre-diabetic individuals. *J. Funct. Foods* **2013**, *5*, 1057–1064. [CrossRef]

48. Bremer Boaventura, B.C.; da Silva, E.L.; Liu, R.H.; Prudêncio, E.S.; Di Pietro, P.F.; Becker, A.M.; Amboni, R.D.d.M.C. Effect of yerba mate (*Ilex paraguariensis* a. St. Hil.) infusion obtained by freeze concentration technology on antioxidant status of healthy individuals. *LWT Food Sci. Technol.* **2015**, *62*, 948–954. [CrossRef]

49. Baeza, G.; Sarria, B.; Mateos, R.; Bravo, L. Dihydrocaffeic acid, a major microbial metabolite of chlorogenic acids, shows similar protective effect than a yerba mate phenolic extract against oxidative stress in HepG2 cells. *Food Res. Int.* **2016**, *87*, 25–33. [CrossRef] [PubMed]

50. Zhao, X.; Song, J.L.; Yi, R.; Li, G.; Sun, P.; Park, K.Y.; Suo, H. Comparison of antioxidative effects of insect tea and its raw tea (kuding tea) polyphenols in Kunming mice. *Molecules* **2018**, *23*, 204. [CrossRef] [PubMed]

51. de Oliveira, C.C.; Calado, V.M.; Ares, G.; Granato, D. Statistical approaches to assess the association between phenolic compounds and the in vitro antioxidant activity of *Camellia sinensis* and *Ilex paraguariensis* teas. *Crit. Rev. Food Sci. Nutr.* **2015**, *55*, 1456–1473. [CrossRef] [PubMed]

52. Yonny, M.E.; Medina, A.V.; Nazareno, M.A.; Chaillou, L.L. Enhancement in the oxidative stability of green peas by *Ilex paraguariensis* addition in a blanching process before their refrigerated and frozen storage. *LWT* **2018**, *91*, 315–321. [CrossRef]

53. Song, J.L.; Qian, Y.; Li, G.J.; Zhao, X. Anti-inflammatory effects of kudingcha methanol extract (*Ilex kudingcha* c.J. Tseng) in dextran sulfate sodium-induced ulcerative colitis. *Mol. Med. Rep.* **2013**, *8*, 1256–1262. [CrossRef] [PubMed]

54. Luz, A.B.G.; da Silva, C.H.B.; Nascimento, M.; de Campos Facchin, B.M.; Baratto, B.; Frode, T.S.; Reginatto, F.H.; Dalmarco, E.M. The anti-inflammatory effect of *Ilex paraguariensis* a. St. Hil (mate) in a murine model of pleurisy. *Int. Immunopharmacol.* **2016**, *36*, 165–172. [CrossRef] [PubMed]

55. Lanzetti, M.; Bezerra, F.S.; Romana-Souza, B.; Brando-Lima, A.C.; Koatz, V.L.; Porto, L.C.; Valenca, S.S. Mate tea reduced acute lung inflammation in mice exposed to cigarette smoke. *Nutrition* **2008**, *24*, 375–381. [CrossRef] [PubMed]

56. Pimentel, G.D.; Lira, F.S.; Rosa, J.C.; Caris, A.V.; Pinheiro, F.; Ribeiro, E.B.; Oller do Nascimento, C.M.; Oyama, L.M. Yerba mate extract (*Ilex paraguariensis*) attenuates both central and peripheral inflammatory effects of diet-induced obesity in rats. *J. Nutr. Biochem.* **2013**, *24*, 809–818. [CrossRef] [PubMed]

57. Munoz-Culla, M.; Saenz-Cuesta, M.; Guereca-Barandiaran, M.J.; Ribeiro, M.L.; Otaegui, D. Yerba mate (*Ilex paraguariensis*) inhibits lymphocyte activation in vitro. *Food Funct.* **2016**, *7*, 4556–4563. [CrossRef] [PubMed]

58. Puangpraphant, S.; Dia, V.P.; de Mejia, E.G.; Garcia, G.; Berhow, M.A.; Wallig, M.A. Yerba mate tea and mate saponins prevented azoxymethane-induced inflammation of rat colon through suppression of NF-κB p65ser(311) signaling via IκB-α and GSK-3β reduced phosphorylation. *Biofactors* **2013**, *39*, 430–440. [CrossRef] [PubMed]

59. Schinella, G.; Neyret, E.; Console, G.; Tournier, H.; Prieto, J.M.; Rios, J.L.; Giner, R.M. An aqueous extract of *Ilex paraguariensis* reduces carrageenan-induced edema and inhibits the expression of cyclooxygenase-2 and inducible nitric oxide synthase in animal models of inflammation. *Planta Med.* **2014**, *80*, 961–968. [CrossRef] [PubMed]

60. Petrilli, A.A.; Souza, S.J.; Teixeira, A.M.; Pontilho, P.M.; Souza, J.M.P.; Luzia, L.A.; Rondo, P.H.C. Effect of Chocolate and Yerba Mate Phenolic Compounds on Inflammatory and Oxidative Biomarkers in HIV/AIDS Individuals. *Nutrients* **2016**, *8*, 132. [CrossRef] [PubMed]

61. Prado Martin, J.G.; Porto, E.; de Alencar, S.M.; da Glória, E.M.; Corrêa, C.B.; Ribeiro Cabral, I.S. Antimicrobial activity of yerba mate (*Ilex paraguariensis* St. Hil.) against food pathogens. *Rev. Argent. Microbiol.* **2013**, *45*, 93–98. [CrossRef]

62. Burris, K.P.; Davidson, P.M.; Stewart, C.N., Jr.; Harte, F.M. Antimicrobial activity of yerba mate (*Ilex paraguariensis*) aqueous extracts against *Escherichia coli* O157:H7 and *Staphylococcus aureus*. *J. Food Sci.* **2011**, *76*, M456–M462. [CrossRef] [PubMed]

63. Burris, K.P.; Higginbotham, K.L.; Stewart, C.N. Aqueous extracts of yerba mate as bactericidal agents against methicillin-resistant *Staphylococcus aureus* in a microbiological medium and ground beef mixtures. *Food Control.* **2015**, *50*, 748–753. [CrossRef]

64. Correa, V.G.; Goncalves, G.A.; de Sa-Nakanishi, A.B.; Ferreira, I.; Barros, L.; Dias, M.I.; Koehnlein, E.A.; de Souza, C.G.M.; Bracht, A.; Peralta, R.M. Effects of in vitro digestion and in vitro colonic fermentation on stability and functional properties of yerba mate (*Ilex paraguariensis* a. St. Hil.) beverages. *Food Chem.* **2017**, *237*, 453–460. [CrossRef] [PubMed]

65. Rempe, C.S.; Burris, K.P.; Woo, H.L.; Goodrich, B.; Gosnell, D.K.; Tschaplinski, T.J.; Stewart, C.N., Jr. Computational ranking of yerba mate small molecules based on their predicted contribution to antibacterial activity against methicillin-resistant *Staphylococcus aureus*. *PLoS ONE* **2015**, *10*, e0123925. [CrossRef] [PubMed]

66. Rempe, C.S.; Lenaghan, S.C.; Burris, K.P.; Stewart, C.N. Metabolomic analysis of the mechanism of action of yerba mate aqueous extract on *Salmonella enterica* serovar Typhimurium. *Metabolomics* **2017**, *13*. [CrossRef]

67. Song, C.; Yu, Q.; Li, X.; Jin, S.; Li, S.; Zhang, Y.; Jia, S.; Chen, C.; Xiang, Y.; Jiang, H. The hypolipidemic effect of total saponins from kuding tea in high-fat diet-induced hyperlipidemic mice and its composition characterized by UPLC-QTOF-MS/MS. *J. Food Sci.* **2016**, *81*, H1313–H1319. [CrossRef] [PubMed]

68. Balzan, S.; Hernandes, A.; Reichert, C.L.; Donaduzzi, C.; Pires, V.A.; Gasparotto, A., Jr.; Cardozo, E.L., Jr. Lipid-lowering effects of standardized extracts of *Ilex paraguariensis* in high-fat-diet rats. *Fitoterapia* **2013**, *86*, 115–122. [CrossRef] [PubMed]

69. de Resende, P.E.; Kaiser, S.; Pittol, V.; Hoefel, A.L.; D'Agostini Silva, R.; Vieira Marques, C.; Kucharski, L.C.; Ortega, G.G. Influence of crude extract and bioactive fractions of *Ilex paraguariensis* a. St. Hil. (yerba mate) on the Wistar rat lipid metabolism. *J. Funct. Foods* **2015**, *15*, 440–451. [CrossRef]

70. Gao, H.; Long, Y.; Jiang, X.; Liu, Z.; Wang, D.; Zhao, Y.; Li, D.; Sun, B.L. Beneficial effects of yerba mate tea (*Ilex paraguariensis*) on hyperlipidemia in high-fat-fed hamsters. *Exp. Gerontol.* **2013**, *48*, 572–578. [CrossRef] [PubMed]

71. de Morais, E.C.; Stefanuto, A.; Klein, G.A.; Boaventura, B.C.; de Andrade, F.; Wazlawik, E.; Di Pietro, P.F.; Maraschin, M.; da Silva, E.L. Consumption of yerba mate (*Ilex paraguariensis*) improves serum lipid parameters in healthy dyslipidemic subjects and provides an additional LDL-cholesterol reduction in individuals on statin therapy. *J. Agric. Food Chem.* **2009**, *57*, 8316–8324. [CrossRef] [PubMed]

72. Messina, D.; Soto, C.; Mendez, A.; Corte, C.; Kemnitz, M.; Avena, V.; Del Balzo, D.; Perez Elizalde, R. Lipid—Lowering effect of mate tea intake in dyslipidemic subjects. *Nutr. Hosp.* **2015**, *31*, 2131–2139. [CrossRef] [PubMed]

73. Chaves, G.; Britez, N.; Oviedo, G.; Gonzalez, G.; Italiano, C.; Blanes, M.; Sandoval, G.; Mereles, D. Heavy drinkers of *Ilex paraguariensis* beverages show lower lipid profiles but higher body weight. *Phytother. Res.* **2018**, *32*, 1030–1038. [CrossRef] [PubMed]

74. Feng, R.B.; Fan, C.L.; Liu, Q.; Liu, Z.; Zhang, W.; Li, Y.L.; Tang, W.; Wang, Y.; Li, M.M.; Ye, W.C. Crude triterpenoid saponins from *Ilex latifolia* (Da Ye Dong Qing) ameliorate lipid accumulation by inhibiting SREBP expression via activation of AMPK in a non-alcoholic fatty liver disease model. *Chin. Med.* **2015**, *10*, 23. [CrossRef] [PubMed]

75. Che, Y.Y.; Wang, Q.H.; Xiao, R.Y.; Zhang, J.Y.; Zhang, Y.Q.; Gu, W.; Rao, G.X.; Wang, C.F.; Kuang, H.X. Kudinoside-d, a triterpenoid saponin derived from *Ilex kudingcha* suppresses adipogenesis through modulation of the AMPK pathway in 3T3-L1 adipocytes. *Fitoterapia* **2018**, *125*, 208–216. [CrossRef] [PubMed]

76. Arcari, D.P.; Santos, J.C.; Gambero, A.; Ribeiro, M.L. The in vitro and in vivo effects of yerba mate (*Ilex paraguariensis*) extract on adipogenesis. *Food Chem.* **2013**, *141*, 809–815. [CrossRef] [PubMed]

77. Gonzalez-Gil, F.; Diaz-Sanchez, S.; Pendleton, S.; Andino, A.; Zhang, N.; Yard, C.; Crilly, N.; Harte, F.; Hanning, I. Yerba mate enhances probiotic bacteria growth in vitro but as a feed additive does not reduce *Salmonella enteritidis* colonization in vivo. *Poult. Sci.* **2014**, *93*, 434–440. [CrossRef] [PubMed]

78. Chen, G.; Xie, M.; Dai, Z.; Wan, P.; Ye, H.; Zeng, X.; Sun, Y. Kudingcha and fuzhuan brick tea prevent obesity and modulate gut microbiota in high-fat diet fed mice. *Mol. Nutr. Food Res.* **2018**, *62*, e1700485. [CrossRef] [PubMed]

79. Xie, M.; Chen, G.; Hu, B.; Zhou, L.; Ou, S.; Zeng, X.; Sun, Y. Hydrolysis of dicaffeoylquinic acids from *Ilex kudingcha* happens in the colon by intestinal microbiota. *J. Agric. Food Chem.* **2016**, *64*, 9624–9630. [CrossRef] [PubMed]

80. Dasanayake, A.P.; Silverman, A.J.; Warnakulasuriya, S. Mate drinking and oral and oro-pharyngeal cancer: A systematic review and meta-analysis. *Oral. Oncol.* **2010**, *46*, 82–86. [CrossRef] [PubMed]

81. Amigo-Benavent, M.; Wang, S.; Mateos, R.; Sarria, B.; Bravo, L. Antiproliferative and cytotoxic effects of green coffee and yerba mate extracts, their main hydroxycinnamic acids, methylxanthine and metabolites in different human cell lines. *Food Chem. Toxicol.* **2017**, *106*, 125–138. [CrossRef] [PubMed]

82. Gomez-Juaristi, M.; Martinez-Lopez, S.; Sarria, B.; Bravo, L.; Mateos, R. Absorption and metabolism of yerba mate phenolic compounds in humans. *Food Chem.* **2018**, *240*, 1028–1038. [CrossRef] [PubMed]

83. Murad, L.D.; Soares Nda, C.; Brand, C.; Monteiro, M.C.; Teodoro, A.J. Effects of caffeic and 5-caffeoylquinic acids on cell viability and cellular uptake in human colon adenocarcinoma cells. *Nutr. Cancer* **2015**, *67*, 532–542. [CrossRef] [PubMed]

84. Ronco, A.L.; De Stefani, E.; Mendoza, B.; Deneo-Pellegrini, H.; Vazquez, A.; Abbona, E. Mate intake and risk of breast cancer in uruguay: A. case-control study. *Asian Pac. J. Cancer Prev.* **2016**, *17*, 1453–1461. [CrossRef] [PubMed]

85. Puangpraphant, S.; Berhow, M.A.; Vermillion, K.; Potts, G.; Gonzalez de Mejia, E. Dicaffeoylquinic acids in yerba mate (*Ilex paraguariensis* St. Hilaire) inhibit NF-κB nucleus translocation in macrophages and induce apoptosis by activating caspases-8 and -3 in human colon cancer cells. *Mol. Nutr. Food Res.* **2011**, *55*, 1509–1522. [CrossRef] [PubMed]

86. Zhai, X.; Ren, D.; Luo, Y.; Hu, Y.; Yang, X. Chemical characteristics of an *Ilex kuding* tea polysaccharide and its protective effects against high fructose-induced liver injury and vascular endothelial dysfunction in mice. *Food Funct.* **2017**, *8*, 2536–2547. [CrossRef] [PubMed]

87. Cardozo Junior, E.L.; Morand, C. Interest of mate (*Ilex paraguariensis* a. St.-Hil.) as a new natural functional food to preserve human cardiovascular health—A review. *J. Funct. Foods* **2016**, *21*, 440–454. [CrossRef]

88. Yu, S.; Yue, S.; Liu, Z.; Zhang, T.; Xiang, N.; Fu, H. Yerba mate (*Ilex paraguariensis*) improves microcirculation of volunteers with high blood viscosity: A. randomized, double-blind, placebo-controlled trial. *Exp. Gerontol.* **2015**, *62*, 14–22. [CrossRef] [PubMed]

89. da Veiga, D.T.A.; Bringhenti, R.; Copes, R.; Tatsch, E.; Moresco, R.N.; Comim, F.V.; Premaor, M.O. Protective effect of yerba mate intake on the cardiovascular system: A *post hoc* analysis study in postmenopausal women. *Braz. J. Med. Biol. Res.* **2018**, *51*, e7253. [CrossRef] [PubMed]

90. Wu, H.; Chen, Y.L.; Yu, Y.; Zang, J.; Wu, Y.; He, Z. *Ilex latifolia* thunb protects mice from HFD-induced body weight gain. *Sci. Rep.* **2017**, *7*, 14660. [CrossRef] [PubMed]

91. Silva, R.D.; Bueno, A.L.; Gallon, C.W.; Gomes, L.F.; Kaiser, S.; Pavei, C.; Ortega, G.G.; Kucharski, L.C.; Jahn, M.P. The effect of aqueous extract of gross and commercial yerba mate (*Ilex paraguariensis*) on intra-abdominal and epididymal fat and glucose levels in male Wistar rats. *Fitoterapia* **2011**, *82*, 818–826. [CrossRef] [PubMed]

92. Lima Nda, S.; Franco, J.G.; Peixoto-Silva, N.; Maia, L.A.; Kaezer, A.; Felzenszwalb, I.; de Oliveira, E.; de Moura, E.G.; Lisboa, P.C. *Ilex paraguariensis* (yerba mate) improves endocrine and metabolic disorders in obese rats primed by early weaning. *Eur. J. Nutr.* **2014**, *53*, 73–82. [CrossRef] [PubMed]

93. Gambero, A.; Ribeiro, M.L. The positive effects of yerba mate (*Ilex paraguariensis*) in obesity. *Nutrients* **2015**, *7*, 730–750. [CrossRef] [PubMed]

94. de Oliveira, E.; Lima, N.S.; Conceicao, E.P.S.; Peixoto-Silva, N.; Moura, E.G.; Lisboa, P.C. Treatment with *Ilex paraguariensis* (yerba mate) aqueous solution prevents hepatic redox imbalance, elevated triglycerides, and microsteatosis in overweight adult rats that were precociously weaned. *Braz. J. Med. Biol. Res.* **2018**, *51*, e7342. [CrossRef] [PubMed]

95. Kang, Y.R.; Lee, H.Y.; Kim, J.H.; Moon, D.I.; Seo, M.Y.; Park, S.H.; Choi, K.H.; Kim, C.R.; Kim, S.H.; Oh, J.H.; et al. Anti-obesity and anti-diabetic effects of yerba mate (*Ilex paraguariensis*) in C57BL/6J mice fed a high-fat diet. *Lab. Anim. Res.* **2012**, *28*, 23–29. [CrossRef] [PubMed]

96. Hussein, G.M.E.; Matsuda, H.; Nakamura, S.; Hamao, M.; Akiyama, T.; Tamura, K.; Yoshikawa, M. Mate tea (*Ilex paraguariensis*) promotes satiety and body weight lowering in mice: Involvement of glucagon-like peptide-1. *Biol. Pharm. Bull.* **2011**, *34*, 1849–1855. [CrossRef] [PubMed]

97. Kim, S.Y.; Oh, M.R.; Kim, M.G.; Chae, H.J.; Chae, S.W. Anti-obesity effects of yerba mate (*Ilex paraguariensis*): A randomized, double-blind, placebo-controlled clinical trial. *BMC Complement Altern. Med.* **2015**, *15*, 338. [CrossRef] [PubMed]

98. De Oliveira, E.P.; Torezan, G.A.; Goncalves, L.D.; Corrente, J.E.; McLellan, K.C.P.; Burini, R.C. Acute intake of yerba mate increases energy expenditure of health young men: A. pilot study. *Rbone-Rev. Bras. Obes.* **2016**, *10*, 242–249.

99. Maufrais, C.; Sarafian, D.; Dulloo, A.; Montani, J.P. Cardiovascular and metabolic responses to the ingestion of caffeinated herbal tea: Drink it hot or cold? *Front. Physiol.* **2018**, *9*, 315. [CrossRef] [PubMed]

100. Wang, Z.; Clifford, M.N.; Sharp, P. Analysis of chlorogenic acids in beverages prepared from Chinese health foods and investigation, in vitro, of effects on glucose absorption in cultured Caco-2 cells. *Food Chem.* **2008**, *108*, 369–373. [CrossRef]

101. Riachi, L.G.; De Maria, C.A.B. Yerba mate: An overview of physiological effects in humans. *J. Funct. Foods* **2017**, *38*, 308–320. [CrossRef]

102. Kim, J.Y.; Lee, H.K.; Hwang, B.Y.; Kim, S.; Yoo, J.K.; Seong, Y.H. Neuroprotection of *Ilex latifolia* and caffeoylquinic acid derivatives against excitotoxic and hypoxic damage of cultured rat cortical neurons. *Arch. Pharm. Res.* **2012**, *35*, 1115–1122. [CrossRef] [PubMed]

103. Kim, J.Y.; Lee, H.K.; Jang, J.Y.; Yoo, J.K.; Seong, Y.H. *Ilex latifolia* prevents amyloid beta protein (25–35)-induced memory impairment by inhibiting apoptosis and tau phosphorylation in mice. *J. Med. Food* **2015**, *18*, 1317–1326. [CrossRef] [PubMed]

104. Kim, J.Y.; Jeong, H.Y.; Lee, H.K.; Yoo, J.K.; Bae, K.; Seong, Y.H. Protective effect of *Ilex latifolia*, a major component of "kudingcha", against transient focal ischemia-induced neuronal damage in rats. *J. Ethnopharmacol.* **2011**, *133*, 558–564. [CrossRef] [PubMed]

105. Gatto, E.M.; Melcon, C.; Parisi, V.L.; Bartoloni, L.; Gonzalez, C.D. Inverse association between yerba mate consumption and idiopathic Parkinson's disease. A case-control study. *J. Neurol. Sci.* **2015**, *356*, 163–167. [CrossRef] [PubMed]

106. Conforti, A.S.; Gallo, M.E.; Saravi, F.D. Yerba mate (*Ilex paraguariensis*) consumption is associated with higher bone mineral density in postmenopausal women. *Bone* **2012**, *50*, 9–13. [CrossRef] [PubMed]

107. Brasilino, M.D.S.; Stringhetta-Garcia, C.T.; Pereira, C.S.; Pereira, A.A.F.; Stringhetta, K.; Leopoldino, A.M.; Crivelini, M.M.; Ervolino, E.; Dornelles, R.C.M.; de Melo Stevanato Nakamune, A.C.; et al. Mate tea (*Ilex paraguariensis*) improves bone formation in the alveolar socket healing after tooth extraction in rats. *Clin. Oral. Investig.* **2018**, *22*, 1449–1461. [CrossRef] [PubMed]

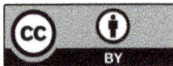

nutrients

MDPI

Article

Colon Bioaccessibility and Antioxidant Activity of White, Green and Black Tea Polyphenols Extract after In Vitro Simulated Gastrointestinal Digestion

Giuseppe Annunziata *,†**, Maria Maisto** †**, Connie Schisano, Roberto Ciampaglia, Patricia Daliu, Viviana Narciso, Gian Carlo Tenore and Ettore Novellino**

Department of Pharmacy, University of Naples "Federico II", Via Domenico Montesano 49, 80131 Naples, Italy; maria.maisto@unina.it (M.M.); connie.schisano@unina.it (C.S.); roberto.ciampaglia@unina.it (R.C.); patricia.daliu@unina.it (P.D.); viviana.narciso@gmail.com (V.N.); giancarlo.tenore@unina.it (G.C.T.); ettore.novellino@unina.it (E.N.)
* Correspondence: giuseppe.annunziata@unina.it; Tel.: +39-081-678-606
† These authors contributed equally to this work.

Received: 15 October 2018; Accepted: 5 November 2018; Published: 8 November 2018

Abstract: The beneficial effects of the tea beverage are well-known and mainly attributed to polyphenols which, however, have poor bioaccessibility and bioavailability. The purpose of the present study was the evaluation of colon bioaccessibility and antioxidant activity of tea polyphenolic extract. An 80% methanolic extract (v/v) of tea polyphenols was obtained from green (GT), white (WT) and black tea (BT). Simulated gastrointestinal (GI) digestion was performed on acid-resistant capsules containing tea polyphenolic extract. The main tea polyphenols were monitored by HPLC-diode-array detector (DAD) method; in addition, Total Phenol Content (TPC) and antioxidant activity were evaluated. After GI digestion, the bioaccessibility in the colon stage was significantly increased compared to the duodenal stage for both tea polyphenols and TPC. Similarly, the antioxidant activity in the colon stage was significantly higher than that in the duodenal stage. Reasonably, these results could be attributable in vivo to the activity of gut microbiota, which is able to metabolize these compounds, generating metabolites with a greater antioxidant activity. Our results may guide the comprehension of the colon digestion of polyphenols, suggesting that, although poorly absorbed in the duodenum, they can exert their antioxidant and anti-inflammatory activities in the lower gut, resulting in a novel strategy for the management of gut-related inflammatory diseases.

Keywords: tea; polyphenols; bioaccessibility; nutraceutical; microbiota

---

1. Introduction

Tea is historically recognized as the typical beverage consumed in the oriental tradition, used for more than 5000 years in diet and folk medicine, especially in Asian countries [1]. However, its consumption has increased all over the world, becoming one of the most popular beverages [2]. This spreading is mainly due to the widely accepted beneficial effects of tea on human health, which have been attributed to polyphenols [3], the largest group of phytochemical compounds which includes about 8000 different structures [4]. These compounds are largely contained in several plant-based foods, such as fruits, nuts, tea, coffee and cocoa [5,6], suggesting the pivotal role of their consumption in prevention and management of several diseases, including type 2 diabetes mellitus (T2DM) [6] and cardiovascular disease (CVD) [7]. Most of the main beneficial effects of the Mediterranean Diet, which is recognized as the best health-promoting dietary style, indeed, are attributed to the elevated amount of polyphenols present in its main food constituents [6–10]. Evidence, indeed, suggests that polyphenols, in addition to their well-known antioxidant activity, exert a number of other beneficial effects on human health contributing to preventing and/or managing several pathological conditions, including neurodegenerative diseases, inflammation, cancer, CVD, T2DM and obesity, as recently reviewed by Cory et al. [11]. Among polyphenols, catechins are the most representative in tea (more than 30% of leaf dried weight) [12]. After their synthesis, catechins undergo several esterification reactions with gallic acid, resulting in a number of other bioactive compounds, including (−)-catechin-3-gallate (CG), (−)-epicatechin-3-gallate (ECG), (−)-epigallocatechin (EGC), (−)-epigallocatechin-3-gallate (EGCG), and (−)-gallocatechin-3-gallate (GCG). The EGCG is the most abundant polyphenol in green, white and black tea; ECG and EGC levels are high in white tea, where gallic acid, caffeine and theobromine are also present [13].

Although a number of studies have reported several beneficial effects of tea, it is important to consider that gastrointestinal (GI) digestion is a complex physiological process, which strongly affects structure and activity of diet-derived bioactive compounds, resulting in decreased bioaccessibility and bioavailability. Tenore et al. [14] evaluated in vitro bioaccessibility and bioavailability of polyphenols in black, white and green tea infusions (0.5 g of tea in 20 mL of hot water, 90 °C). Bioaccessibility was investigated using a simulated GI digestion protocol; bioavailability was assessed by a monolayer of Caco-2 human colon carcinoma cell line, as intestinal epithelium experimental model. Results showed a very low intestinal bioaccessibility (about 8%) and bioavailability (2–15% of the intestinal content). The low bioaccessibility is mainly ascribed to the neutral intestinal pH, which causes epimerization and auto-oxidation of catechins. Furthermore, the low catechin transepithelial permeation is probably due to polyphenol instability at neutral pH values and/or the presence of efflux transporters on the apical membrane of intestinal cells [14]. Similar results were obtained by Peters et al. [15] who highlighted that both duodenal bioaccessibility and bioavailability of catechins from green tea were reduced compared to non-digested samples. Interestingly, the same authors demonstrated that these two parameters were enhanced using a formulation of green tea extract with sucrose and ascorbic acid, alone or in combination [15].

Jilani et al. [16] also demonstrated that in vitro GI digestion reduces intestinal bioaccessibility of polyphenols from green and black tea infusions; however, total antioxidant capacity was reduced only in green tea samples, while increased in black tea samples. Additionally, biosorption with *S. cerevisiae* has been proposed as a useful approach to increase polyphenol bioaccessibility. In general, yeast fermentation enhanced both bioaccessibility and antioxidant capacity of tea polyphenols. Specifically, fermented infusions exhibited a lower bioaccessibility than not-fermented; however, in the suspension of *S. cerevisiae* (the pellet obtained after centrifugation of fermented samples) a certain amount of polyphenols was detected. Interestingly, both bioaccessibility and antioxidant capacity of polyphenols in the yeast suspension significantly increased after in vitro GI digestion, suggesting that yeast acted as a good strategy for extracting polyphenols and as delivery system protecting phytochemicals during the GI digestion. This is mainly due to the ability of polyphenols to bind wall components of yeast cells forming complexes with affinities depending on several factors, including chemical structure of polyphenols, protein or polysaccharides concentrations, temperature and pH. According to the authors, the affinity between polyphenols and wall components of yeast cells was higher in black tea samples; this is due to a higher specificity toward high molecular weight polyphenols, such as thearubigins and theaflavins, which also present a high affinity for milk proteins [17,18]. This suggest that food components may also affect bioaccessibility of polyphenols. The formation of complexes between polyphenols and food components may represent a delivery system that protects bioactive compounds from the activity of GI digestion; in turn, changes in pH (in particular, the middle-alkaline pH), variating the affinity of polyphenols, may increase their bioaccessibility.

On the contrary, Coe et al. [19] demonstrated that bioaccessibility of polyphenols from green, white and black tea infusions increased both in gastric and duodenal stages after in vitro GI digestion.

Overall, these data provide information about the metabolic fate of diet-derived bioactive compounds and suggest that, although diet is the main source of bioactive substances, the single or sporadic consumption of foods rich in these compounds is not sufficient to obtain the claimed beneficial effects. The use of nutraceutical products, thus, might represent the best approach to take benefit from their properties.

However, taking into account the physiology of the GI system, a further interpretation of tea polyphenol metabolic fate should be proposed. The prolonged permanence of polyphenols in the intestinal lumen leads to the assumption that these compounds may exert, in situ, their beneficial effects, including the actions on glucose and lipid metabolism [12,13]. Moreover, the non-absorbed polyphenols reach the lower intestine where, before being excreted, they might also exert their antioxidant activity. Interestingly, evidence showed that non-absorbed polyphenols could be metabolized by the microbiota in the colon, resulting in the production of several metabolites, which have higher antioxidant activity [20–22].

A limited number of studies have investigated the metabolic fate of tea polyphenols in the large intestine. The purpose of the present study is to investigate the bioaccessibility and antioxidant activity of tea polyphenols in an experimental model of large intestine. Bioaccessibility and antioxidant activity were evaluated using a nutraceutical formulation based on acid-resistant capsules containing 80% methanolic extract (*v/v*) of green (GT), white (WT) and black tea (BT). After in vitro simulated GI digestion, significant increases in tea polyphenols and antioxidant activity were observed in the colon stage, as compared to the duodenal stage, suggesting a possible role of gut microbiota in metabolising these compounds in vivo.

2. Materials and Methods

2.1. Reagents

All chemicals and reagents used were either analytical or HPLC-grade reagents. The water was treated in a Milli-Q water purification system (Millipore, Bedford, MA, USA) before use. Chemicals and reagents used to simulate the gastrointestinal digestion: potassium chloride (KCl), potassium thiocyanate (KSCN), monosodium phosphate (NaH_2PO_4), sodium sulphate (Na_2SO_4), sodium chloride (NaCl), sodium bicarbonate ($NaHCO_3$), hydrochloric acid (HCl) and also the enzymes pepsin ($\geq$250 U/mg solid) from porcine gastric mucosa, pancreatin (4 × USP) from porcine pancreas, protease from Streptomyces griseus, called also Pronase E ($\geq$3.5 U/mg solid), and Viscozyme L were purchased from Sigma-Aldrich (Milan, Italy).

2.2. Tea Polyphenolic Extraction

Three variety of tea samples (*C. sinensis*) were purchased in a local market. These were green, white and black tea. All samples were obtained from the same tea cultivar Chun Mee 41022 (Vicony Teas Company, Huangshan, China). For the preparation of the tea polyphenolic extract, 75 mL of 80% methanol was added to 15 g of each dry tea samples, homogenized for 1 min by ultra-turrax (T25-digital, IKA, Staufen im Breisgau, Germania), shaken on orbital shaker (Sko-DXL, Argolab, Carpy, Italy) at 300 rpm for 10 min; the samples were placed in ultrasonic bath for other 10 min and then centrifuged at 6000 rpm for 10 min. The supernatants were collected and stored in the darkness, at 4 °C. The pellets obtained, were re-extracted with other 35 mL of the same mixture, following the procedure previously described. Finally, the extracts were filtered under vacuum, the methanol fraction was eliminated, and the water fraction was lyophilized. The powders obtained were used for the capsules' formulation. In particular, capsules contained 1000 mg GT, WT or BT polyphenolic extract. The capsules used were acid-resistant (hydroxypropyl cellulose E464, gellan gum E418, hioxide titanium E171).

2.3. In Vitro Simulated Gastrointestinal Digestion

The in vitro digestion experiments were performed according to the procedure described by Raiola et al. (2012) [23] and by Tenore et al. (2013) [24], with few modifications. For GI digestion, a capsule was mixed with 6 mL of artificial saliva composed of KCl (89.6 g/L), KSCN (20 g/L),

NaH$_2$PO$_4$ (88.8 g/L), Na$_2$SO$_4$ (57.0 g/L), NaCl (175.3 g/L), NaHCO$_3$ (84.7 g/L), urea (25.0 g/L) and 290 mg of α-amylase. The pH of the solution was adjusted to 6.8 with HCl 0.1 N. The mixture was introduced in a plastic bag containing 40 mL of water and homogenized in a Stomacher 80 Microbiomaster (Seward, Worthing, UK) for 3 min. Immediately, 0.5 g of pepsin (14,800 U) dissolved in HCl 0.1 N was added, the pH was adjusted to 2.0 with HCl 6 N, and the solution was incubated at 37 °C in a Polymax 1040 orbital shaker (250 rpm) (Heidolph, Schwabach, Germany) for 2 h. Then the pH was increased to 6.5 with NaHCO$_3$ 0.5 N and 5 mL of a mixture of pancreatin (8.0 mg/mL) and bile salts (50.0 mg/ mL) (1:1; *v/v*), dissolved in 20 mL of water, was added and incubated at 37 °C in an orbital shaker (250 rpm) for 2 h. Finally, the mixture was centrifuged at 6000 rpm and the remaining pellets were treated first with 5 mL of 1 mg/mL Pronase E solution (pH 8 for 1 h), and then, with 150 μL of Viscozyme L (pH 4 for 16 h), in order to simulate the colon digestion process, as previously described by Papillo et al. (2014) [25]. Each of the supernatants collected during the different digestion phases simulated were lyophilized, and then dissolved in methanol for the analysis.

2.4. Total Phenol Content (TPC)

Total phenol content (TPC) was determined through Folin-Ciocalteau's method, using gallic acid as standard (Sigma-Aldrich, St. Louis, MO, USA). In brief, 0.1 mL of samples (properly diluted with water in order to obtain an absorbance value within the linear range of the spectrophotometer) underwent an addition of: 0.5 mL of Folin-Ciocalteau's (Sigma-Aldrich, St. Louis, MO, USA) reagent and 0.2 mL of an aqueous solution of Na$_2$CO$_3$ (20%; *w/v* %), bringing the final volume to 10 mL with water. After mixing, the samples were kept in the dark for 90 min. After the reaction period, the absorbance was measured at 760 nm. Each sample was analyzed in triplicate and the concentration of total polyphenols was calculated in terms of gallic acid equivalents (GAE) [26].

2.5. HPLC-DAD Analysis of Tea Polyphenols

The main tea polyphenols were assessed by HPLC/diode-array detector (DAD) analysis, performed using a HPLC system Jasco Extrema LC-4000 system (Jasco Inc., Easton, MD, USA) fitted with an auto sampler, a binary solvent pump, and a diode-array detector (DAD). The separation and quantification were achieved using Synergy Polar-RP C18 column (150 × 4.6 mm I.D., 4 μm particle size, Phenomenex, Torrance, CA, USA) preceded by a Polar RP security guard cartridge. The column temperature was set at 40 °C. The PDA acquisition wavelength was set in the range of 200–400 nm. The mobile phase consisted of water-acetic acid, (97:3 *v/v*) (A) and methanol (B). Injection volume was 20 μL and flow rate was kept at 1 mL/min. The gradient program was: 0–1 min %(A), followed by a linear increase of solvent B to 63% in 27 min; then the phase composition was brought back to the initial conditions in 2 min [27]. Calibration curves were obtained at detection wavelength of 280 nm for all catechins using a series of standard dilutions in MeOH, over the concentration range of 0.20–80.0 mg/L.

2.6. Antioxidant Activity

2.6.1. DPPH Assay

The antioxidant activity of tea samples was measured with respect to the radical scavenging ability of the antioxidants present in the sample using the stable radical 2,2-diphenyl-1-picrylhydrazyl (DPPH) (Sigma-Aldrich St. Louis, MO, USA). The analysis was performed by adding 100 μL of each sample to 1000 μL of a methanol solution of DPPH (153 mmol L^{-1}). The decrease in absorbance was determined with a UV-visible spectrophotometer (Beckman, Los Angeles, CA, USA). The absorbance of DPPH radical without antioxidant, i.e., the control, was measured as basis. All determinations were in triplicate. Inhibition was calculated according to the formula:

$$[(Ai - Af)/Ac] \times 100, \tag{1}$$

where Ai is absorbance of sample at t = 0, Af is the absorbance after 6min, and Ac is the absorbance of the control at time zero [28]. Trolox was used as standard antioxidant. Results were expressed in mmol Trolox Equivalent (TE).

2.6.2. ABTS Assay

The ABTS assay was performed according to the method described by Rufino et al. (2010) [26] with slight modifications. ABTS solution was prepared [2,20 -azinobis(3-ethylbenzotiazoline-6-sulfonate)] by mixing 5 mL of ABTS 7.0 mM solution and 88 µL of potassium persulfate 2.45 mM solution, which was left to react for 12 h, at 5 °C in the dark. Then, ethanol water was added to the solution until an absorbance value of 0.700 (0.05) at 754 nm (Beckman, Los Angeles, CA, USA). The determination of sample absorbance was accomplished at room temperature and after 6 min of reaction. All determinations were in triplicate. Inhibition was calculated according to the formula:

$$[(Ai - Af)/Ac] \times 100, \tag{2}$$

where Ai is absorbance of sample at t = 0, Af is the absorbance after 6 min, and Ac is the absorbance of the control at time zero [29]. Trolox was used as standard antioxidant. Results were expressed in mmol Trolox Equivalent (TE).

2.7. Statistics

Unless otherwise stated, all the experimental results were expressed as mean ± standard deviation (SD) of three determinations. Statistical analysis of data was performed by the Student's *t* test or two-way ANOVA (SPSS 13.0) followed by the Tukey-Kramer multiple comparison test to evaluate significant differences between a pair of means. P values less than 0.05 were regarded as significant. The degree of linear relationship between two variables was measured using the Pearson product moment correlation coefficient (R). Correlation coefficients (R) were calculated by using Microsoft Office Excel application.

3. Results

3.1. In Vitro Bioaccessibility of Tea Polyphenols

Tea polyphenol bioaccessibility was evaluated by using a simulated GI digestion. The use of acid-resistant capsule allowed us to avoid the effects of gastric conditions on the bioactive compounds. For each sample, the gastric bioaccessibility was 0% (Table 1). Equally, the oral bioaccessibility was also 0% (Table 1).

In order to obtain an overview of the bioaccessibility of the tea polyphenols in the various stages of the GI digestion, we firstly evaluated the TPC by Folin-Ciocalteu assay. Table 1 shows the mean values (mg GAE/g) of TPC for GT, WT and BT in each stage of the in vitro GI digestion. In the duodenal stage, TPC was significantly lower than in the not digested samples ($p < 0.0001$ for all samples). On the contrary, in the colon stage TPC significantly increased compared to the duodenal stage ($p < 0.001$, 0.0005 and 0.0001 for GT, WT and BT, respectively). In particular, despite the initial TPC measured in not-digested samples, after in vitro GI digestion WT renders the higher colon bioaccessibility (WT > BT > GT).

Table 1. Total Phenol Content (TPC) evaluated by Folin-Ciocalteu method. Data are expressed as mean value (mg gallic acid equivalents (GAE)/g extract) $\pm$ SD of three repetitions.

Sample		TPC (mg/g) $\pm$ SD
Tea Variety	Digestion Stage	
Green	Not digested	1005.703 $\pm$ 28.784
	Oral stage	n.d.
	Gastric stage	n.d.
	Duodenal stage	62.507 $\pm$ 2.254 [a,*]
	Pronase E stage	210.448 $\pm$ 24.479
	Viscozyme L stage	42.180 $\pm$ 10.939
	Total colon stage	252.628 $\pm$ 35.048 [b,**]
White	Not digested	650.654 $\pm$ 15.848
	Oral stage	n.d.
	Gastric stage	n.d.
	Duodenal stage	82.053 $\pm$ 15.294 [c,*]
	Pronase E stage	402.221 $\pm$ 17.794
	Viscozyme L stage	120.760 $\pm$ 38.581
	Total colon stage	522.981 $\pm$ 55.831 [d,***]
Black	Not digested	814.600 $\pm$ 6.968
	Oral stage	n.d.
	Gastric stage	n.d.
	Duodenal stage	42.111 $\pm$ 1.751 [e,*]
	Pronase E stage	340.196 $\pm$ 15.132
	Viscozyme L stage	78.432 $\pm$ 6.288
	Total colon stage	418.628 $\pm$ 21.375 [f,**]

Statistical significance is calculated by Student's *t*-test analysis: * $p < 0.0001$ Not digested vs. Duodenal stage; ** $p < 0.001$ Duodenal stage vs. Colon stage (Pronase E + Viscozyme L stages); *** $p < 0.0005$ Duodenal stage vs. Colon stage (Pronase E + Viscozyme L stages). [a,b,c,d,e,f] Mean values with different superscript letters are significantly different by Tukey-Kramer multiple comparison test. n.d.: not detected.

The most representative tea polyphenols were then monitored by HPLC-DAD analysis before and after in vitro GI digestion. HPLC-DAD chromatograms of not digested samples with the identification of the different catechins are reported in Figure 1. Mean values of the main tea polyphenols are reported in Table 2.

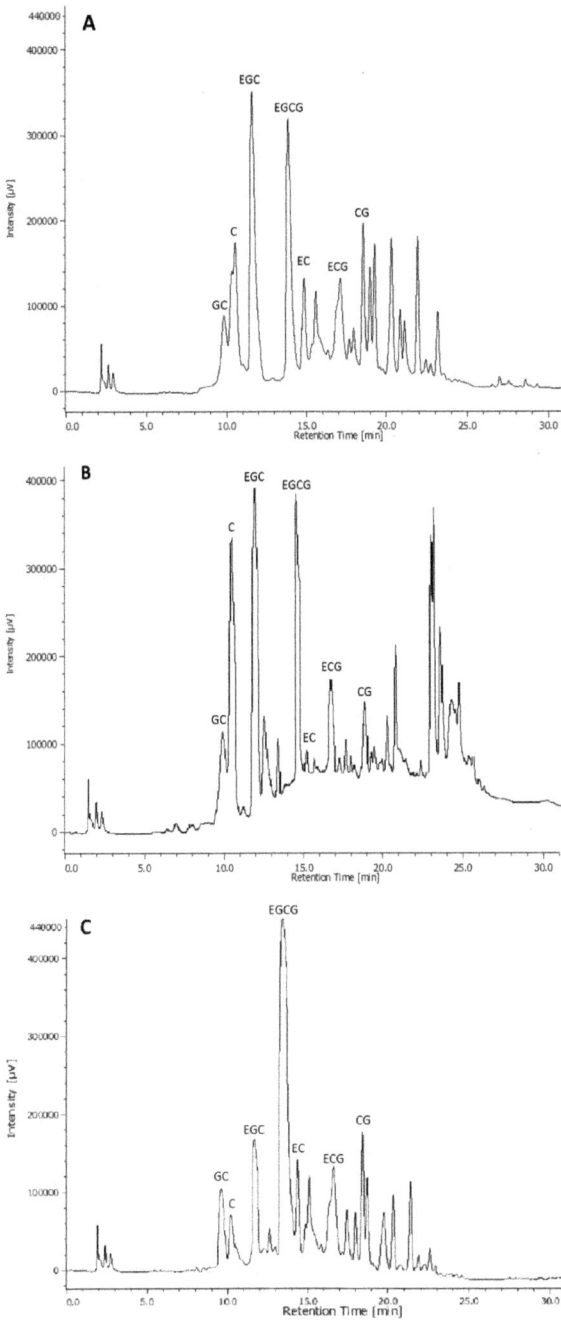

Figure 1. HPLC-diode-array detector (DAD) chromatograms of not digested green tea (GT) (**A**), black tea (BT) (**B**) and white tea (WT) (**C**) with identifying observed catechins. C: (+)-catechin; EC: (−)-epicatechin; ECG: (−)-epicatechingallate; EGC: (−)-epigallocatechin; EGCG: (−)-epigallocatechingallate; GC: (−)-gallocatechin; CG: (−)-catechingallate.

Table 2. HPLC-DAD analysis of the main tea polyphenols.

| Sample | | | | | | | | | Main Tea Polyphenols, Mean Values (mg/g) ± SD |
Tea Variety	Digestion Stage	C	EC	EGCG	ECG	EGC	GC	CG	Tot.
Green	Not digested	112.016 ± 1.493	56.361 ± 0.620	213.260 ± 1.337	101.010 ± 1.322	280.430 ± 0.149	33.735 ± 1.294	84.106 ± 0.146	880.924 ± 6.309
	Duodenal stage	26.618 ± 1.617	13.314 ± 0.153	50.769 ± 0.535	24.085 ± 0.521	66.597 ± 0.100	7.980 ± 0.278	20.012 ± 0.018	209.377 ± 3.151
	Pronase E stage	79.894 ± 1.747	39.823 ± 0.399	152.95 ± 0.889	71.910 ± 1.847	199.8 ± 0.163	25.099 ± 1.016	59.987 ± 0.122	629.466 ± 3.885
	Viscozyme L stage	41.979 ± 1.617	20.833 ± 0.417	79.675 ± 0.429	37.894 ± 0.432	105.010 ± 0.287	12.545 ± 0.881	31.527 ± 0.141	329.469 ± 4.158
White	Not digested	88.646 ± 1.456	33.776 ± 0.539	382.790 ± 1.404	96.294 ± 1.849	98.594 ± 0.522	40.711 ± 1.420	67.486 ± 0.396	808.294 ± 6.662
	Duodenal stage	17.085 ± 1.541	6.432 ± 0.229	74.152 ± 0.369	18.539 ± 0.573	19.017 ± 0.185	7.981 ± 0.528	13.095 ± 0.024	156.302 ± 3.430
	Pronase E stage	56.687 ± 1.902	21.283 ± 0.475	254.32 ± 1.585	61.615 ± 1.630	62.890 ± 0.187	25.856 ± 1.682	43.272 ± 0.290	516.925 ± 7.696
	Viscozyme L stage	34.055 ± 1.564	12.654 ± 0.737	146.580 ± 1.559	36.856 ± 1.406	37.443 ± 0.349	15.848 ± 1.563	25.826 ± 0.278	309.259 ± 7.393
Black	Not digested	231.918 ± 2.085	26.266 ± 1.010	267.080 ± 1.254	92.348 ± 1.423	287.53 ± 0.583	45.322 ± 1.382	18.678 ± 0.483	969.143 ± 8.176
	Duodenal stage	30.177 ± 1.300	3.329 ± 0.297	34.749 ± 0.131	12.010 ± 0.120	37.447 ± 0.177	5.898 ± 0.115	2.423 ± 0.014	126.035 ± 2.147
	Pronase E stage	170.548 ± 2.326	19.353 ± 0.920	196.540 ± 1.562	67.882 ± 1.704	211.710 ± 0.503	33.283 ± 1.634	13.720 ± 0.320	713.038 ± 8.966
	Viscozyme L stage	89.895 ± 1.674	10.133 ± 0.796	103.090 ± 1.392	35.787 ± 0.290	111.420 ± 0.280	17.478 ± 0.639	7.164 ± 0.252	374.968 ± 5.274

Polyphenolic content is expressed as mean value (mg/g tea extract) ± SD ($n = 3$). C: (+)-catechin; EC: (−)-epicatechin; ECG: (−)-epicatechingallate; EGC: (−)-epigallocatechin; EGCG: (−)-epigallocatechingallate; GC: (−)-gallocatechin; CG: (−)-catechingallate.

As shown in Table 3, interesting data regarding the intestinal bioaccessibility were obtained. In particular, the bioaccessibility in the duodenal stage was significantly reduced compared to not digested samples ($p < 0.0001$ for all samples). On the other hand, the colon bioaccessibility (considered as Pronase E stage + Viscozyme L stage) was significantly higher than duodenal stage ($p < 0.005$ for all samples).

Table 3. Intestinal bioaccessibility of tea polyphenols evaluated by HPLC-DAD method after the simulated in vitro digestion.

Sample	Duodenal Bioaccessibility		Colon Bioaccessibility	
	Total Polyphenols (mg/g)	%	Total Polyphenols (mg/g)	%
Green tea	209.377 *	23.77	958.933 **	108.85
White tea	156.302 *	19.33	826.185 **	102.21
Black tea	126.035 *	13.00	1088.007 **	112.26

Statistical significance is calculated by Student's *t*-test analysis: * $p < 0.0001$ Not digested vs. Duodenal stage; ** $p < 0.005$ Duodenal stage vs. Colon stage (Pronase E + Viscozyme L stages).

Data obtained by HPLC-DAD and Folin-Ciocalteu methods were compared (Figure 2). An almost equivalent trend was observed, suggesting that these two methods, although the well-known differences and limitations, provided similar results.

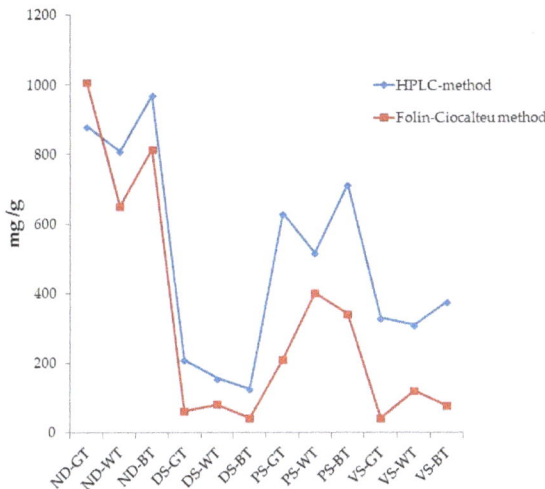

Figure 2. Comparison between the data obtained by the HPLC-DAD method and the spectrophotometric Folin-Ciocalteu method, expressed as mg/g total polyphenols and mg/g gallic acid, respectively.

3.2. Antioxidant Activity of Tea Polyphenolic Extract after In Vitro Digestion

The antioxidant activity was evaluated by using both DPPH and ABTS assays; results were expressed as mmol of Trolox Equivalent (TE) per g of dried extract. The mean values are reported in Table 4 for each sample in different stages of the in vitro GI digestion.

Table 4. Antioxidant activity of digested samples evaluated by DPPH and ABTS assays. Data are expressed as mean value in mmol TE/g extract ± SD (of three repetitions).

Sample		Antioxidant Activity (mmol TE/g ± SD)	
Tea Variety	Digestion Stage	DPPH Assay	ABTS Assay
Green	Not digested	3.649 ± 0.342	4.269 ± 0.274
	Duodenal stage	0.325 ± 0.013	0.469 ± 0.187
	Pronase E stage	1.339 ± 0.336	1.335 ± 0.403
	Viscozyme L stage	0.098 ± 0.006	0.108 ± 0.046
White	Not digested	3.961 ± 0.453	4.085 ± 0.213
	Duodenal stage	0.338 ± 0.102	0.344 ± 0.140
	Pronase E stage	2.244 ± 0.743	2.421 ± 0.779
	Viscozyme L stage	0.684 ± 0.073	0.375 ± 0.139
Black	Not digested	2.322 ± 0.206	2.971 ± 0.274
	Duodenal stage	0.093 ± 0.014	0.283 ± 0.039
	Pronase E stage	1.793 ± 0.094	2.129 ± 0.302
	Viscozyme L stage	0.100 ± 0.006	0.564 ± 0.115

For all samples, in both assays, the antioxidant activity in the colon stages was higher than in duodenum. The variation of the antioxidant activity expressed as % inhibition and mmol TE/g in duodenal and colon stages are represented in Figure 3. In particular, a significant increase of the antioxidant activity was observed in the colon stage for both DPPH ($p < 0.005$, 0.01 and 0.0001 for GT, WT and BT, respectively) and ABTS ($p < 0.05$, 0.01 and 0.001 for GT, WT and BT, respectively) assays.

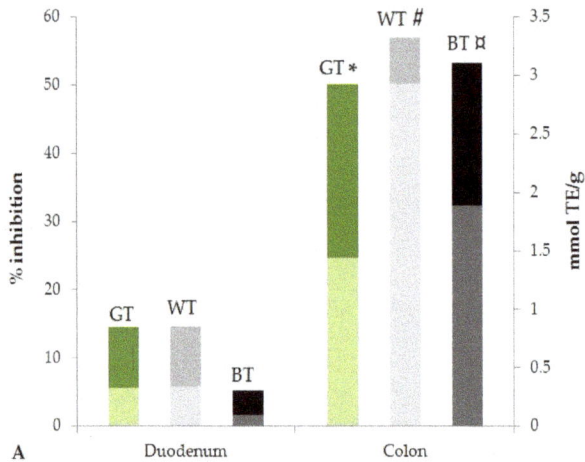

Figure 3. *Cont.*

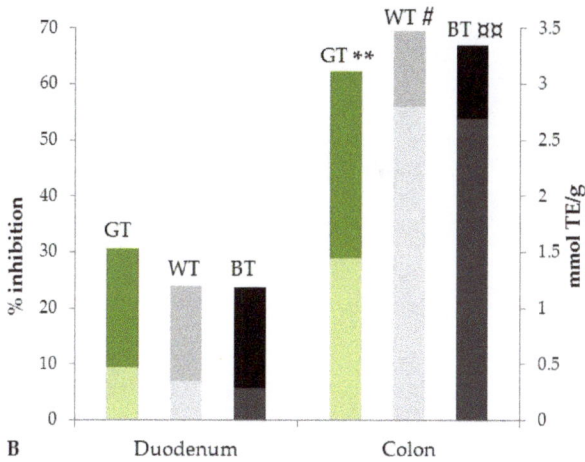

Figure 3. Antioxidant activity evaluated by (**A**) DPPH and (**B**) ABTS methods after simulated in vitro digestion. Statistical significance is calculated by Student's *t*-test analysis of data expressed in mmol TE/g extract: * $p < 0.005$; # $p < 0.01$; ¤ $p < 0.0001$; ** $p < 0.05$; ¤¤ $p < 0.001$, for all Duodenal stage vs. Colon stage (Pronase E + Viscozyme L stages).

A linear correlation between the TPC evaluated by Folin-Ciocalteu (mg GAE/g) and antioxidant activity (mmol TE/g) evaluated by DPPH and ABTS methods were performed (Figure 4). A significant correlation was observed between the two spectrophotometric assays (R^2 = 0.975 and 0.969 for Folin-Ciocalteu vs. DPPH and Folin-Ciocalteu vs. ABTS, respectively).

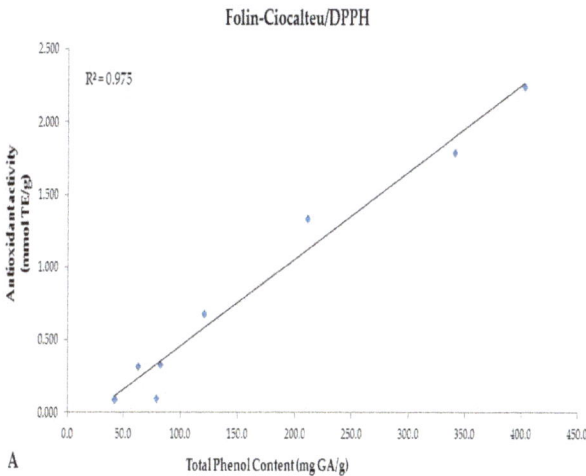

Figure 4. *Cont.*

Folin-Ciocalteu/ABTS

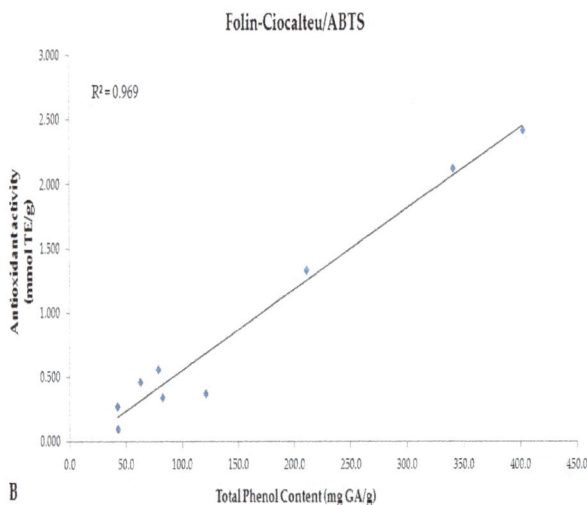

B

Figure 4. Linear correlation between TPC evaluated by Folin-Ciocalteu (mg GA/g) and antioxidant activity (mmol TE/g) evaluated by (**A**) DPPH and (**B**) ABTS methods.

4. Discussion

The present study aimed to evaluate the bioaccessibility and antioxidant activity of tea polyphenols after in vitro GI digestion. The digestion protocol was performed on acid-resistant capsules containing 80% methanolic extract (v/v) of GT, BT and WT. The use of acid-resistant capsules for the formulation of nutraceutical products represents a useful strategy in order to move bioactive compounds to the intestine, where they can be absorbed or can exert their activities in their active form. Specifically, acid-resistant capsules protect bioactive substances from degradation or alteration of their chemical structure caused by changes in pH or the action of digestive enzymes. A previous study [14] demonstrated that on average 44.4% of native catechin in tea infusions were lost due to gastric digestion and 91.8% after intestinal digestion. Additionally, in the same study, tea polyphenol bioavailability was reported to be very low, suggesting that, overall, GI digestion strongly affects the nutraceutical potential of tea. Thus, taking into account both of these aspects, and the well-established susceptibility of polyphenols to the mild-alkaline conditions, the use of delivery systems is recognized as a novel strategy to increase the amount of bioactive compounds that reach the small intestine, resulting in an increased permeation degree. Data reported in this study might be useful for the formulation of tea polyphenol-based nutraceutical products, which should be formulated under acid-resistant conditions.

As expected, the gastric bioaccessibility was 0%, suggesting that capsules did not decompose during this digestion stage, and polyphenols were not lost Table 1. Similarly, the oral bioaccessibility was 0%, although the oral stage was performed for 3 min. This timing is commonly used for the in vitro digestion of food matrices which undergo chewing, and it seems unrealistic for capsule intake; however, it was performed in order to respect the digestion protocol. Nevertheless, our data suggest that polyphenols are not lost during the oral digestion as well as in vivo when mastication process does not occur after capsule intake, and swallowing is immediate.

The protocol we used for the simulated GI intestinal digestion has been previously performed in our labs and published in various studies [20,21]. In general, it is not too much different from the Infogest method [30] that is recognized as the most eligible method for a comparison of results among different labs using similar and close conditions. In particular, equal timing was kept for each digestive stage (oral stage: 2 min vs. 3 min, Infogest method vs. our method; gastric stage: 2 h; intestinal stage: 2 h). The pH conditions of each stage were similar between the two methods (oral stage 7 vs. 6.8; gastric stage: 3 vs. 2; intestinal stage: 7 vs. 6.5, Infogest method vs. our method).

Differences were present among the saline solutions simulating the digestive fluids. The Infogest method uses simulated salivary, gastric and intestinal fluids with standard ions concentrations and volume; on the contrary, we used an artificial saliva that, however, contains several components used in the Infogest method. Similarly, slight differences were among the concentrations of digestive enzymes, although we used the same (α-amylase for the oral stage, pepsin for the gastric stage, pancreatin for the intestinal stage). Nevertheless, these differences may appear as a limitation, it is important to consider that two of the three digestion stages (oral and gastric) were only performed in order to respect the protocol, but variation in the studied matrix or particular results were not expected. As the simulated GI digestion was performed on acid-resistant capsules, oral and gastric digestion did not affect the digested components; thus, these two stages were not relevant. Moreover, during the intestinal stage, the composition of pancreatin we used was similar to that described by the Infogest method. In addition, the main aim of this study was the evaluation of colon digestion that is not contemplate in the Infogest method.

Our main finding in this study is that, after in vitro GI digestion, both bioaccessibility and antioxidant activity of tea polyphenols significantly increased in the colon stage compared to the duodenal stage. Although TPC in not-digested WT was the lowest, our results demonstrate that after simulated GI digestion this kind of tea extract renders the highest duodenal and colonic bioaccessibility, confirming the role of GI digestion in affecting the nutraceutical potential of food-derived extracts. These data suggest that WT extract would benefit the higher polyphenols delivery in both upper and lower intestine.

Bioaccessibility is defined as the amount of polyphenols contained in the water-soluble fraction of each digestion stage, which, in vivo, may be considered as potentially absorbable. As GI digestion is a complex physiological process, in vitro approaches should appear limiting, in particular for the study of digestion in the large intestine, where the activity of microbiota plays a pivotal role. However, the protocol herein used reproductions which were as close as possible to the physiological GI digestion process, as concern chemical, chemical-physical and enzymatic conditions, as well as the average duration of all of the individual stages.

During the simulated GI digestion, a low duodenal bioaccessibility was found for each tea sample (Table 3). This is in agreement with the studies of Tenore et al. [14], Peters et al. [15] and Jilani et al. [16], suggesting that, despite of the fact that polyphenols can be assumed as food or nutraceutical products, their intestinal absorption is low, mainly due to the neutral pH, as mentioned above. This consideration supports the use of delivery systems as strategy to increase the duodenal bioaccessibility.

Physiologically, non-absorbed polyphenols reach the lower gut where they undergo microbial activity [31,32]. This action is due to specific enzymes expressed by bacteria, including carbohydrases which are responsible for both the release of fiber-bound polyphenols and their metabolism [32]. In food matrices polyphenols should exist in the form of glycosides [33]; the presence of a glucose residue strongly reduces both bioaccessibility and bioavailability of phytochemicals. Additionally, some classes of polyphenols, such as catechins, can form oligomers, also called proanthocyanidins or condensed tannins [21]. Simplest catechin (such as monomeric, dimeric and trimeric catechins) are readily absorbed in the small intestine, while catechins with high molecular weight (such as oligomers) have a really poor bioavailability [34], as well as insoluble-bound phenols [35]. In vivo, during the colonic digestion polyphenols may be subjected to hydrolyses by gut microbiota enzymes which are responsible for hydrolytic release of aglycones from *O*-glucoside and carbon-carbon cleavage in the heterocycle and in the aromatic rings [21], resulting in several modifications of the native chemical structures and generation of smaller metabolites with higher antioxidant activity than native compounds [20–22]. It is well-established that techniques using fecal inoculum are the most accurate for the study of colonic digestion, mimicking the activity of microbiota. Previous studies proposed further methods based on the use of mix of bacterial enzymes, such as Pronase E and Viscozyme L [25,36]. Pronase E contains a mix of bacterial protease, whereas Viscozyme L is a preparation containing several carbohydrases, including cellulase, arabanase, hemicellulase, β-glucanase and xylanase [25]. The combination of Pronase E and Viscozyme L reproduces the biochemical conditions physiologically occurring in the colon, simulating the action of microbiota on the digested dietary matrix [36]. According to these studies, thus, the increased bioaccessibility and antioxidant activity observed in our experimental model of colon digestion appears not so far from what may occur in vivo for the activity of gut microbiota.

The protocol herein performed to obtain the methanolic extract is not fully selective for polyphenols and, probably, further components from the food matrix may be extracted, including cell-wall polysaccharides, sugar, alcohols or amines which were not investigated in our study. We hypothesized that in our extracts a certain amount of polyphenols were present in the glycoside form, thus, not detectable through the HPLC-DAD method we used. After the in vitro GI digestion, polyphenols might be released from glucose residues by the activities of Pronase and Viscozyme, showing the increase of free polyphenols observed by both Folin-Ciocalteu and HPLC-DAD methods. This is our hypothesis to explain both relative and total increases of polyphenols in the colon stage observed through these two methods, but no further experiments were performed in order to prove it.

Although a comparison between Folin-Ciocalteu and HPLC-DAD methods was performed (Figure 2), indicating the existence of an almost overlapping trend, discrepancies are notable among the values of TPC and tea catechins chromatographically monitored. This is justified by the different approaches used. Folin-Ciocalteu is a simple and highly efficient method which quantifies TPC as gallic acid [37,38]. Several molecules, however, do not react with the Folin-Ciocalteu reagent. This is due to the absence of functional groups, including catechol moieties [39]. Folin-Ciocalteu method, thus, appears useful to approximately determine the TPC, while through HPLC-DAD selected molecules can be monitored. A heterogeneous pattern of phytochemicals may occur in food matrices, and most of them are extractable by the method we used. As indicated by Folin-Ciocalteu method, our samples have a rich phenolic profile; however, the number of catechins we monitored are limited. Data from Folin-Ciocalteu, thus, does not necessarily reflect the levels of catechins chromatographically monitored. Accordingly, during the in vitro GI digestion, polyphenols should be metabolized by the combined activity of Pronase and Viscozyme, resulting in release of smaller molecules (more reactive to Folin reagents) and which are responsible for the increased antioxidant activity. Specifically, variations in the antioxidant activity have been observed during each stages of the in vitro GI digestion. The percentage of decrease in antioxidant activity from not-digested to duodenal stage was almost similar in all samples (DPPH: −91%, −91.5% and −96% for GT, WT and BT, respectively; ABTS: −89%, −91.6% and −90.5% for GT, WT and BT, respectively). After colon digestion, the percentage of decrease followed a different trend (BT < WT < GT), suggesting that, despite the antioxidant activities of not-digested samples, colonic digestion may affect and/or improve the nutraceutical properties of single extract by enhancing its antioxidant capacity (% of decrease from not-digested to colon stage - DPPH: −60.6%, −26.1% and −18.5% for GT, WT and BT, respectively; ABTS: −66.2%, −31.5% and −9.3% for GT, WT and BT, respectively). As mentioned above, the digestion performed in our experimental model of colon would cause metabolism of native polyphenols contained in the extracts and release of both smaller molecules with higher antioxidant activity and polyphenols from components of the food matrix (i.e., cell wall polysaccharides), resulting in variations in antioxidant activities during the GI digestion. Interestingly, data obtained from both DPPH and ABTS tests correlate well with TPC values, as shown in Figure 4 (R^2 = 0.975 and 0.969, respectively). After the colon digestion, the highest percentage of decrease in TPC was observed in GT (−74.8%); this is perfectly in line with data regarding the colon antioxidant activity.

Interestingly, beside the potential role of gut microbiota in metabolism of phytochemicals, a 'two-way' relationship has been previously described between microbiota and polyphenols [40,41]. Evidences reported that polyphenols are able to modulate the gut microbiota [40–43], acting as bactericidal and bacteriostatic agents [44]. This is mainly due to the ability of polyphenols to bind bacterial membrane proteins, inhibit the glucose inward transport and complex free iron [44,45]. These effects of polyphenols on gut microbiota, however, seem to be strain-specific.

Van Duynhoven et al. [44] described a *'bifidogenic effect'* of black tea and its extract, whereas a *'prebiotic-like effect'* of polyphenols has been recently reported, showing the ability of polyphenols to favour the growth of specific bacteria, mainly beneficial strains, and reduce the incidence of pathogens [46]. Recent studies reported that GT polyphenols efficiently modulate gut microbiota composition [47,48]; in particular, a reduction of the *Bacteroidetes* to *Firmicutes* ratios was observed in mice fed with high-fat-diet after administration of GT polyphenols [47], suggesting that these phytochemicals may play a pivotal role in managing metabolic diseases through a different mechanism of action from those previously established [47,48].

5. Conclusions

In summary, our results show that, after in vitro GI digestion, tea polyphenol bioaccessibility and antioxidant activity are higher in the colon than in the duodenum, suggesting that, in vivo, the gut microbiota might be able to metabolize dietary polyphenols, resulting in an increase of their beneficial effects in the large intestine. This potential effect appears relevant considering that the large intestine is a physiological site of oxidative stress and, in certain instances, inflammation. The use of nutraceutical formulations, thus, represents a novel and useful strategy in order to vehicle a high amount of bioactive compounds to the intestine, where they can exert their beneficial effects. However, although we used an experimental model of colon, according to previous published evidence, we are conscious that our result is not sufficient to directly attribute these actions to the gut microbiota; however, they do represent a starting point for further investigations. Further studies, thus, are needed to identify the metabolites generated after microbiota metabolism in colon, and evaluate their actions on human health.

Author Contributions: Conceptualization, G.A. and M.M.; methodology, C.S., R.C., P.C., V.N.; validation, G.C.T and E.N.; formal analysis, G.A.; investigation, G.A. and M.M.; writing—original draft preparation, G.A.; writing—review and editing, G.A.; supervision, G.C.T. and E.N.

Funding: This research received no external funding.

Acknowledgments: The assistance of the staff is gratefully appreciated.

Conflicts of Interest: The authors declare no conflict of interest.

References

1. Nie, S.P.; Xie, M.Y. A review on the isolation and structure of tea polysaccharides and their bioactivities. *Food Hydrocoll.* **2011**, *25*, 144–149. [CrossRef]
2. Yang, C.S.; Zhang, J.; Zhang, L.; Huang, J.; Wang, Y. Mechanisms of body weight reduction and metabolic syndrome alleviation by tea. *Mol. Nutr. Food Res.* **2016**, *60*, 160–174. [CrossRef] [PubMed]
3. Malongane, F.; McGaw, L.J.; Mudau, F.N. The synergistic potential of various teas, herbs and therapeutic drugs in health improvement: A review. *J. Sci. Food Agric.* **2017**, *97*, 4679–4689. [CrossRef] [PubMed]
4. Curin, Y.; Andriantsitohaina, R. Polyphenols as potential therapeutical agents against cardiovascular diseases. *Pharmacol. Rep.* **2005**, *52*, 97–100.
5. Gormaz, J.G.; Valls, N.; Sotomayor, C.; Turner, T.; Rodrigo, R. Potential role of polyphenols in the prevention of cardiovascular diseases: Molecular bases. *Curr. Med. Chem.* **2016**, *23*, 115–128. [CrossRef] [PubMed]
6. Guasch-Ferré, M.; Merino, J.; Sun, Q.; Fitò, M.; Salas-Salvadò, J. Dietary polyphenols, Mediterranean Diet, prediabetes, and type 2 diabetes: A narrative review of the evidence. *Oxid. Med. Cell. Longev.* **2017**, *2017*, 6723931. [CrossRef] [PubMed]
7. Nadtochiy, S.M.; Redman, E.K. Mediterranean diet and cardioprotection: The role of nitrite, polyunsaturated fatty acids, and polyphenols. *Nutrition* **2011**, *27*, 733–744. [CrossRef] [PubMed]
8. Carluccio, M.A.; Siculella, L.; Ancora, M.A.; Massaro, M.; Scoditti, E.; Storelli, C.; Visioli, F.; Distante, A.; De Caterina, R. Olive oil and red wine antioxidant polyphenols inhibit endothelial activation: Antiatherogenic properties of Mediterranean diet phytochemicals. *Arterioscler. Thromb. Vasc. Biol.* **2003**, *23*, 622–629. [CrossRef] [PubMed]

9. Massaro, M.; Scoditti, E.; Carluccio, M.A.; De Caterina, R. Nutraceuticals and prevention of atherosclerosis: Focus on omega-3 polyunsaturated fatty acids and Mediterranean diet polyphenols. *Cardiovasc. Ther.* **2010**, *28*, e13–e19. [CrossRef] [PubMed]

10. Scoditti, E.; Capurso, C.; Capurso, A.; Massaro, M. Vascular effects of the Mediterranean diet-part II: Role of omega-3 fatty acids and olive oil polyphenols. *Vascul. Pharmacol.* **2014**, *63*, 127–134. [CrossRef] [PubMed]

11. Cory, H.; Passarelli, S.; Szeto, J.; Tamez, M.; Mattei, J. The Role of Polyphenols in Human Health and Food Systems: A Mini-Review. *Front Nutr.* **2018**, *5*, 87. [CrossRef] [PubMed]

12. Tenore, G.C.; Stiuso, P.; Campiglia, P.; Novellino, E. In vitro hypoglycaemic and hypolipidemic potential of white tea polyphenols. *Food Chem.* **2013**, *141*, 2379–2384. [CrossRef] [PubMed]

13. Tenore, G.C.; Daglia, M.; Ciampaglia, R.; Novellino, E. Exploring the nutraceutical potential of polyphenols from black, green and white tea infusion—An overview. *Curr. Pharm. Biotechnol.* **2015**, *16*, 265–271. [CrossRef] [PubMed]

14. Tenore, G.C.; Campiglia, P.; Giannetti, D.; Novellino, E. Simulated gastrointestinal digestion, intestinal permeation and plasma protein interaction of white, green, and black tea polyphenols. *Food Chem.* **2015**, *169*, 320–326. [CrossRef] [PubMed]

15. Peters, C.M.; Green, R.J.; Janle, E.M.; Ferruzzi, M.G. Formulation with ascorbic acid and sucrose modulates catechin bioavailability from green tea. *Food Res. Int.* **2010**, *43*, 95–102. [CrossRef] [PubMed]

16. Jilania, H.; Cilla, A.; Barberá, R.; Hamdia, M. Biosorption of green and black tea polyphenols into Saccharomyces cerevisiae improves their bioaccessibility. *J. Funct. Foods* **2015**, *17*, 11–21. [CrossRef]

17. Dubeau, S.; Samson, G.; Tajmir-Riahi, H.A. Dual effect of milk on the antioxidant capacity of green, Darjeeling, and English breakfast teas. *Food Chem.* **2010**, *122*, 539–545. [CrossRef]

18. Ye, J.; Fan, F.; Xu, X.; Liang, Y. Interactions of black and green tea polyphenols with whole milk. *Food Res. Int.* **2013**, *53*, 449–455. [CrossRef]

19. Coe, S.; Fraser, A.; Ryan, L. Polyphenol Bioaccessibility and Sugar Reducing Capacity of Black, Green, and White Teas. *Int. J. Food Sci.* **2013**, *2013*, 238216. [CrossRef] [PubMed]

20. Han, X.; Shen, T.; Lou, H. Dietary polyphenols and their biological significance. *Int. J. Mol. Sci.* **2007**, *8*, 950–988. [CrossRef]

21. Stevens, J.K.; Maier, C.S. The chemistry of gut microbial metabolism of polyphenols. *Phytochem. Rev.* **2016**, *15*, 425–444. [CrossRef] [PubMed]

22. Tomás-Barberán, F.A.; Selma, M.V.; Espín, J.C. Interactions of gut microbiota with dietary polyphenols and consequences to human health. *Curr. Opin. Clin. Nutr. Metab. Care* **2016**, *19*, 471–476. [CrossRef] [PubMed]

23. Raiola, A.; Meca, G.; Mañes, J.; Ritieni, A. Bioaccessibility of deoxynivalenol and its natural co-occurrence with ochratoxin A and aflatoxin B1 in Italian commercial pasta. *Food Chem. Toxicol.* **2012**, *50*, 280–287. [CrossRef] [PubMed]

24. Tenore, G.C.; Campiglia, P.; Ritieni, A.; Novellino, E. In vitro bioaccessibility, bioavailability and plasma protein interaction of polyphenols from Annurca apple (M. pumila Miller cv Annurca). *Food Chem.* **2013**, *141*, 3519–3524. [CrossRef] [PubMed]

25. Papillo, V.A.; Vitaglione, P.; Graziani, G.; Gokmen, V.; Fogliano, V. Release of antioxidant capacity from five plant foods during a multistep enzymatic digestion protocol. *J. Agric. Food Chem.* **2014**, *62*, 4119–4126. [CrossRef] [PubMed]

26. Di Lorenzo, A.; Nabavi, S.F.; Sureda, A.; Moghaddam, A.H.; Khanjani, S.; Arcidiaco, P.; Nabavi, S.M.; Daglia, M. Antidepressive-like effects and antioxidant activity of green tea and GABA green tea in a mouse model of post-stroke depression. *Mol. Nutr. Food Res.* **2015**, *60*, 566–579. [CrossRef] [PubMed]

27. Zuo, Y.; Chen, H.; Deng, Y. Simultaneous determination of catechins, caffeine and gallic acids in green, Oolong, black and pu-erh teas using HPLC with a photodiode array detector. *Talanta* **2002**, *57*, 307–316. [CrossRef]

28. Brand-Williams, W.; Cuvelier, M.E.; Berset, C. Use of free radical method to evaluate antioxidant activity. *LWT-Food Sci. Technol.* **1995**, *28*, 25–30. [CrossRef]

29. Rufino, M.S.M.; Alves, R.E.; de Brito, E.S.; Perez-Jimenez, J.; Saura-Calixto, F.D.; Mancini-Filho, J. Bioactive compounds and antioxidant capacities of eighteen non-traditional tropical fruits from Brazil. *Food Chem.* **2010**, *121*, 996–1002. [CrossRef]

30. Minekus, M.; Alminger, M.; Alvito, P.; Balance, S.; Bohn, T.; Bourlieu, C.; Carrière, F.; Boutrou, R.; Corredig, M.; Dupont, D. A standardised static in vitro digestion method suitable for food—An international consensus. *Food Funct.* **2014**, *5*, 1113–1124. [CrossRef] [PubMed]

31. Liu, A.B.; Tao, S.; Lee, M.J.; Hu, Q.; Meng, X.; Lin, Y.; Yang, C.S. Effects of gut microbiota and time of treatment on tissue levels of green tea polyphenols in mice. *Biofactors* **2018**. [CrossRef] [PubMed]

32. Pasinetti, G.M.; Singh, R.; Westfall, S.; Herman, F.; Faith, J.; Ho, L. The Role of the Gut Microbiota in the Metabolism of Polyphenols as Characterized by Gnotobiotic Mice. *J. Alzheimers Dis.* **2018**, *63*, 409–421. [CrossRef] [PubMed]

33. Masisi, K.; Beta, T.; Moghadasian, M.H. Antioxidant properties of diverse cereal grains: A review on in vitro and in vivo studies. *Food Chem.* **2016**, *196*, 90–97. [CrossRef] [PubMed]

34. Rasmussen, S.E.; Frederiksen, H.; Struntze Krogholm, K.; Poulsen, L. Dietary proanthocyanidins: Occurrence, dietary intake, bioavailability, and protection against cardiovascular disease. *Mol. Nutr. Food Res.* **2005**, *49*, 159–174. [CrossRef] [PubMed]

35. Chandrasekara, A.; Shahidi, F. Bioaccessibility and antioxidant potential of millet grain phenolics as affected by simulated in vitro digestion and microbial fermentation. *J. Funct. Foods* **2012**, *4*, 226–237. [CrossRef]

36. Fogliano, V.; Corollaro, M.L.; Vitaglione, P.; Napolitano, A.; Ferracane, R.; Travaglia, F.; Arlorio, M.; Costabile, A.; Klinder, A.; Gibson, G. In vitro bioaccessibility and gut biotransformation of polyphenols present in the water-insoluble cocoa fraction. *Mol. Nutr. Food Res.* **2011**, *55*, S44–S55. [CrossRef] [PubMed]

37. Rosenblat, M.; Volkova, N.; Coleman, R.; Almagor, Y.; Aviram, M. Antiatherogenicity of extra virgin olive oil and its enrichment with green tea polyphenols in the atherosclerotic apolipoprotein-E-deficient mice: Enhanced macrophage cholesterol efflux. *J. Nutr. Biochem.* **2008**, *19*, 514–523. [CrossRef] [PubMed]

38. Gimeno, E.; Castellote, A.I.; Lamuela-Raventós, R.M.; De la Torre, M.C.; López-Sabater, M.C. The effects of harvest and extraction methods on the antioxidant content (phenolics, α-tocopherol, and β-carotene) in virgin olive oil. *Food Chem.* **2002**, *78*, 207–211. [CrossRef]

39. Alessandri, S.; Ieri, F.; Romani, A. Minor polar compounds in extra virgin olive oil: Correlation between HPLC-DAD-MS and the Folin-Ciocalteu spectrophotometric method. *J. Agric. Food Chem.* **2014**, *62*, 826–835. [CrossRef] [PubMed]

40. Nash, V.; Ranadheera, C.S.; Georgousopoulou, E.N.; Mellor, D.D.; Panagiotakos, D.B.; McKune, A.J.; Kellett, J.; Naumovski, N. The effects of grape and red wine polyphenols on gut microbiota—A systematic review. *Food Res. Int.* **2018**, *113*, 277–287. [CrossRef] [PubMed]

41. Cardona, F.; Andrés-Lacueva, C.; Tulipani, S.; Tinahones, F.J.; Queipo-Ortuño, M.I. Benefits of polyphenols on gut microbiota and implications in human health. *J. Nutr. Biochem.* **2013**, *24*, 1415–1422. [CrossRef] [PubMed]

42. Duda-Chodak, A.; Tarko, T.; Satora, P.; Sroka, P. Interaction of dietary compounds, especially polyphenols, with the intestinal microbiota: A review. *Eur. J. Nutr.* **2015**, *54*, 325–341. [CrossRef] [PubMed]

43. Hervert-Hernández, D.; Goñi, I. Dietary Polyphenols and Human Gut Microbiota: A Review. *Food Rev. Int.* **2011**, *27*, 154–169. [CrossRef]

44. Van Duynhoven, J.; Vaughan, E.E.; van Dorsten, F.; Gomez-Roldan, V.; de Vos, R.; Vervoort, J.; van der Hooft, J.J.; Roger, L.; Draijer, R.; Jacobs, D.M. Interactions of black tea polyphenols with human gut microbiota: Implications for gut and cardiovascular health. *Am. J. Clin. Nutr.* **2013**, *98*, 1631S–1641S. [CrossRef] [PubMed]

45. Daglia, M. Polyphenols as antimicrobial agents. *Curr. Opin. Biotechnol.* **2012**, *23*, 174–181. [CrossRef] [PubMed]

46. Filosa, S.; Di Meo, F.; Crispi, S. Polyphenols-gut microbiota interplay and brain neuromodulation. *Neural Regen. Res.* **2018**, *13*, 2055–2059. [CrossRef] [PubMed]

47. Wang, L.; Zeng, B.; Liu, Z.; Liao, Z.; Zhong, Q.; Gu, L.; Wei, H.; Fang, X. Green Tea Polyphenols Modulate Colonic Microbiota Diversity and Lipid Metabolism in High-Fat Diet Treated HFA Mice. *J. Food Sci.* **2018**, *83*, 864–873. [CrossRef] [PubMed]

48. Zhou, J.; Tang, L.; Shen, C.L.; Wang, J.S. Green tea polyphenols modify gut-microbiota dependent metabolisms of energy, bile constituents and micronutrients in female Sprague-Dawley rats. *J. Nutr. Biochem.* **2018**, *61*, 68–81. [CrossRef] [PubMed]

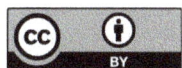

nutrients

MDPI

Article

Rosmarinic Acid, a Component of Rosemary Tea, Induced the Cell Cycle Arrest and Apoptosis through Modulation of HDAC2 Expression in Prostate Cancer Cell Lines

Yin-Gi Jang, Kyung-A Hwang and Kyung-Chul Choi *

Laboratory of Biochemistry and Immunology, College of Veterinary Medicine, Chungbuk National University, Cheongju 28644, Chungbuk, Korea; mingue32@naver.com (Y.-G.J.); hka9400@naver.com (K.-A.H.)
* Correspondence: kchoi@cbu.ac.kr; Tel.: +82-43-261-3664; Fax: +82-43-267-3150

Received: 13 October 2018; Accepted: 15 November 2018; Published: 16 November 2018

Abstract: Rosmarinic acid (RA), a main phenolic compound contained in rosemary which is used as tea, oil, medicine and so on, has been known to present anti-inflammatory, anti-oxidant and anti-cancer effects. Histone deacetylases (HDACs) are enzymes that play important roles in gene expression by removing the acetyl group from histone. The aberrant expression of HDAC in human tumors is related with the onset of human cancer. Especially, HDAC2, which belongs to HDAC class I composed of HDAC 1, 2, 3 and 8, has been reported to be highly expressed in prostate cancer (PCa) where it downregulates the expression of p53, resulting in an inhibition of apoptosis. The purpose of this study is to investigate the effect of RA in comparison with suberoylanilide hydroxamic acid (SAHA), an HDAC inhibitor used as an anti-cancer agent, on survival and apoptosis of PCa cell lines, PC-3 and DU145, and the expression of HDAC. RA decreased the cell proliferation in cell viability assay, and inhibited the colony formation and tumor spheroid formation. Additionally, RA induced early- and late-stage apoptosis of PC-3 and DU145 cells in Annexin V assay and terminal deoxynucleotidyl transferase dUTP nick end labeling (TUNEL) assay, respectively. In western blot analysis, RA inhibited the expression of HDAC2, as SAHA did. Proliferating cell nuclear antigen (PCNA), cyclin D1 and cyclin E1 were downregulated by RA, whereas p21 was upregulated. In addition, RA modulated the protein expression of intrinsic mitochondrial apoptotic pathway-related genes, such as Bax, Bcl-2, caspase-3 and poly (ADP-ribose) polymerase 1 (*PARP-1*) (cleaved) via the upregulation of p53 derived from HDAC2 downregulation, leading to the increased apoptosis of PC-3 and DU145 cells. Taken together, treatment of RA to PCa cell lines inhibits the cell survival and induces cell apoptosis, and it can be used as a novel therapeutic agent toward PCa.

Keywords: Rosmarinic acid; suberoylanilide hydroxamic acid (SAHA); histone deacetylase 2 (HDAC2); p53; cell cycle arrest and apoptosis

---

1. Introduction

Phenolic compounds found in tea are known to have anti-oxidant and anti-cancer effects [1]. Rosmarinic acid (RA) is a main phenolic compound in *Rosmarinus officinalis* L. (called rosemary) which is a common herb cultivated in many parts of the world and has been consumed as tea, oil, medicine and so on [2,3]. Previous studies on RA have reported its biological effects such as anti-inflammation [4], anti-diabetes [5] and especially anti-cancer effect against colorectal [6], gastric [7], ovarian [8], skin [9], liver [10] and breast cancer [11].

Prostate cancer (PCa) is the most leading type of cancer occurring in men and the second most common cause of cancer-related death worldwide [12]. Though chemotherapies, such as docetaxel, cabazitaxel, doxorubicin, mitoxantrone, and estramustine, have been used in treatment of PCa, these chemotherapies have some adverse side effects such as hair loss, nausea, vomiting, and fatigue [13]. Moreover, using the chemotherapeutic drugs in the long term allows aggressive PCa cells to experience mutations in the gene of beta-tubulin and activation of drug efflux pumps, leading to increased survival and the drug resistance [14–16].

Histone deacetylases (HDACs) are enzymes that play important roles in gene expression by removing the acetyl group from histone [17,18]. Based on their sequence homology, HDACs are classified into four classes such as class I (HDAC1, 2, 3 and 8), class II (HDAC4, 5, 6, 7, 9 and 10) and class IV (HDAC11) [19]. A number of studies related with HDACs have proved that the aberrant expression of HDAC is related with the onset of human cancer [20]. In diverse types of cancers, such as prostate [21], colorectal [22], breast [23], lung [24], liver [25] and gastric cancer [26], overexpression of HDACs is associated with a poor cancer prognosis and disease outcome, and can help to predict the tumor type and disease progression. Furthermore, the overexpression of HDACs has been highly associated with critical cancer-related phenomena such as the epigenetic repression of tumor suppressor genes like CDKN1A (encoding the cyclin-dependent kinase inhibitor p21) [27,28], and p53 resulting in its decreased transcriptional activity [29], and upregulation of oncogenes such as B-cell lymphoma-2 (BCL-2) [30]. Especially, high expression of HDAC2 which belongs to HDAC class I is observed in human epithelial cancer such as PCa, and downregulation of HDAC2 is related with growth arrest and apoptosis of PCa [21]. HDAC inhibitors, as a new class of anti-tumor agents, such as trichostatin A (TSA), suberoylanilide hydroxamic acid (SAHA), valproic acid, depsipeptide and sodium butyrate, are useful for the downregulation and inhibition of cancer growth [31,32].

The recent studies regarding the therapeutic properties of RA have shown that RA inhibits the cell proliferation via induction of the cell cycle arrest and apoptosis in colorectal cancer [6]. However, the detailed mechanisms underlying anti-cancer effects of RA on PCa has been not yet known. Therefore, based on the previous studies, we investigated the anti-PCa mechanisms of RA in association with its activity regulating HDAC2 expression. The abilities of RA to induce cell cycle arrest and apoptosis of PCa cells through HDAC inhibition were also identified in comparison with SAHA, a chemical inhibitor of HDAC2. By doing this, we examined the anti-PCa potential of RA as a novel phytochemical that can be substituted for the existing chemotherapeutic drugs including HDAC inhibitors.

2. Materials and Methods

2.1. Reagents and Chemicals

SAHA was purchased from Santa Cruz Biotechnology (Dallas, TX, USA) and RA (≥98% (HPLC)) was purchased from Sigma-Aldrich (St. Louis, MO, USA). All chemicals were dissolved in 100% dimethyl sulfoxide (DMSO, Junsei Chemical Co., Tokyo, Japan) which was used as a negative control (NC) and stocked at 10^{-1} M.

2.2. Cell Culture and Media

The human PCa cell lines, PC-3 and DU145, were purchased from the Korean Cell Line Bank (Seoul, Korea). Both cell lines were cultured using a medium (DMEM, HyClone Laboratories, Chicago, IL, USA) supplemented with 10% fetal bovine serum (FBS; RMBIO, Missoula, MT, USA), 1% penicillin G/streptomycin (Bio west, San Marcos, TX, USA), 1% HEPES (Gibco by Life Technologies, Gaithersburg, MD, USA) and 0.05% cell maxin (GenDEPOT, Katy, TX, USA) in cell culture dishes (SPL Life Science, Pocheon, Korea) at 37 °C in a humidified atmosphere containing 95% air and 5% CO_2. Both cell lines were detached by using 0.05% Trypsin-EDTA (Gibco by Life Technologies, Gaithersburg, MD, USA).

2.3. Cell Viability Assay

Cell viability assay was performed to find the proper concentrations of SAHA and RA to inhibit viability of PCa cells. Both cell lines were seeded at 1×10^4 cells per well in 96-well plates (SPL Life Science) in a humidified atmosphere of 5% CO_2 at 37 °C. After the cells were incubated with medium for 24 h, the medium containing DMSO, SAHA (1, 2.5, 5, 10, 25 and 50 µM) and RA (25, 50, 100, 200, 250 and 300 µM) were treated for 48 h. Cell viability was determined using a EZ-Cytox cell viability assay kit (iTSBiO, Seoul, Korea). The medium in 96-well plates was gently removed, and then, EZ-Cytox reagent was dispensed to each well and incubated for 1 h under the standard cell culture condition. At last, 96-well plates were gently shaken and the absorbance at 450 nm of each well was measured by using an ELISA reader (Epoch, BioTek, Winooski, VT, USA).

2.4. Colonogenic Survival Assay

Colonogenic assay or colony formation assay is normally performed to estimate the in vitro cell survival activity based on the ability of single cells to grow into a colony [33–35]. Both cell lines were seeded at 5×10^3 cells per well in 6-well plates (SPL Life Science) for 24 h, and then, the medium containing DMSO, SAHA (1 µM) and RA (200 µM) were added into plates and incubated for 2 weeks. Each medium was replaced every 4 days. After 2 weeks, all cells were fixed with 4% methanol-free formalin (Sigma-Aldrich) for 10 min and permeabilized with methanol (Sigma-Aldrich) for 10 min. After that, cells were stained with 0.5% crystal violet (hexamethylpararosaniline chloride; Sigma-Aldrich) for 10 min, and then washed with Dulbecco's Phosphate-Buffered Saline (DPBS, WELGENE, Gyeongsan, Korea). The attached cells stained with crystal violet were pictured by using the camera (Samsung, Seoul, Korea) and counted by using the Image J program (National Institutes of Health, Bethesda, MD, USA).

2.5. Hanging Drop Assay Detecting for Tumor Spheroid Formation

Hanging drop assay allows for the formation of spheroid shaped tumors by self-assembly of tumor colonies, which can be used to evaluate chemotherapeutic drugs in a biological environment closer to in vivo models [36,37]. Both cell lines in media containing DMSO, SAHA (1 µM) and RA (200 µM) were seeded on petri dish covers (SPL Life Science) at 3×10^3 cells in 25 µL each medium by using a multi-pipette to form spheroids. After a week, the droplets were gently gathered in 6-well plates (SPL Life Science) and photographed by using the IX-73 inverted microscope (Olympus, Tokyo, Japan). The size of tumor spheroids in each droplet was measured by using the Image J program (National Institutes of Health).

2.6. Annexin V Assay

Firstly, to confirm whether SAHA and RA are effective to induce early and late apoptosis, Annexin V assay was performed following the protocol of Alexa Fluor 488 annexin V/Dead Cell Apoptosis kit (Invitrogen, Carlsbad, CA, USA). Concisely, both cell lines were seeded in cell culture dishes at 7×10^5 cells/10 mL for 24 h and cultured in medium containing DMSO, SAHA (1 µM) and RA (200 µM) for 48 h. Then, cells of each group were detached by trypsin and centrifuged. The cells were placed in $1\times$ annexin-binding buffer containing Alexa Fluor 488 annexin V (Alexa), propidium iodide (PI) and Alexa + PI under dark condition at room temperature for 15 min. The apoptotic cells at each stage were analyzed by using the flow cytometry (Sony SH800 Cell sorter, Tokyo, Japan).

2.7. TUNEL Assay

To examine whether SAHA and RA affect DNA fragmentation occurring at a stage of late apoptosis, TUNEL assay was performed by using a DeadEnd™ fluorometric terminal deoxynucleotidyl transferase (TdT)-mediated deoxyuridine triphosphate (dUTP) nick-end labeling (TUNEL) system (Promega, Madison, WI, USA) following the manufacturer instructions. Both cell lines were seeded at 3×10^5 cells per well in 24-well plates with media and incubated for 24 h. Next day, the medium containing DMSO, SAHA (1 μM) and RA (200 μM) were added into plates. After treatment for 48 h, the cells were fixed with 4% methanol-free formalin (Sigma-Aldrich) for 25 min at 4 °C, and washed by DPBS for 5 min. Permeabilization was done by using a lysis buffer (1% Triton X-100 in 1% sodium citrate) for 5 min, and then treated with 50 μL TdT enzyme buffers composed of equilibration buffer, nucleotide mix and rTdT enzyme which were bound to DNA strand breaks. Finally, labeled strand breaks were confirmed through the attachment of fluorescein isothiocyanate-5-dUTP. After staining apoptotic cells with TUNEL assay kit, every well was counterstained with a 4, 6-diamidino-2-phenylindole (DAPI; Invitrogen) and observed by using a fluorescence microscope (IX-73 Inverted Microscopy, Olympus). The apoptotic activity of SAHA and RA on PC3-3 and DU145 cells was quantified and analyzed using the Cell Sens Dimension software 1.13 (Build 13479, Olympus).

2.8. Western Blot Analysis

To determine the protein expression of HDAC2 and of genes involved in cell cycle and apoptosis regulation, western blot analysis was performed. Both cell lines were seeded at 1×10^6 in cell culture dishes for 24 h and treated with DMSO, SAHA (1 μM) and RA (200 μM) for 48 h. Then, whole cell lysates were prepared by RIPA buffer which was composed of 50 mM Tris, 150 mM NaCl, 1% Triton X-100 (Sigma-Aldrich), 0.5% deoxycholic acid (Sigma-Aldrich), and 0.1% SDS and protease inhibitor (GenDEPOT, Katy, TX, USA). Total proteins that were extracted from the cell lysates were quantified using bicinchoninic acid (BCA; Sigma-Aldrich). Protein mixtures (protein, distilled water (DW) and dye) were then loaded and separated in SDS-polyacrylamide gel electrophoresis (SDS-PAGE), and then transferred to polyvinylidene difluoride (PVDF) membranes (Bio-Rad, Hercules, CA, USA). Finally, the membranes were blocked in 5% skim milk (Blotting-Grade Blocker; Bio-Rad) for an hour at 4 °C on a shaker. The membranes were incubated overnight at 4 °C in BCA containing primary antibodies shown in Table 1. Washing steps were performed by using 1X Tris-buffered saline Tween (TBS-T; 50 mM Tris and 150 mM NaCl with 0.1% Tween 20 (GenDEPOT), pH: 7.6). Primary antibodies bound to membrane were detected with horse radish peroxidase (HRP)-conjugated anti-mouse IgG or anti-rabbit IgG (1:2000, Thermo Scientific, Waltham, MA, USA) incubated for 2 h at room temperature. Targeted bands were detected by using the Ez west-Lumi plus (ATTO, Tokyo, Japan) and Lumino graph II (ATTO). The expression levels were quantified and normalized by using the CS Analyzer4 (ATTO).

Table 1. Information of antibodies used in this study.

Antibody Name	Company	Description	Dilution
HDAC2	Santa cruz (Dallas, TX, USA)	Mouse monoclonal	1:1000
p53			1:200
PARP-1 (cleaved)			1:200
Caspase-3	Flarebio (College Park, Maryland)	Rabbit polyclonal	1:1000
PCNA		Mouse monoclonal	1:10,000
Cyclin D1		Mouse monoclonal	1:2000
Cyclin E1	Abcam	Rabbit polyclonal	1:2000
Bax	(Cambridge, UK)	Mouse monoclonal	1:1000
Bcl-2		Mouse monoclonal	1:1000
GAPDH		Mouse monoclonal	1:12,000

HDAC2: histone deacetylase 2; PCNA: proliferating cell nuclear antigen; PARP-1: poly (ADP-ribose) polymerase 1; GAPDH: glyceraldehyde-3-phosphate dehydrogenase.

2.9. Statistical Analysis

All experiments were conducted at least three times, and all data were statistically analyzed with the Graph-pad Prism software (Graph-pad software Inc, San Diego, CA, USA). Data were expressed as the means ± standard deviation (SD) and analyzed by one-way analysis of variance (ANOVA) followed by Dunnett's multiple comparison test. *p*-Values of <0.05 indicates statistical difference versus control.

3. Results

3.1. RA Decreased the Viability of PCa Cell Lines in a Dose-Dependent Manner

To select the inhibition concentrations of SAHA and RA on PCa cell viability, the cell viability assay was done in PC-3 and DU145 cells. The culture medium containing 0.2% DMSO was used as NC because the same concentration of DMSO was employed as a vehicle to dissolve SAHA or RA. SAHA and RA were administered to both cell lines for 48 h and the cell viability of PCa cells was confirmed by Water Soluble Tetrazolium (WST) salt assay. As a result, SAHA significantly decreased the cell viability of both cell lines in a dose-dependent manner in the concentration range tested (1–50 μM) (Figure 1A). For RA, it slightly decreased cell viability of both cell lines at 25, 50, and 100 μM, but significantly inhibited cell viability (>50%) at the concentrations of higher than 200 μM (Figure 1B). Based on these results, 1 μM SAHA and 200 μM RA were selected for further experiments.

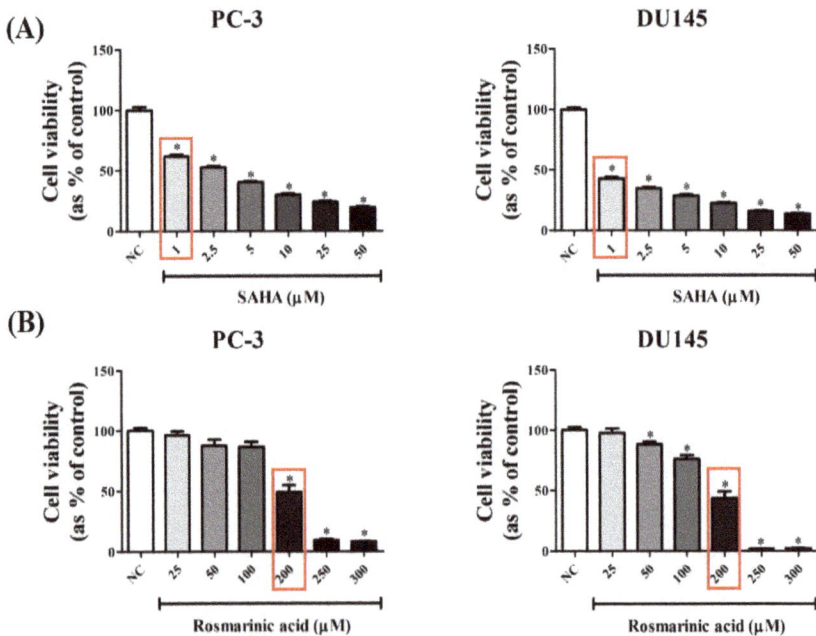

Figure 1. Effects of suberoylanilide hydroxamic acid (SAHA) and Rosmarinic acid (RA) on cell viability in PC-3 and DU145 cell lines. After PC-3 and DU145, cell lines were seeded at 1×10^4 cells per well in 96-well plates and treated with media containing negative control (NC; DMSO), SAHA (1, 2.5, 5, 10, 25, 50 μM) and RA (25, 50, 100, 200, 250, 300 μM), cell viability of each cell line was evaluated. The data showed (**A**) the effect of SAHA and (**B**) the effect of RA on cell viability of both cell lines. The results are expressed as means ± standard deviation (SD). * *p* < 0.05: a significant difference versus control.

3.2. RA Inhibited the Formation of Colonies of PCa Cell Lines

The inhibition ability of RA against PCa cell survival was confirmed by colony formation assay. After treatment with NC (DMSO), SAHA and RA for 2 weeks, colonies formed by each cell line were stained and quantified. The results showed a high number of colonies in NC, but only few colonies in SAHA and RA treatments as the almost cells were dead (Figure 2A). According to these results, SAHA and RA significantly inhibited the formation of colonies. It was shown that RA considerably decreased the survival activity of PCa cell lines, as SAHA did.

In addition to colony formation assay, hanging drop assay was conducted to examine the effects of SAHA and RA on tumor spheroid formation of PCa cells. The results showed that the larger tumor spheroids were formed in NC, while small-size spheroids were detected in SAHA and RA treatments. The inhibition effect of SAHA and RA on tumor spheroid formation was more conspicuous for PC-3 than for DU145 (Figure 2C,D). Referring to the results of tumor spheroid formation assay, RA effectively interrupted 3 dimensional (3D) tumor formation of PCa cells, as SAHA did.

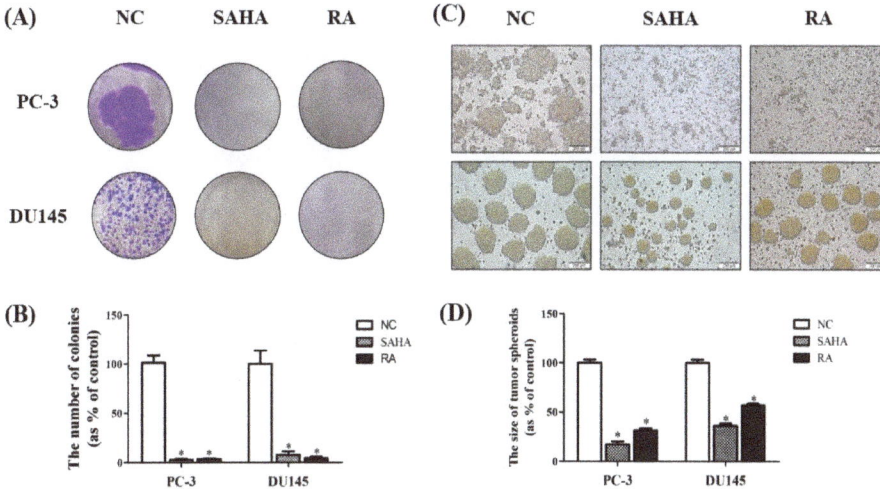

Figure 2. Effects of SAHA and RA on formation of colonies and tumor spheroids in PC-3 and DU145 cell lines. (**A**) After both cell lines were seeded at 5×10^3 cells per well in 6-well plates and treated with media containing NC (DMSO), SAHA (1 µM) and RA (200 µM), colonogenic assay was performed to measure the colony formation. (**B**) The number of colonies was quantified by using the Image J program. (**C**) Both cell lines in media containing NC (DMSO), SAHA (1 µM) and RA (200 µM) were seeded on petri dish covers at 3×10^3 cells in 25 µL. (**D**) The size of tumor spheroids was measured by using the Image J program. The results are expressed as means ± SD. * $p < 0.05$: a significant difference versus control.

3.3. RA Induced Apoptosis in PCa Cell Lines

To check which phase of apoptosis is mainly induced by RA, Annexin V assay was performed after treatment with NC, SAHA and RA. In this assay, the protein Annexin V detects early and late stages of apoptosis. The cells undergoing apoptosis or not are detected by flow cytometry and divided into 4 groups (Q1, Q2, Q3 and Q4), which indicate necrosis (Annexin V-negative/PI-positive), late apoptosis (Annexin V-positive/PI-positive), live state (Annexin V-negative/PI-negative) and early apoptosis (Annexin V-positive/PI-negative). The results showed that RA mainly increased the number of cells in late apoptosis and necrosis, while SAHA mainly increased the number of cells in early apoptosis in DU-145 cells. For PC-3 cells, RA increased the number of early apoptotic cells, and SAHA increased the number of late apoptotic cells compared to NC (Figure 3).

3.4. RA Induced the DNA Fragmentation in PCa Cell Lines

To investigate whether RA is effective in DNA fragmentation related with induction of late apoptosis, compared to SAHA in PC-3 and DU145 cell lines, TUNEL assay was performed after treatment with NC, SAHA and RA. Cell nuclei were stained in blue with DAPI, and DNA fragmentation occurring in apoptotic cells was detected as green fluorescence by TUNEL. As shown in Figure 4, apoptotic cells were rarely detected in NC, but in case of SAHA and RA treatment, the apoptotic cells observed by DNA fragmentation were significantly increased in comparison with NC in both cell lines (Figure 4).

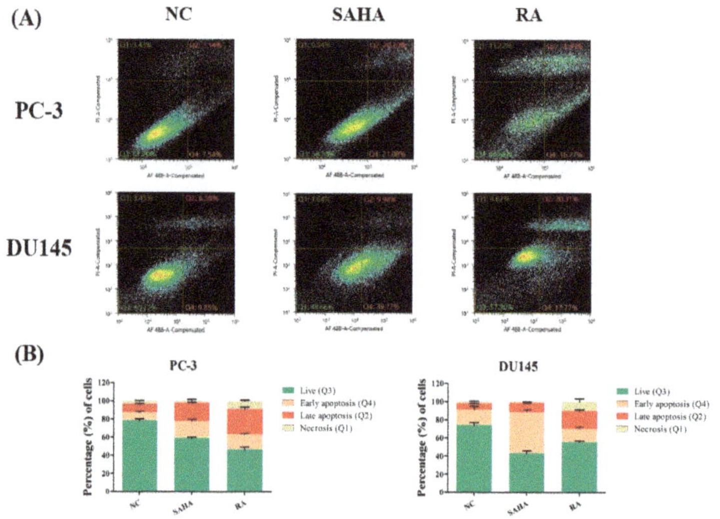

Figure 3. Effects of SAHA and RA on the apoptotic events in PC-3 and DU145 cell lines. (**A**) After both cell lines were seeded at 7×10^5 cells in cell culture dishes and treated with media containing NC (DMSO), SAHA (1 μM) and RA (200 μM), Annexin V assay was conducted. (**B**) The apoptotic cells at each stage were analyzed and quantified by using the flow cytometry. Q1, Q2, Q3 and Q4 indicate necrosis, late apoptosis, live and early apoptosis, respectively.

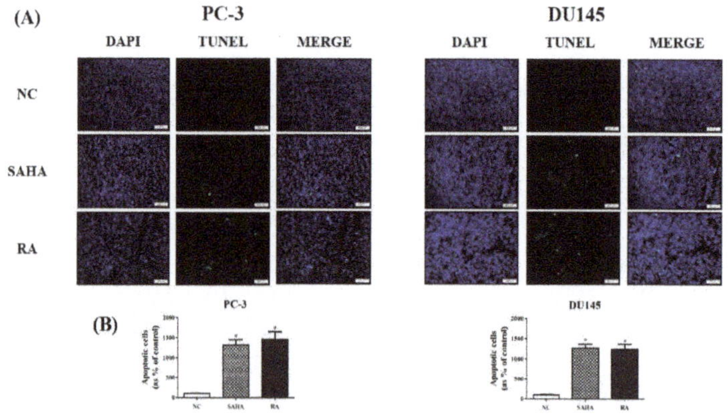

Figure 4. Effects of SAHA and RA on DNA fragmentation in PC-3 and DU145 cell lines. After both cell lines were seeded at 3×10^5 cells per well in 24-well plates and treated with media containing NC (DMSO), SAHA (1 μM) and RA (200 μM), terminal deoxynucleotidyl transferase dUTP nick end labeling (TUNEL) assay was performed. (**A**) The data indicated that nuclei were stained with 4′,6-diamidino-2-phenylindole (DAPI), and DNA fragmentation was stained with TUNEL. DAPI and TUNEL were merged to observe apoptotic nuclei. (**B**) The apoptotic cells presenting DNA fragmentation were quantified separately. The results are expressed as means ± SD. * $p < 0.05$: a significant difference versus control. MERGE means the combined picture of DAPI and TUNEL pictures.

3.5. RA Downregulated the Expression of HDAC2 and p53 in PCa Cell Lines

To confirm the effects of RA on HDAC2 and p53 expression at the protein level, western blot analysis was performed. As shown in Figure 5, RA significantly reduced the protein expression of HDAC2, similarly to SAHA in PC-3 cells, by half as much as SAHA in DU145 cells. In case of p53, RA significantly increased its protein expression in both cell lines, and SAHA significantly increased the p53 expression only in PC-3 cells, but decreased its expression in DU145 cells as compared to NC. These data suggested that RA effectively reduced the protein expression of HDAC2 and p53 in both PCa cell lines. For SAHA, it displayed a similar result to that of RA in PC-3 cells, but a significant decrease of p53 in DU145, although it apparently decreased the HDAC2 protein expression (Figure 5).

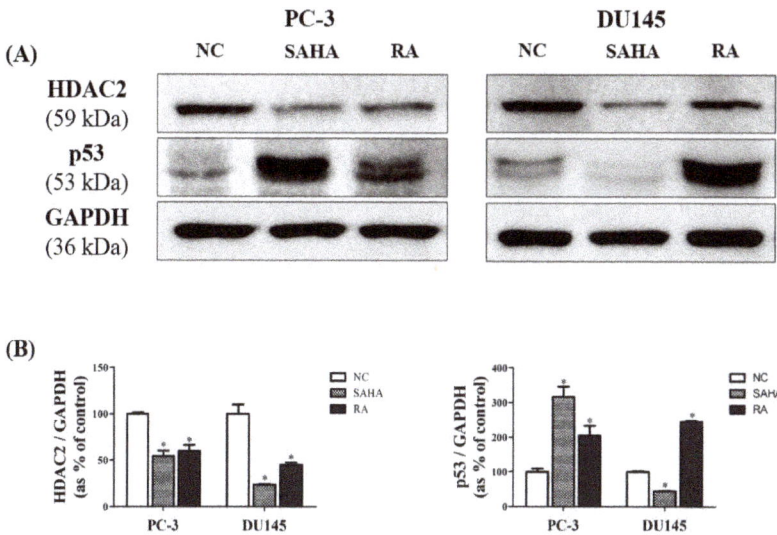

Figure 5. Effects of SAHA and RA on expression of histone deacetylase 2 (HDAC2) and p53 in PC-3 and DU145 cell lines. After both cell lines were seeded at 1×10^6 in cell culture dishes and treated with media containing NC (DMSO), SAHA (1 μM) and RA (200 μM), the western blot analysis was performed. (**A**) The expressions of HDAC2 and p53 at the protein level were confirmed by western blot analysis. (**B**) The expression levels of HDAC2 and p53 were quantified and normalized to glyceraldehyde-3-phosphate dehydrogenase (GAPDH). The results are expressed as means ± SD. * $p < 0.05$: a significant difference versus control.

3.6. RA Regulated the Expression of Cell Cycle-Related Genes in PCa Cell Lines

To further confirm the mechanisms related with modulation of HDAC2 and p53 by RA treatment, western blot analysis pertaining to the expression of cell cycle-related genes was done. Based on these results, RA significantly increased the expression of p21 only in PC-3 cells, but there was no change in DU145 cells. Despite this situation, RA significantly decreased the expression of cell cycle-related genes, such as *PCNA*, cyclin D1 and cyclin E1 in both cell lines, as SAHA did. These data suggested that RA inhibited the cell proliferation via the induction of cell cycle arrest, similar to SAHA (Figure 6).

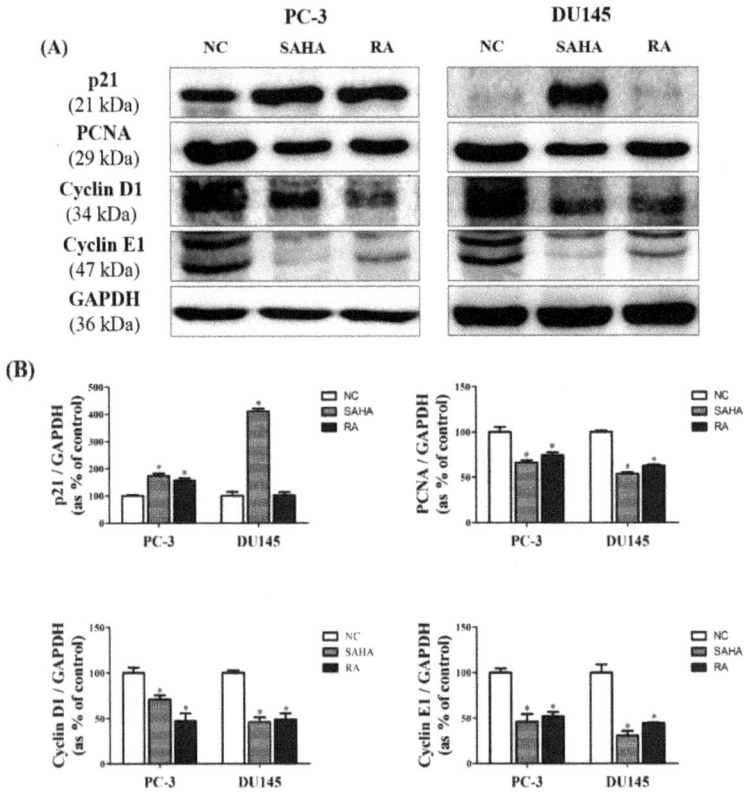

Figure 6. Effects of SAHA and RA on expression of cell cycle related genes in PC-3 and DU145 cell lines. After both cell lines were seeded at 1×10^6 in cell culture dishes and treated with media containing NC (DMSO), SAHA (1 μM) and RA (200 μM), the western blot analysis was performed. (**A**) The expressions of p21, proliferating cell nuclear antigen (PCNA), cyclin D1 and cyclin E1 at the protein level were confirmed by western blot analysis. (**B**) The expression levels of each gene were quantified and normalized to GAPDH. The results are expressed as means ± SD. * $p < 0.05$: a significant difference versus control.

3.7. RA Regulated the Expression of Apoptosis-Related Genes in PCa Cell Lines

The protein expression of genes related with apoptosis was confirmed by conducting the western blot analysis. The expression of Bcl-2-associated X (Bax) protein was greatly upregulated by SAHA and RA in PC-3 cells, but only upregulated by RA in DU145 cells, likewise the expression of p53. The expression of Bcl-2 was significantly downregulated by treatment with SAHA and RA in both cell lines. The expression of Caspase-3 was upregulated by SAHA and RA in both cell lines, but PARP-1was cleaved in the cells treated with RA only. These results indicated that RA can promote apoptosis of PCa cells by regulating the protein expression of apoptosis-related genes. However, SAHA did not stimulate the expression of apoptotic genes, which RA did (Figure 7).

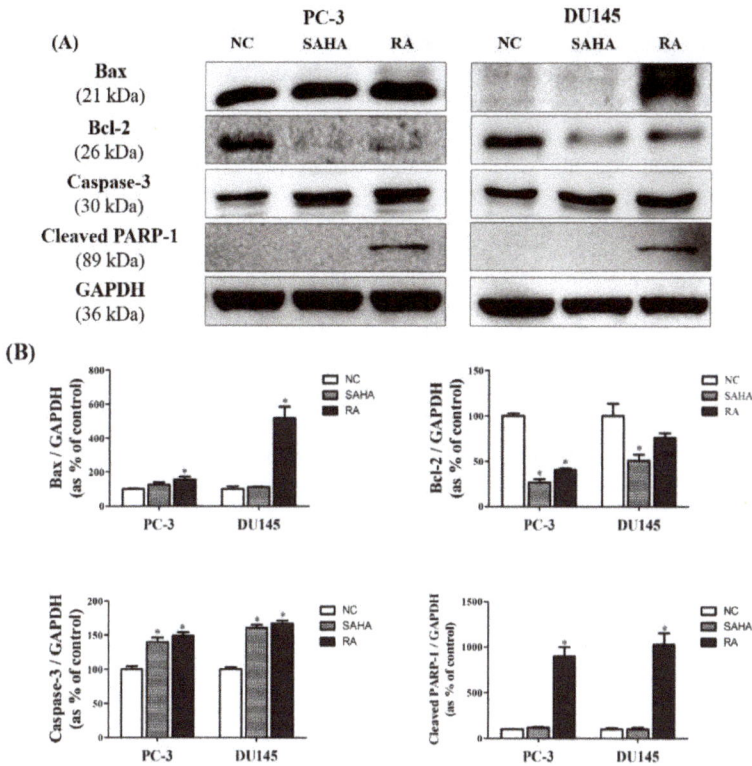

Figure 7. Effects of SAHA and RA on expression of apoptosis related genes in PC-3 and DU145 cell lines. After both cell lines were seeded at 1×10^6 in cell culture dishes and treated with media containing NC (DMSO), SAHA (1 µM) and RA (200 µM), the western blot analysis was performed. (**A**) The expressions of Bax, Bcl-2, caspase-3 and poly [ADP-ribose] polymerase 1 (PARP-1) (cleaved) at the protein level were confirmed by western blot analysis. (**B**) The expression levels of each gene were quantified and normalized to GAPDH. The results are expressed as means ± SD. * $p < 0.05$: a significant difference versus control.

4. Discussion

RA, which is easily taken from tea and vegetables, is a dietary phytochemical that has diverse bioactivities, such as anti-bacterial, anti-oxidative, and anti-inflammatory effects [38]. Recently, RA has been getting attention because it is known to have anticancer property with relatively low toxicity compared with conventional chemotherapies that have severe side effects and drug resistance [14–16]. However, its anti-cancer effect and related mechanisms on PCa have not yet been known, despite the fact that the chemopreventive effects of several phytochemicals including genistein, resveratrol, kaempferol and catechin on PCa have been identified [39–42]. In this study, we tried to discover the anti-cancer effect of RA on PCa, along with its underlying mechanism associated with HDAC2 inhibition and apoptosis induction.

Firstly, RA and SAHA were found to significantly inhibit the cell viability of PC-3 and DU145 cell lines (Figure 1). RA decreased the cell viability of both PCa cell lines by about 50% at 200 µM and sharply decreased the cell viability at higher concentrations than that. For SAHA, it inhibited the cell viability of both PCa cell lines in a dose-dependent manner in the concentration range of 1–50 µM and significantly decreased the cell viability even at 1 µM (a 40% decrease for PC-3 and a 60% decrease for DU145). Based on these results, the concentrations of RA and SAHA for the next experiments were selected as 200 µM and 1 µM, respectively. It was also found that RA and SAHA regulated the protein expression of cell cycle-related genes in the direction of cell cycle arrest at these concentrations (Figure 6).

In addition, the effects of RA and SAHA on the colony formation and tumor spheroid formation were displayed to correspond with the results of cell viability; RA and SAHA remarkably suppressed the colony and tumor spheroid formation of both PCa cell lines at these concentrations (Figure 2). Colony formation capacity of cells reflects their survival and proliferation abilities, and spheroid formation is associated with the ability of cells that can grow in all directions by interacting with themselves or their surroundings, as in the in vivo culture [43,44]. Therefore, these findings indicate that RA can inhibit the viability and proliferation of PCa cells as well as blocking the formation of tumor spheroids that resemble the condition of in vivo tumor tissue, like SAHA.

Secondly, apoptotic activity of RA and SAHA on PCa cells were identified in Annexin V assay and flow cytometry; RA mainly induced the late apoptosis and necrosis in PC-3 and DU145 cell lines, unlike SAHA which was effective in induction of early apoptosis in both cell lines (Figure 3). However, in PC-3 cells, RA also induced early apoptosis, and SAHA also induced late apoptosis. Meanwhile, RA and SAHA significantly induced DNA fragmentation in both PCa cell lines, which was identified by TUNEL assay (Figure 4). Although there were differences in the individual effect of RA and SAHA on the protein expression of apoptosis-related genes in both PCa cell lines, RA and SAHA were found to induce apoptosis of PCa cells by upregulating caspase-3 and downregulating Bcl-2 (Figure 7). For RA, it additionally increased the protein expression of Bax and cleaved form of PARP-1. Pro-apoptotic protein Bax and anti-apoptotic protein Bcl-2 family members bound to the mitochondrial membrane affect the intrinsic mitochondrial pathway of apoptosis by regulating efflux of cytochrome c from mitochondria to cytoplasm and subsequent activation of caspases such as caspase-3, -6, and -7 that are cysteine-aspartic proteases playing important roles in apoptosis [45]. PARP-1 is a poly-(ADP-ribosylating) enzyme necessary for DNA repair processes. During apoptosis, it is cleaved by caspase-3 or -7 and becomes inactive in recovering DNA damage. Thus, cleaved form of PARP-1 is considered as a remarkable marker of apoptosis [46]. As a result, RA was revealed to effectively induce apoptosis of PCa cells by influencing an intrinsic mitochondrial apoptotic pathway.

As an inhibitor of HDAC1 and HDAC2, SAHA, also known as Vorinostat, has a broad spectrum of epigenetic activities through the inhibition of histone acetylation and has been used to treat several diseases including glioblastoma [47] and non-small-cell lung carcinoma [48]. In association with tumor, HDAC1 and HDAC2 enhance the tumorigenesis by decreasing the transcriptional activity of tumor suppressor like p53 through histone deacetylation. In addition, deacetylation of lysine residues of p53 by HDACs leads to ubiquitinylation and proteolysis of p53 by the proteasome. Therefore, HDACs downregulate p53 activity, which cannot block anymore the cell cycle progression and trigger apoptosis [49]. On the other hand, SAHA can have anti-cancer efficacies by inhibiting HDACs and upregulating p53 [50]. In the present study, SAHA was found to effectively suppress the protein expression of HDAC2 in both PCa cell lines, and the protein expression of p53 was dramatically increased as a result of HDAC2 inhibition in PC-3 cells. However, p53 was not upregulated in DU145 cells beyond expectations (Figure 5). Nevertheless, the growth inhibition effects or apoptotic activities of SAHA on DU145 cells were found on PC3 cells, indicating that SAHA may induce apoptosis of DU145 cells through p53-independent pathway. In the previous study on U937 human leukemia cells, SAHA was revealed to induce apoptosis through the pathway independent of p53 [51]. The more detailed mode of apoptotic action of SAHA in DU145 cells needs to be elucidated. In comparison with SAHA, RA inhibited the protein expression of HDAC2 and increased the protein expression of p53 in both PCa cell lines, which was more noticeable in DU145 cells than in PC-3 cells.

p53, as a tumor suppressor protein, has diverse anti-cancer effects such as cell cycle arrest, apoptosis induction, and inhibition of angiogenesis [52]. Cell cycle arrest mediated by p53 is known to be partially achieved through activating p21, which hinders G1/S transition in the cell cycle as an inhibitor of CDK complexes [53,54]. p53 also mediates apoptosis through upregulating the expression of Bax, a pro-apoptotic gene, which prevents the activity of Bcl-2, an anti-apoptotic gene [55]. In the present study, it was confirmed that cell cycle arrest and apoptosis of PCa cells were achieved in parallel by p53, which was upregulated by RA and SAHA as a result of HDAC2 inhibition.

Among numerous anticancer mechanisms of plant-derived phytochemicals, it is known that they are related with apoptotic cell death that is mediated by p53-dependent or -independent pathways. A recent review emphasized the cell death mechanisms of diverse plant-derived anti-cancer polyphenolics, alkaloids, terpenoids, and so on [56]. The present study is considered to firstly identify the cell death mechanism of RA on PCa cells that is relevant to p53-induced apoptosis caused by HDAC2 inhibition.

5. Conclusions

RA, as a dietary phenolic compound ingested from tea, was displayed to have anti-PCa activities by inhibiting viability, colony formation, and spheroid formation of PCa cells via HDAC2 inhibition and the consequential p53-mediated cell cycle arrest and apoptosis Therefore, RA would be used as a novel phytomedicine to act as an HDAC inhibitor targeted to PCa, with the anticipation to decrease the adverse side effects of the existing chemotherapeutical agents. To do this, further studies are necessary to identify eventual cytotoxic effects of RA on normal cells. In addition, supraphysiologic doses of RA should be attained to produce anti-cancer effects on PCa with the formulation containing RA as a dietary additive or a drug containing its effective therapeutic concentration.

Author Contributions: Conceptualization, Y.-G.J. and K.-A.H.; experiments and software, Y.-G.J.; formal analysis, Y.-G.J. and K.-A.H.; writing of the original draft preparation, Y.-G.J.; writing of review and editing, K.-A.H. and K.-C.C.; project administration, K.-C.C.; funding acquisition, K.-C.C.

Funding: This work was also supported by a National Research Foundation of Korea (NRF) grant funded by the Ministry of Education, Science and Technology (MEST) of the Republic of Korea (2017R1D1A1A09000663). In addition, this work was also supported by the Global Research and Development Center (GRDC) Program through the National Research Foundation of Korea (NRF) funded by the Ministry of Education, Science and Technology (2017K1A4A3014959).

Acknowledgments: We would like to thank for Gun-Hwi Lee for his assistance with the flow cytometry assay.

Conflicts of Interest: There are no conflicts of interest in declaration among the authors.

References

1. Lin, Y.W.; Hu, Z.H.; Wang, X.; Mao, Q.Q.; Qin, J.; Zheng, X.Y.; Xie, L.P. Tea consumption and prostate cancer: An updated meta-analysis. *World J. Surg. Oncol.* **2014**, *12*, 38. [CrossRef] [PubMed]
2. Rocha, J.; Eduardo-Figueira, M.; Barateiro, A.; Fernandes, A.; Brites, D.; Bronze, R.; Duarte, C.M.; Serra, A.T.; Pinto, R.; Freitas, M.; et al. Anti-inflammatory effect of rosmarinic acid and an extract of rosmarinus officinalis in rat models of local and systemic inflammation. *Basic Clin. Pharmacol. Toxicol.* **2015**, *116*, 398–413. [CrossRef] [PubMed]
3. Ferlemi, A.V.; Katsikoudi, A.; Kontogianni, V.G.; Kellici, T.F.; Iatrou, G.; Lamari, F.N.; Tzakos, A.G.; Margarity, M. Rosemary tea consumption results to anxiolytic- and anti-depressant-like behavior of adult male mice and inhibits all cerebral area and liver cholinesterase activity; phytochemical investigation and in silico studies. *Chem. Biol. Interact.* **2015**, *237*, 47–57. [CrossRef] [PubMed]
4. Amoah, S.K.; Sandjo, L.P.; Kratz, J.M.; Biavatti, M.W. Rosmarinic acid—Pharmaceutical and clinical aspects. *Planta Med.* **2016**, *82*, 388–406. [CrossRef] [PubMed]
5. Sotnikova, R.; Okruhlicova, L.; Vlkovicova, J.; Navarova, J.; Gajdacova, B.; Pivackova, L.; Fialova, S.; Krenek, P. Rosmarinic acid administration attenuates diabetes-induced vascular dysfunction of the rat aorta. *J. Pharm. Pharmacol.* **2013**, *65*, 713–723. [CrossRef] [PubMed]
6. Han, Y.H.; Kee, J.Y.; Hong, S.H. Rosmarinic Acid Activates AMPK to Inhibit Metastasis of Colorectal Cancer. *Front. Pharmacol.* **2018**, *9*, 68. [CrossRef] [PubMed]
7. Han, S.; Yang, S.; Cai, Z.; Pan, D.; Li, Z.; Huang, Z.; Zhang, P.; Zhu, H.; Lei, L.; Wang, W. Anti-Warburg effect of rosmarinic acid via miR-155 in gastric cancer cells. *Drug. Des. Dev. Ther.* **2015**, *9*, 2695–2703. [PubMed]

8. Zhang, Y.; Hu, M.; Liu, L.; Cheng, X.L.; Cai, J.; Zhou, J.; Wang, T. Anticancer effects of Rosmarinic acid in OVCAR-3 ovarian cancer cells are mediated via induction of apoptosis, suppression of cell migration and modulation of lncRNA MALAT-1 expression. *J. BUON* **2018**, *23*, 763–768. [PubMed]

9. Alcaraz, M.; Alcaraz-Saura, M.; Achel, D.G.; Olivares, A.; LÓPEZ-MORATA, J.A.; Castillo, J. Radiosensitizing effect of rosmarinic acid in metastatic melanoma B16F10 cells. *Anticancer Res.* **2014**, *34*, 1913–1921. [PubMed]

10. Yesil-Celiktas, O.; Sevimli, C.; Bedir, E.; Vardar-Sukan, F. Inhibitory effects of rosemary extracts, carnosic acid and rosmarinic acid on the growth of various human cancer cell lines. *Plant Foods Hum. Nutr.* **2010**, *65*, 158–163. [CrossRef] [PubMed]

11. Xu, Y.; Jiang, Z.; Ji, G.; Liu, J. Inhibition of bone metastasis from breast carcinoma by rosmarinic acid. *Planta Med.* **2010**, *76*, 956–962. [CrossRef] [PubMed]

12. Jemal, A.; Siegel, R.; Xu, J.; Ward, E. Cancer statistics, 2010. *CA Cancer J. Clin.* **2010**, *60*, 277–300. [CrossRef] [PubMed]

13. Galvao, D.A.; Nosaka, K.; Taaffe, D.R.; Spry, N.; Kristjanson, L.J.; McGuigan, M.R.; Suzuki, K.; Yamaya, K.; Newton, R.U. Resistance training and reduction of treatment side effects in prostate cancer patients. *Med. Sci. Sports Exerc.* **2006**, *38*, 2045–2052. [CrossRef] [PubMed]

14. Mahon, K.L.; Henshall, S.M.; Sutherland, R.L.; Horvath, L.G. Pathways of chemotherapy resistance in castration-resistant prostate cancer. *Endocr. Relat. Cancer* **2011**, *18*, R103–R123. [CrossRef] [PubMed]

15. Domingo-Domenech, J.; Vidal, S.J.; Rodriguez-Bravo, V.; Castillo-Martin, M.; Quinn, S.A.; Rodriguez-Barrueco, R.; Bonal, D.M.; Charytonowicz, E.; Gladoun, N.; de la Iglesia-Vicente, J.; et al. Suppression of acquired docetaxel resistance in prostate cancer through depletion of notch- and hedgehog-dependent tumor-initiating cells. *Cancer Cell* **2012**, *22*, 373–388. [CrossRef] [PubMed]

16. Semenas, J.; Allegrucci, C.A.; Boorjian, S.P.; Mongan, N.; Liao Persson, J. Overcoming drug resistance and treating advanced prostate cancer. *Curr. Drug Targets* **2012**, *13*, 1308–1323. [CrossRef] [PubMed]

17. Olsen, C.A. Expansion of the lysine acylation landscape. *Angew. Chem. Int. Ed. Engl.* **2012**, *51*, 3755–3756. [CrossRef] [PubMed]

18. Tan, M.; Luo, H.; Lee, S.; Jin, F.; Yang, J.S.; Montellier, E.; Buchou, T.; Cheng, Z.; Rousseaux, S.; Rajagopal, N.; et al. Identification of 67 histone marks and histone lysine crotonylation as a new type of histone modification. *Cell* **2011**, *146*, 1016–1028. [CrossRef] [PubMed]

19. Abbas, A.; Gupta, S. The role of histone deacetylases in prostate cancer. *Epigenetics* **2008**, *3*, 300–309. [CrossRef] [PubMed]

20. Ozdag, H.; Teschendorff, A.E.; Ahmed, A.A.; Hyland, S.J.; Blenkiron, C.; Bobrow, L.; Veerakumarasivam, A.; Burtt, G.; Subkhankulova, T.; Arends, M.J.; et al. Differential expression of selected histone modifier genes in human solid cancers. *BMC Genom.* **2006**, *7*, 90. [CrossRef] [PubMed]

21. Weichert, W.; Roske, A.; Gekeler, V.; Beckers, T.; Stephan, C.; Jung, K.; Fritzsche, F.R.; Niesporek, S.; Denkert, C.; Dietel, M.; et al. Histone deacetylases 1, 2 and 3 are highly expressed in prostate cancer and HDAC2 expression is associated with shorter PSA relapse time after radical prostatectomy. *Br. J. Cancer* **2008**, *98*, 604–610. [CrossRef] [PubMed]

22. Weichert, W.; Roske, A.; Niesporek, S.; Noske, A.; Buckendahl, A.C.; Dietel, M.; Gekeler, V.; Boehm, M.; Beckers, T.; Denkert, C. Class I histone deacetylase expression has independent prognostic impact in human colorectal cancer: Specific role of class I histone deacetylases in vitro and in vivo. *Clin. Cancer Res.* **2008**, *14*, 1669–1677. [CrossRef] [PubMed]

23. Krusche, C.A.; Wulfing, P.; Kersting, C.; Vloet, A.; Bocker, W.; Kiesel, L.; Beier, H.M.; Alfer, J. Histone deacetylase-1 and -3 protein expression in human breast cancer: A tissue microarray analysis. *Breast Cancer Res. Treat.* **2005**, *90*, 15–23. [CrossRef] [PubMed]

24. Minamiya, Y.; Ono, T.; Saito, H.; Takahashi, N.; Ito, M.; Mitsui, M.; Motoyama, S.; Ogawa, J. Expression of histone deacetylase 1 correlates with a poor prognosis in patients with adenocarcinoma of the lung. *Lung Cancer* **2011**, *74*, 300–304. [CrossRef] [PubMed]

25. Rikimaru, T.; Taketomi, A.; Yamashita, Y.; Shirabe, K.; Hamatsu, T.; Shimada, M.; Maehara, Y. Clinical significance of histone deacetylase 1 expression in patients with hepatocellular carcinoma. *Oncology* **2007**, *72*, 69–74. [CrossRef] [PubMed]

26. Weichert, W.; Roske, A.; Gekeler, V.; Beckers, T.; Ebert, M.P.; Pross, M.; Dietel, M.; Denkert, C.; Rocken, C. Association of patterns of class I histone deacetylase expression with patient prognosis in gastric cancer: A retrospective analysis. *Lancet Oncol.* **2008**, *9*, 139–148. [CrossRef]

27. Glozak, M.A.; Seto, E. Histone deacetylases and cancer. *Oncogene* **2007**, *26*, 5420–5432. [CrossRef] [PubMed]
28. Eot-Houllier, G.; Fulcrand, G.; Magnaghi-Jaulin, L.; Jaulin, C. Histone deacetylase inhibitors and genomic instability. *Cancer Lett.* **2009**, *274*, 169–176. [CrossRef] [PubMed]
29. Luo, J.; Su, F.; Chen, D.; Shiloh, A.; Gu, W. Deacetylation of p53 modulates its effect on cell growth and apoptosis. *Nature* **2000**, *408*, 377–381. [CrossRef] [PubMed]
30. Duan, H.; Heckman, C.A.; Boxer, L.M. Histone deacetylase inhibitors down-regulate bcl-2 expression and induce apoptosis in t (14; 18) lymphomas. *Mol. Cell Biol.* **2005**, *25*, 1608–1619. [CrossRef] [PubMed]
31. Gui, C.Y.; Ngo, L.; Xu, W.S.; Richon, V.M.; Marks, P.A. Histone deacetylase (HDAC) inhibitor activation of p21WAF1 involves changes in promoter-associated proteins, including HDAC1. *Proc. Natl. Acad. Sci. USA* **2004**, *101*, 1241–1246. [CrossRef] [PubMed]
32. Subramanian, S.; Bates, S.E.; Wright, J.J.; Espinoza-Delgado, I.; Piekarz, R.L. Clinical Toxicities of Histone Deacetylase Inhibitors. *Pharmaceuticals* **2010**, *3*, 2751–2767. [CrossRef] [PubMed]
33. Lai, R.H.; Hsiao, Y.W.; Wang, M.J.; Lin, H.Y.; Wu, C.W.; Chi, C.W.; Li, A.F.; Jou, Y.S.; Chen, J.Y. SOCS6, down-regulated in gastric cancer, inhibits cell proliferation and colony formation. *Cancer Lett.* **2010**, *288*, 75–85. [CrossRef] [PubMed]
34. Iseki, H.; Takeda, A.; Andoh, T.; Kuwabara, K.; Takahashi, N.; Kurochkin, I.V.; Ishida, H.; Okazaki, Y.; Koyama, I. ALEX1 suppresses colony formation ability of human colorectal carcinoma cell lines. *Cancer Sci.* **2012**, *103*, 1267–1271. [CrossRef] [PubMed]
35. Franken, N.A.; Rodermond, H.M.; Stap, J.; Haveman, J.; van Bree, C. Clonogenic assay of cells in vitro. *Nat. Protoc.* **2006**, *1*, 2315–2319. [CrossRef] [PubMed]
36. Benien, P.; Swami, A. 3D tumor models: History, advances and future perspectives. *Future Oncol.* **2014**, *10*, 1311–1327. [CrossRef] [PubMed]
37. Griffith, L.G.; Swartz, M.A. Capturing complex 3D tissue physiology in vitro. *Nat. Rev. Mol. Cell Biol.* **2006**, *7*, 211–224. [CrossRef] [PubMed]
38. Petersen, M.; Simmonds, M.S. Rosmarinic acid. *Phytochemistry* **2003**, *62*, 121–125. [CrossRef]
39. Chiyomaru, T.; Yamamura, S.; Fukuhara, S.; Yoshino, H.; Kinoshita, T.; Majid, S.; Saini, S.; Chang, I.; Tanaka, Y.; Enokida, H.; et al. Genistein inhibits prostate cancer cell growth by targeting miR-34a and oncogenic HOTAIR. *PLoS ONE* **2013**, *8*, e70372. [CrossRef] [PubMed]
40. Benitez, D.A.; Pozo-Guisado, E.; Alvarez-Barrientos, A.; Fernandez-Salguero, P.M.; Castellon, E.A. Mechanisms involved in resveratrol-induced apoptosis and cell cycle arrest in prostate cancer-derived cell lines. *J. Androl.* **2007**, *28*, 282–293. [CrossRef] [PubMed]
41. Halimah, E.; Diantini, A.; Destiani, D.P.; Pradipta, I.S.; Sastramihardja, H.S.; Lestari, K.; Subarnas, A.; Abdulah, R.; Koyama, H. Induction of caspase cascade pathway by kaempferol-3-O-rhamnoside in LNCaP prostate cancer cell lines. *Biomed. Rep.* **2015**, *3*, 115–117. [CrossRef] [PubMed]
42. Kumar, N.B.; Pow-Sang, J.; Egan, K.M.; Spiess, P.E.; Dickinson, S.; Salup, R.; Helal, M.; McLarty, J.; Williams, C.R.; Schreiber, F.; et al. Randomized, Placebo-Controlled Trial of Green Tea Catechins for Prostate Cancer Prevention. *Cancer Prev. Res.* **2015**, *8*, 879–887. [CrossRef] [PubMed]
43. Hoffman, R.M. In vitro sensitivity assays in cancer: A review, analysis, and prognosis. *J. Clin. Lab. Anal.* **1991**, *5*, 133–143. [CrossRef] [PubMed]
44. Friedrich, J.; Seidel, C.; Ebner, R.; Kunz-Schughart, L.A. Spheroid-based drug screen: Considerations and practical approach. *Nat. Protoc.* **2009**, *4*, 309–324. [CrossRef] [PubMed]
45. Loreto, C.; La Rocca, G.; Anzalone, R.; Caltabiano, R.; Vespasiani, G.; Castorina, S.; Ralph, D.J.; Cellek, S.; Musumeci, G.; Giunta, S.; et al. The role of intrinsic pathway in apoptosis activation and progression in Peyronie's disease. *Biomed Res. Int.* **2014**, *2014*, 616149. [CrossRef] [PubMed]
46. Soldani, C.; Scovassi, A.I. Poly (ADP-ribose) polymerase-1 cleavage during apoptosis: An update. *Apoptosis* **2002**, *7*, 321–328. [CrossRef] [PubMed]
47. Bezecny, P. Histone deacetylase inhibitors in glioblastoma: Pre-clinical and clinical experience. *Med. Oncol.* **2014**, *31*, 985. [CrossRef] [PubMed]
48. Ramalingam, S.S.; Maitland, M.L.; Frankel, P.; Argiris, A.E.; Koczywas, M.; Gitlitz, B.; Thomas, S.; Espinoza-Delgado, I.; Vokes, E.E.; Gandara, D.R.; et al. Carboplatin and Paclitaxel in combination with either vorinostat or placebo for first-line therapy of advanced non-small-cell lung cancer. *J. Clin. Oncol.* **2010**, *28*, 56–62. [CrossRef] [PubMed]

49. Ropero, S.; Esteller, M. The role of histone deacetylases (HDACs) in human cancer. *Mol. Oncol.* **2007**, *1*, 19–25. [CrossRef] [PubMed]

50. Eckschlager, T.; Plch, J.; Stiborova, M.; Hrabeta, J. Histone Deacetylase Inhibitors as Anticancer Drugs. *Int. J. Mol. Sci.* **2017**, *18*, 1414. [CrossRef] [PubMed]

51. Vrana, J.A.; Decker, R.H.; Johnson, C.R.; Wang, Z.; Jarvis, W.D.; Richon, V.M.; Ehinger, M.; Fisher, P.B.; Grant, S. Induction of apoptosis in U937 human leukemia cells by suberoylanilide hydroxamic acid (SAHA) proceeds through pathways that are regulated by Bcl-2/Bcl-XL, c-Jun, and p21CIP1, but independent of p53. *Oncogene* **1999**, *18*, 7016–7025. [CrossRef] [PubMed]

52. Wang, Z.; Sun, Y. Targeting p53 for Novel Anticancer Therapy. *Transl. Oncol.* **2010**, *3*, 1–12. [CrossRef] [PubMed]

53. El-Deiry, W.S.; Tokino, T.; Velculescu, V.E.; Levy, D.B.; Parsons, R.; Trent, J.M.; Lin, D.; Mercer, W.E.; Kinzler, K.W.; Vogelstein, B. WAF1, a potential mediator of p53 tumor suppression. *Cell* **1993**, *75*, 817–825. [CrossRef]

54. Harper, J.W.; Adami, G.R.; Wei, N.; Keyomarsi, K.; Elledge, S.J. The p21 Cdk-interacting protein Cip1 is a potent inhibitor of G1 cyclin-dependent kinases. *Cell* **1993**, *75*, 805–816. [CrossRef]

55. Oltvai, Z.N.; Milliman, C.L.; Korsmeyer, S.J. Bcl-2 heterodimerizes in vivo with a conserved homolog, Bax, that accelerates programmed cell death. *Cell* **1993**, *74*, 609–619. [CrossRef]

56. Gali-Muhtasib, H.; Hmadi, R.; Kareh, M.; Tohme, R.; Darwiche, N. Cell death mechanisms of plant-derived anticancer drugs: Beyond apoptosis. *Apoptosis* **2015**, *20*, 1531–1562. [CrossRef] [PubMed]

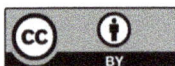

nutrients

MDPI

Review

Molecular Targets of Epigallocatechin—Gallate (EGCG): A Special Focus on Signal Transduction and Cancer

Aide Negri [1,†], Valeria Naponelli [1,2,*,†], Federica Rizzi [1,2,3] and Saverio Bettuzzi [1,2,3]

1   Department of Medicine and Surgery, University of Parma, Via Gramsci 14, 43126 Parma, Italy;
    aide.negri@unipr.it (A.N.); federica.rizzi@unipr.it (F.R.); saverio.bettuzzi@unipr.it (S.B.)
2   National Institute of Biostructure and Biosystems (INBB), Viale Medaglie d'Oro 305, 00136 Rome, Italy
3   Centre for Molecular and Translational Oncology (COMT), University of Parma, Parco Area delle Scienze
    11/a, 43124 Parma, Italy
*   Correspondence: valeria.naponelli@unipr.it; Tel.: +39-0521-033790
†   These authors contributed equally to this work.

Received: 7 November 2018; Accepted: 4 December 2018; Published: 6 December 2018

Abstract: Green tea is a beverage that is widely consumed worldwide and is believed to exert effects on different diseases, including cancer. The major components of green tea are catechins, a family of polyphenols. Among them, epigallocatechin-gallate (EGCG) is the most abundant and biologically active. EGCG is widely studied for its anti-cancer properties. However, the cellular and molecular mechanisms explaining its action have not been completely understood, yet. EGCG is effective in vivo at micromolar concentrations, suggesting that its action is mediated by interaction with specific targets that are involved in the regulation of crucial steps of cell proliferation, survival, and metastatic spread. Recently, several proteins have been identified as EGCG direct interactors. Among them, the trans-membrane receptor 67LR has been identified as a high affinity EGCG receptor. 67LR is a master regulator of many pathways affecting cell proliferation or apoptosis, also regulating cancer stem cells (CSCs) activity. EGCG was also found to be interacting directly with Pin1, TGFR-II, and metalloproteinases (MMPs) (mainly MMP2 and MMP9), which respectively regulate EGCG-dependent inhibition of NF-kB, epithelial-mesenchimal transaction (EMT) and cellular invasion. EGCG interacts with DNA methyltransferases (DNMTs) and histone deacetylases (HDACs), which modulates epigenetic changes. The bulk of this novel knowledge provides information about the mechanisms of action of EGCG and may explain its onco-suppressive function. The identification of crucial signalling pathways that are related to cancer onset and progression whose master regulators interacts with EGCG may disclose intriguing pharmacological targets, and eventually lead to novel combined treatments in which EGCG acts synergistically with known drugs.

Keywords: green tea catechins; epigallocatechin-gallate (EGCG); 67LR; cancer apoptosis; cell death; chemoprevention; gene expression

1. Introduction

Green tea is produced from Camellia sinensis and it represents the second most consumed beverage in the world after water, being used primarily in Asia and in the Middle East [1].

Several observational and intervention studies have demonstrated that green tea consumption has beneficial effects on many human diseases, including obesity, metabolic syndrome, neurodegenerative disorders inflammatory diseases, and cancer [2–6]. The major polyphenolic component of dried green tea extracts is epigallocatechin-gallate (EGCG) EGCG is the most abundant and biologically active catechin from green tea, accounting for at least 50% of the total catechin content in green tea leaves [7].

The biological effects of green tea were initially ascribed to pro- or anti-oxidative properties of catechins. Most of the studies have been conducted administrating green tea extracts or pure EGCG. A typical weakness of many studies is related to data collected in vitro and cell culture systems, following the administration of doses of green tea extracts (or EGCG) much higher than those that were reached in human plasma after green tea consumption. In vivo, administration of the equivalent of two or three cups of green tea leads to a peak in the plasma levels of tea catechins in the sub-micromolar range in humans [8,9].

Several in vitro, in vivo, and clinical studies have shown multiple EGCG anticancer actions. Among them there are anti-proliferative, pro-apoptotic, anti-angiogenic, and anti-invasive functions [10]. Furthermore, EGCG has been observed to impair other processes that are involved in carcinogenesis as inflammation, oxidative stress and hypoxia and to target tumor microenviroment components (e.g., cancer stem cells, fibroblasts, macrophages, and microvasculature) [11]. In several in vitro and in vivo cancer types, EGCG has been shown to act synergistically with other natural compounds (e.g., curcumin, ascorbic acid, quercetin, genestein, caffeine) [10,12] and it has also been testing in combination with currently used chemotherapeutic drugs (e.g., doxorubicin, cisplatin, sunitinib) [13–16]. Furthermore, in order to improve EGCG bioavailability and stability, novel formulations of the catechin encapsulated in nanoparticles have been developed [17–20].

Even if the anti-tumoural effect of green tea catechins (and specifically EGCG) has been extensively demonstrated in vitro, their molecular and cellular mechanisms are not yet completely understood [21,22].

The anti-cancer effect of EGCG and green tea extracts is mediated through several mechanisms, including stimulation of anti-oxidant activity and activation of detoxification system [23,24], alteration of the cell cycle [25], suppression of mitogen-activated protein kinase (MAPK) and receptor protein kinase (RTKs) pathways [26,27], inhibition of clonal expansion of the tumour-initiating stem cell population [28], and production of epigenetic changes in gene expression [29]. These mechanisms (reviewed recently in [30–32]) are not completely understood yet. Green tea catechins are thought to function both as powerful radical scavengers, in particular, under increased oxidative stress conditions [33], and as ROS generators leading to the inhibition of cancer cell growth through the induction of apoptotis [24,34]. Moreover, they have been shown to induce apoptosis in several ways, such as modulating pro- and anti-apoptotic protein (Bax, Bcl-2, Bcl-XL) and cell cycle regulator proteins (cyclins, CDKs) [35]. Green tea catechins are also able to target genes and proteins that are associated with cell proliferation and apoptosis, including RTKs (receptor tyrosine kinases). Several studies described the inhibitory effect of green tea catechins on these receptors and on Ras/extracellular signal-regulated kinase (ERK)/MAPK and phosphatidylinositol 3-kinase (PI3K)/Akt, which are RTKs-related downstream pathways that are often constitutively activated in tumor cells. EGCG negatively modulates the expression of various transcription factors, including Sp1, AP-1, and NF-kB preventing cancer formation [36,37]. Another mechanism that can explain the pleiotropic effects exerted by green tea catechins is represented by the epigenetic changes in gene expression and chromatin organization. The major epigenetic mechanisms are DNA methylation, histone modifications, and expression of noncoding regulatory micro RNA (miRNAs). Green tea catechins can induce an epigenetic reactivation of genes silenced during carcinogenesis or an epigenetic downregulation of oncogenes through the inhibition of DNA methyltransferases (DNMTs) or histone deacetylases (HDACs) activity and the reduction of their expression [38,39].

Micromolar concentrations of EGCG have been shown to exert a wide array of different effects in a cancer cell. The current understanding is that catechins may either interact with a single critical regulator affecting the activity of key enzymes that are involved in important pathways, or by hitting multiple targets in parallel, thereby modulating different pathways simultaneously [40,41].

First it is necessary to identify proteins that bind to catechins with high affinity, which may represent the master regulators controlling one or multiple pathways. Using in vitro models, several research teams have identified proteins that are targeted by EGCG. Among these are vimentin, Fyn,

ZAP70, insulin-like growth factor 1 receptor, and glucose regulated protein 78 kDa [42–46]. However, the functional effect of green tea catechins on the target protein activity has been demonstrated only at much higher concentrations of EGCG than Kd values, probably because of the non-specific binding of EGCG to other proteins competing for the target [47]. In Table 1 are listed the principal EGCG molecular targets that were identified in cancer cells.

We think that EGCG-protein binding can be important for the beneficial effect of green tea catechins. Green tea catechins bind to a plethora of proteins and the process of the interaction is highly dependent on the folding status and on the conformational properties of the target protein. In this review, we decided to take into consideration only few proteins that, after direct binding to EGCG, alter and affect their downstream pathways promoting anti-cancer effects. These data could be used for a rational drug design of green tea catechins derivatives exploitable for more specific and effective anti-cancer therapies. We will focus particularly on the onset and progression of cancer, describing and discussing the possible molecular mechanisms through which catechins exert their action.

Table 1. Epigallocatechin-gallate (EGCG) molecular targets that are involved in cancer onset and progression.

Cell Cycle, Proliferation & Survival	Apoptosis & Cell Death	Motility, Invasion and Metastatization	Inflammation	Epigenetic Control	Others
p16 [48]	Bax [49]	MMP-2 * [50]	FcεRI [51]	DNMT1 * [39]	DAPK1 [52]
p18 [35]	Bad [53]	MMP-9 * [50]	IL-8 [54]	DNMT3A [48]	MRLC [55]
p21 [48]	Bak [56]	MMP-14 [57]	IGF-1R * [45]	DNMT3B * [39]	MYPT1 [55]
p27 [56]	Bcl-2 * [58]	uPA [59]	VEGF [60]	HDAC1 * [39]	eEF1a [61]
Cyclin D [56]	Bcl-xl [53]	PAI-1 [59]	CSF-1 [62]	HDAC2 [63]	ID1 [64]
Cyclin E [35]	Bcl-xs [56]	E-cadherine [39]	CCL-2 [62]	HAT [65]	RAR-β [39]
Cyclin A [66]	Caspase3 [56]	SLUG [67]	COX-2 [60]	hTERT [68]	HSP70 [53]
Cyclin B [66]	Caspase8 [69]	SNAIL1 [70]	iNOS [71]	EZH2 [72]	HSP90 * [73]
CDK4 [56]	Caspase9 [56]	Vimentin * [42]	eNOS [74–78]		GRP78 * [46]
CDK6 [56]	Apaf-1 [53]	Twist [79]			PECAM-1 [80]
CDK2 [35]	Puma [56]	N-cadherine [79]			miR-16 [62]
CDK1 [66]	XIAP [53]	HIF-1α [60]			let-7b miRNA [81]
Erk1/2 [56]	Cytochrome C [56]	β-catenin [54]			miR-210 [82]
Pin * [83]	p53 [84]	Wnt [54]			miR34a [85]
PPA2 [86]	Survivin [87]	TIMP-3 [72]			miR145 [85]
PKA [86]	Fas [69]				miR200c [85]
STAT [12]	DR5 [69]				ZAP70 * [44]
AR [65]	PARP [88]				TRAF-6 * [89]
67LR * [90]					Oct4 [85]
FcεRI [51]					Sox2 [91]
EGFR [92]					Notch1 [85]
HGFR [93]					Nanog [85]
TGFR-II * [94]					CD133 [95]
cGMP [74] [96]					
cAMP [86]					
P-glycoprotein [88]					
NF-kB [97]					
c-Myc [98]					
FOXO3a [99]					
GSK-3β [98]					
PI3K [100]					
AKT [100]					
PKC-δ [74]					
JAK-1/2 [12]					
Src [57]					
CK1α [98]					
p38 MAPK [56]					
JNK [56]					

* EGCG direct interactors.

2. 67-kDa Laminin Receptor Signalling Pathways

One of the most interesting targets of EGCG action is the 67-kDa laminin receptor (67LR), a non-integrin cell surface receptor whose expression has been shown to be increased in several cancers, such as blood, prostate, breast, gastric, and colon [101–106]. The receptor expression is usually correlated with drug resistance, and it contributes positively to cancer cells viability, tumour progression, metastatic diffusion, and neo-angiogenesis [101,102,107,108].

In 2004, Tachibana et al. identified for the first time the 67LR as a specific EGCG membrane receptor using surface plasmon resonance. The study revealed that 67LR was able to bind EGCG with a Kd value of 39.9 nM. This interaction enabled EGCG to reduce the growth of the lung cancer cell line A549 [90], thus exerting anticancer activity. Other green tea components, such as caffeine, quercetin, epicatechin (EC), and epigallocatechin (EGC) were tested for binding to 67LR, but none were specific ligands of the receptor or showed tumour suppressive effects [90]. Therefore, EGCG appears to be the only catechin able to bind 67LR. Subsequently, a putative EGCG binding site corresponding to the region between the residues 161 and 170 of the receptor has been identified [109]. The direct binding between EGCG and 67LR has been confirmed in prostate cancer cells by Yu et al. [104]. Using MVD (Molegro Virtual Docker, an integrated platform for predicting protein ligand interactions), these authors identified a binding site for EGCG with the same sequence of the laminin tyrosine-isoleucine-glycine-serine-arginine (YIGSR) peptide, corresponding to the 929–933 sequence of β1 chain of 67LR [104].

Many studies have explored the signalling cascades that are triggered by EGCG-67LR interaction, some of which will be discussed in this review. In many cases, the tumour suppression pathway affected ordered microdomains of the cell membrane known as lipid rafts, where the 67LR has been located [110]. Lipid rafts differ from the surrounding membrane, because their composition is enriched in specific lipids (sphingomyelins and glycosphingolipids) and cholesterol, which are tightly packed to form liquid ordered assemblies [111]. Lipid rafts are dynamic, heterogeneous structures whose composition is extremely variable, not only in relation to the lipid and sterols content, but also because of the several proteins that can be recruited (e.g., BCR, FcεRI) or harboured (e.g., Scr tyrosin kinases) [112–115]. Lipid rafts are rich in tyrosine kinase receptors (RTKs), such as EGFR [116–118], IGF1R [119], and HER2 [120]. These receptors have been found to be inhibited by EGCG in several in vitro and in vivo cancer models (e.g., colon, lung, liver and breast cancers) [92,121–123]. The functional proteins recruited by lipid rafts allow these structures to play complex roles. Lipid rafts can float within the plasma membrane or can cluster in larger and stabilized platforms in response to different stimuli. In most cases, the lipid rafts clustering allows for the activation of the proteins [124]. Furthermore, modifications in lipid rafts/protein interaction can lead to alterations in lipid and sterol content, which can, in turn, influence lipid raft functions. Thanks to their capability to interact with several cellular and molecular factors as caveolae [111], viruses [125], bacteria, inflammatory molecules [126,127], and growth factors [128–130], these microdomains are involved in a plethora of biological functions, like cell polarization, membrane trafficking [111], pathogen internalization [126], and regulation of a wide spectrum of signal transduction pathways [131]. Because most of these pathways can control cancer development, progression, rate of cell proliferation [114], migration, invasion [132,133], and apoptosis [134], lipid rafts composition and functions have received much attention. In addition, many anti-cancer agents (e.g., edelfosine, avicin D, resveratrol) exert their anti-tumour activity, at least in part, by altering or disrupting the structure of lipid rafts [135,136].

EGCG has been found to bind to the plasma membrane by interacting with the lipid rafts. The first evidence of this association was shown in the basophilic cell line KU812, where the suppressive action of EGCG on the expression of the high-affinity immunoglobulin E receptor (FcεRI) was triggered by direct binding to lipid rafts. This was mediated by the inhibition of Erk1/2 kinases phosphorylation and activation [51]. Shortly after, the same research team observed that the down-regulation of FcεRI was driven by EGCG through binding to 67LR, a receptor associated with lipid rafts [110]. Others reported that the EGCG inhibitory effect on EGFR in colon cancer cell line HT29 [92], and on HGFR in prostate cancer cell line DU145 [93] was mediated by the alteration of lipid rafts. The collection of signalling pathways affected by lipid rafts structure/function via EGCG/67LR quickly increased in number, as reported in several tumour models, such as multiple myeloma, mammary and epidermiod carcinoma, and chronic myeloid leukemia [52,137–139].

2.1. Lipid Rafts-Mediated Apoptosis

2.1.1. EGCG/67LR/Akt/eNOS/NO/cGMP/PKCδ/aSMase Pathway

Together with the inhibition of cell proliferation, migration, and angiogenesis, induction of apoptosis is one of the main mechanisms through which EGCG exerts its anti-tumour activity [140,141]. Several studies reported that EGCG is able to affect the expression and function of anti-apoptotic factors (e.g., Bcl-2, Bcl-xl) and to up-regulate pro-apoptotic molecules (e.g., Bax, caspase-3) in several cancer models [58,142–144]. However, the mechanisms through which EGCG modulates key cell death regulators are not completely understood. Some studies reported that 67LR plays a relevant role in triggering apoptosis after binding its ligand, EGCG, in haematological malignancies, such as acute myeloid leukemia and multiple myeloma [145,146]. More recently, a signalling pathway inducing EGCG/67LR-dependent apoptosis through the activation of protein kinase Cδ (PKCδ), acid sphingomyelinase (aSMase), and lipid rafts clustering has been described in multiple myeloma models [137] (Figure 1). The enzyme aSMase is responsible for the catabolism of sphingomyelin (SM) and is known to be part of the signalling cascades that mediates lipid raft-dependent apoptosis [147]. It can be activated in response to external pro-apoptotic stimuli as physical agents (e.g., radiation, UVA light) [148,149], anti-cancer drugs (e.g., cisplantin, doxorubicin) [150,151], and pro-apoptotic receptors (e.g., Fas, TNF-R) [147,152]. One of the best described mechanisms of aSMase activation is triggered by Fas receptor. The binding between death receptor Fas, harboured in lipid rafts [153], and its ligand FasL lead to the recruitment of adaptor Fas-associated protein with death domain FADD, which in turn recruits and activates pro-caspase 8. The final death-inducing signalling complex (DISC) then activates aSMase, which migrates from the cytoplasmic compartment to lipid rafts, where it generates the sphingolipid ceramide from SM [154–156]. In response to ceramide generation, cholesterol is displaced from lipid rafts, thus leading to an increase of membrane fluidity [157]. Ceramide plays a role as second messenger in the signal transduction, inducing lipid raft clustering and the stabilization of DISC complex, amplification of Fas/FasL signalling, finally leading to apoptosis [155,158,159]. A similar mechanism has been hypothesized in the case of cervical, prostate and colon cancer, where EGCG administration induces cell apoptosis through aSMase activation and ceramide increase [160–162].

Studies on multiple myeloma cell lines in vitro and in vivo, in patients or murine models, showed that the activation of 67LR through EGCG binding induces the activation of PKCδ after phosphorylation of Ser664. Activation of PKCδ leads, in turn, to aSMase activation, and finally to cell apoptosis [137]. These authors pointed out that treatment with 5 μM EGCG led to an increase of nitric oxide (NO) [74]. NO is an inorganic signalling messenger triggering a wide range of cellular pathways. The increase in NO levels is due to the activation of endothelial nitric oxide synthase (eNOS), after phosphorylation in the residue Ser1177 by Akt kinase [74]. Production of NO causes an increase of cGMP, produced by NO-dependent soluble guanylate cyclase (sGC) activation, and then the phosphorylation of PKCδ [74] (Figure 1). Furthermore, more recently, it has been observed that the anticancer agent coptisine induces apoptosis in hepatocellular carcinoma (HCC) cells via the 67LR/cGMP pathway [163]. Conversely, several studies reported that EGCG negatively regulates eNOS/NO production in different cancer types [75–78] and also sGC/cGMP amount [96].

However, the fact that administration of 5 μM EGCG was sufficient to enhance NO production, but not a significant increase of cGMP levels to induce cell apoptosis, gives rise to the question of whether other factors might interfere with cGMP-mediated aSMase activation (Figure 1). Enzyme phosphodiesterase 5 (PDE5), one of the major cGMP negative regulators, was found to be highly expressed in multiple myeloma patients as compared to healthy donors, suggesting that PDE5 could be a target for a possible combinatorial therapy with 5 μM EGCG [74]. This experimental approach has been implemented. The combined treatment of PDE5 inhibitor Vardenafil and 5 μM EGCG caused a strong reduction of cell viability not only in multiple myeloma, but also in other models as prostate, gastric, pancreatic, breast cancer, and in acute myeloid and chronic lymphocytic leukemia cell lines [74,164,165]. Vardenafil and EGCG synergistic action has been found to cause a significant reduction of IC_{50} of EGCG [74,164,165]. The tumour suppressive effects of the combinatorial therapy have also been confirmed in vivo in xenograft murine models of multiple myeloma, treatment that resulted in the reduction of tumour volume and increased survival without hepatotoxicity, a possible side effect of high EGCG administration [74]. In this model, controls (namely cell lines and primary cultures, as well as healthy animal models), were not affected by EGCG alone or in combination with Vardenafil.

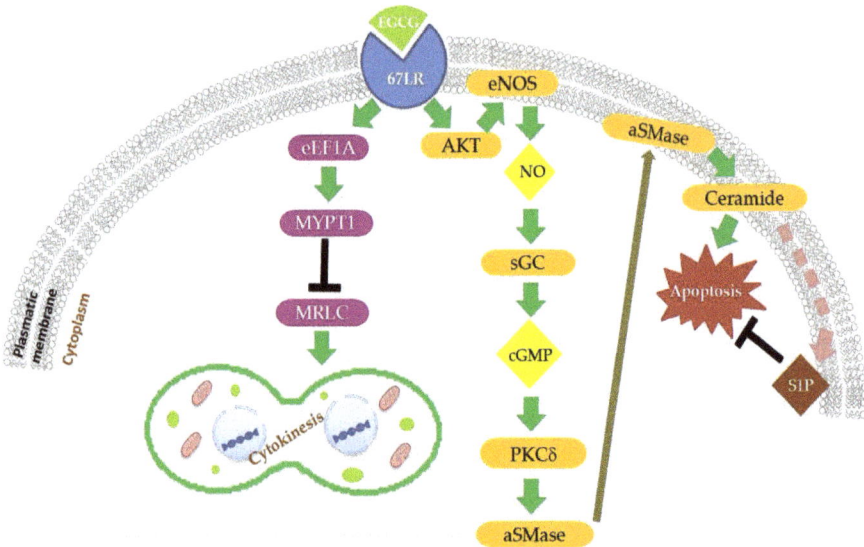

Figure 1. EGCG modulates cell division and apoptosis via 67LR. EGCG binding to 67-kDa laminin receptor (67LR) activates apoptosis program through enhanced nitric oxide (NO) and cGMP production, acid sphingomyelinase (αSMase) activation and ceramide generation. Ceramide metabolization in sphingosine-1-phosphate (S1P) reduces cell apoptosis. EGCG binding to 67LR inhibits via eukaryotic translation elongation factor 1a (eEF1A) cell cytokinesis inducing myosin phosphatase target subunit (MYPT1) dephosphorylation and activation and myosin II regulatory light chain (MRLC) dephosphorylation and inactivation.

2.1.2. EGCG/67LR/Ceramide/SphK1/S1P Pathway

The formation of larger platforms of cholesterol-enriched lipid rafts in cancer cells is often associated with aberrant activation of RTKs, resulting in increased proliferation, survival, and metastatic spread [166]. Instead, ceramide causes cholesterol displacement from lipid rafts, formation of ceramide-enriched lipid rafts, and induction of cell apoptosis [147]. Therefore, ceramide catabolism/degradation may produce anti-apoptotic effects. Ceramide can be deacetylazed and converted to sphingosine, which can be phosphorylated to sphingosine-1-phosphate (S1P) by the sphingosine kinase 1 (SphK1), an enzyme that is highly expressed in several cancers. The S1P can activate protein G-coupled receptors that can in turn activate pro-survival and anti-apoptotic signalling. In prostate cancer models, treatment with high doses of EGCG (75 μM) suppressed tumour growth in vitro and in vivo through the inhibition of SphK1/S1P signalling [167] (Figure 1).

The lesson from these data is that, in a particular cell system, a correct balance between ceramide synthesis and catabolism is fundamental [168,169]. Treatment with 1 µM and 5 µM EGCG in the multiple myeloma cell line U266 caused the induction of aSMase activity [52]. However, ceramide accumulation has been observed only after giving high concentrations of EGCG (10 µM and 20 µM EGCG) [52]. Treatment with these high doses of EGCG leads to the disruption of cholesterol-enriched lipid rafts and the inhibition of phosphorylation and the activation of several RTKs (e.g., EGFR, ErbB2, ErbB3, HGFR, IGF1R, Mer, and Flt3). IGFR inhibition has been demonstrated to be dependent on 67LR and aSMase expression [52]. Because the amount of SphK1 has been found to be increased in multiple myeloma cell lines and specimens from patients, the combinatorial treatment of 5 µM EGCG and SphK1 inhibitor Safingol was tested. The data demonstrate that the combination of the two drugs caused an increase in ceramide content, the disruption of cholesterol-enriched lipid rafts, inhibition of RTKs phosphorylation, and finally an increase of cell apoptosis [52]. Furthermore, the combination treatment also affected another cell death mediator that was activated by ceramide, the death-associated protein kinase 1 (DAPK1), causing the de-phosphorylation of DAPK1 inhibitory residue Ser308 and leading to its activation [52].

Thus, like the inhibition of PDE5 with Vardenafil, the simultaneous action on two related pathways employing two agents in combination, produced a synergistic effect that strongly reduced the IC_{50} of EGCG [52]. The onco-suppressive action of the double treatment (EGCG plus Safingol) has been found effective in vitro in acute myeloid leukemia, chronic myeloid leukemia, and in chronic lymphocytic leukemia models [170]. Absence of toxicity of the combined therapy has also been shown in vivo [52].

2.2. Cancer Cell Growth Inhibition

2.2.1. EGCG/67LR/eEF1a/MYPT1/MRLC Pathway

EGCG can exert anticancer functions inducing cell cycle arrest. Several studies reported the blockade of the cell division cycle by EGCG administration in G0, G1, S, and G2 phases. EGCG may act through the indirect downregulation of pro-proliferative factors, such as cyclin D1, cyclin E, cyclin A, cyclin B, CDK4, CDK6, CDK2, and CDK1, as well as by the upregulation of anti-proliferative effectors, such as CDK inhibitors p27, p21, p16, and p18 [35,48,56,66,171,172]. In addition, EGCG has been found to act on cytokinesis, a critic step of cell division, by interacting with 67LR receptor [55,61,173].

Cytokinesis is the final step of cell division, leading a mother cell to be divided into two daughter cells. Early events of the process require the formation of an actomyosin ring, also known as contractile ring, that allows the formation of the cleavage furrow at the equator of mitotic cells [174,175]. Generation of the furrow enables the equal division of genetic material between the two forming cells and their subsequent separation. The interaction between actin filaments (F-actin) and myosin motors is controlled by different processes among which is the phosphorylation/dephosphorylation of the myosin II regulatory light chain (MRLC). Myosin II is one of the main motors involved in cytokinesis, activated through MRLC phosphorylation at Ser19/Thr18 by kinases, such as MLCK, ROCK, and Citron kinase [176]. Ser19 phosphorylation favours the interaction with F-actin, the contractile ring formation, and filaments assembly. A di-phosphorylation seems to be involved in the assembly of filaments, but the role of phosphorylation in Thr18 alone is less clear [177–179]. Conversely, MRLC dephosphorylation in Ser19 or Ser19/Thr18 by the myosin phosphatase leads to myosin inactivation. The MRLC activity is also indirectly regulated through the phosphorylation of myosin phosphatase itself. When the largest region of myosin phosphatase, called myosin phosphatase target subunit (MYPT1), is phosphorylated in at least one of the inhibitory sites (e.g., Thr696, Thr853), its activity is inhibited, and, as a consequence, MRLC remains active, thus providing a positive signal triggering cytokinesis [180].

EGCG has been found to be able to interfere with the cytokinesis of HeLa cells through its action on MRLC phosphorylation status, thereby affecting the cellular growth [55]. EGCG activates the signalling cascade that is responsible for the impaired MRLC phosphorylation through binding to its membrane receptor 67LR [55] (Figure 1). At first, it was reported that the treatment of HeLa cells with 10, 20, and 50 μM EGCG resulted in the disruption of stress fibers, reduction of the contractile ring formation, increment of cells blocked in G2/M phases, and inhibition of cell growth [55]. Further analyses revealed that EGCG treatment also caused, via 67LR, a reduction in single Ser19 and in double Ser19/Thr18 MRLC phosphorylation, which effects on MRLC phosphorylation might reasonably trigger the effects shown on cell division and growth [55]. Under similar conditions, EGCG was also found to decrease the phosphorylation of MYTP1 at inhibitory site Thr696 both in vitro and in vivo, thus preventing myosin phosphatase inactivation. According to the literature, the ability of EGCG to interfere with MRLC phosphorylation could be the indirect consequence of MYPT1 loss of inhibition [55]. Recently, another factor has been added to the members of the EGCG signalling pathway, believed to be responsible for impaired cancer cell cytokinesis: the eukaryotic translation elongation factor 1a (eEF1a), which has been found to be necessary to enable EGCG to alter MYPT1 phosphorylation status [61]. eEF1a is mainly known as a component of the eukaryotic translation machinery, but it also takes part in other cellular processes, such as senescence, oncogenic transformation, and cell proliferation [181–183]. eEF1a is able to bind to MYPT1 and F-actin [184]. In vitro and in vivo experiments demonstrated that no significant reduction in MYPT1 and MRLC phosphorylation, actin disassembly and cell proliferation was observed after EGCG administration in eEF1a knockout models [61]. This evidence has been further corroborated by the observation that when eEF1a levels are restored and 67LR is absent, the effects that are described above disappear as well. Thereby, eEF1a is thought to be downstream of 67LR and upstream of MYPT1 in the signalling pathway that is triggered by EGCG [61] (Figure 1).

2.2.2. EGCG/67LR/cAMP/PKA/PP2A Pathway

67LR surface receptor is involved in the selective anti-tumour activity exerted by EGCG in melanomas. Tsukamoto et al. identified protein phosphatase 2A (PP2A) as a downstream target of 67LR in melanoma cells [86]. PP2A is a Ser/Thr phosphatase that is involved in important cellular processes, such as proliferation, signal transduction, and apoptosis, and it is considered to be a tumor suppressor that is functionally inactivated in cancer [185,186].

By performing functional genetic screening, Tsukamoto and colleagues showed that EGCG binding to 67LR receptor induces PP2A activation mediated by the cAMP/PKA pathway [86], which led to the suppression of melanoma tumor cell growth. Even though the direct interaction between EGCG and PP2A was demonstrated using very high EGCG concentrations [84,187,188], 1 μM EGCG was sufficient to activate 67LR/PP2A pathway. PP2A directly interacts with p70S6k and down-regulates mTOR signaling [189], which is usually aberrantly activated in melanomas. Therefore, it represents an important contribution to chemotherapeutic resistance of commonly used BRAF inhibitor treatment. The EGCG-activating 67LR/PP2A pathway exerts a strong synergistic effect with PLX4720, a BRAF inhibitor, in drug-resistant melanomas.

Another effect that is mediated by the 67LR/PP2A signaling is the activation of Merlin, a tumor suppressor protein that is encoded by the NF2 gene at physiological concentrations of EGCG, as low as 1 μM [86]. Merlin activity seems to target cell surface RTKs and adhesion/extracellular matrix receptors, regulating cell proliferation, survival and motility [190]. PKA, p21-activated kinase 1 and 2 (PAK 1/2), or MYPT can activate Merlin by dephosphorylation at Ser-518. In the study by Tsukamoto et al. [86], EGCG was demonstrated to be an activator of Merlin via 67LR/PP2A pathway. In prostate cancer cell lines the absence or inactivation of Merlin contributes to tumor development and progression toward a highly invasive and chemo-resistant state [191–193].

Recently published data show that 10 μM EGCG up-regulates let-7b miRNA expression not only in melanoma cell lines, but also in metastatic melanoma tumours in vivo [81]. miRNAs are non-coding RNAs transcripts that are able to regulate fundamental biological activities related to mRNA degradation or translational inhibition [194]. Yamada et al. demonstrated that 67LR is involved in the EGCG-elicited let-7b increase, which leads to the inhibition of melanoma tumor progression [81].

Let-7b recognizes multiple target genes that are related to tumor progression, such as the high mobility group A2 (HMGA2), decreased in EGCG-treated melanoma cells [81], or Ras [195,196].

Furthermore, the data indicated that PP2A inactivation caused the induction of let-7b, which is generally down-regulated in cancer (including melanoma and prostate cancer) [81,197], even if it is not clear whether let-7b transcription or let-7b processing is modulated by EGCG-induced PP2A activation.

Zhou et al. confirmed that EGCG induced miRNAs profile changes in a mouse model of lung tumor. They highlighted that the miRNAs affected by EGCG and target genes are different from those that were previously identified by in vivo studies [198].

2.3. Modulation of Cancer Stem Cells Properties

EGCG was shown to affect the survival of cancer stem cells (CSCs). EGCG inhibits CSCs growth and stemness in several malignancies, such as breast [199], lung [54,200], colorectal cancer [85], osteosarcoma [14], and neuroblastoma [201].

Kumazoe M. et al. [202] describe the effects of EGCG on the features of pancreatic CSCs (i.e., the capability to form colonies and spheroids) through the activation of the EGCG/67LR/cGMP axis. The same research team had observed that spheroid formation in pancreatic CSCs colonies was inhibited by cGMP targeting of the Forkhead box O3 (FOXO3)/CD44 axes [203]. Transcriptional factor FOXO3 is known to be a cancer suppressor, but it also induces the high expression of CD44, a master regulator (and also a marker) of CSCs [202]. FOXO3 has been shown to be a direct target of EGCG in tumours, like pancreatic and breast cancer. In pancreatic cancer treatment with EGCG suppressed tumour growth, accompanied by FOXO3 downregulation [99]. By contrast, in breast cancer, a positive regulation of FOXO3 exerted by the EGCG has been described [70,204,205]. Although the reported modulations seem to be opposite, the action of EGCG on FOXO3 seems to lead to cancer suppression altogether. Recently, the role of EGCG in inhibiting cancer stem cells (CSC) growth and altering their features is emerging [54,95,199]. According to this literature, EGCG seems to act by downregulating CD44 expression in tumours, like non-small cell lung cancer and pancreatic cancer [200,202]. In pancreatic cancer cell lines expressing CD44, the isoform 3A of the enzyme phosphodiesterase (PDE3A) is highly expressed [202]. Like other members of the same family, PDE3A is a negative regulator of cGMP [206]. In pancreatic cancer cells, low EGCG administration did not lead to a significant increase in cGMP amount, or to the reduction of colony and spheroid formation [202]. Further experiments were conducted using low doses of EGCG combined with the administration of a PDE3A inhibitor, Trequinsin. The combination therapy decreased the protein levels of FOXO3 and CD44, caused an increase of cGMP, and a strong reduction in the CSCs capability to form both colonies and spheroids. The combination of EGCG and Trequinsin is synergistic and it reduces the IC_{50} of EGCG, thus allowing for its use at physiological concentration. These observations have also been confirmed in vivo [202]. Surprisingly, as for the other signalling pathway that is discussed above, the effects of EGCG alone, or in combination with other agents, are always specific for cancer cells, and they do not affect normal cells. This highly specific effect of EGCG is still waiting for an explanation.

3. Other EGCG-Interacting Proteins

Another interesting protein that was shown to interact directly with green tea catechins is the human peptidyl prolyl *cis*/*trans* isomerase (Pin1). Pin is a protein with two domains: an N-terminal WW-domain and a C-terminal PPIase domain; both are necessary for its function. Although many PPIases have been identified some with an established role in cancer, only Pin1 acts distinctively and specifically on phosphorylated proteins. Pin1 catalyzes the *cis*/*trans* isomerization of the peptidyl proline bond of proteins. This activity causes major changes in the conformation of the target protein, with a consequent alteration of its function or stability. In this way, Pin1 affects and modulatse different pathways involving kinase-dependent signaling, such as NF-kB, activator-protein 1 (AP-1), nuclear factor of activated T cells (NFAT), or b-catenin [207]. Pin1 has been demonstrated to have a major role in oncogenic signaling [208,209] and is highly expressed in several cancers [210,211], including prostate cancer [212].

Urusova et al. used crystallographic and biochemical data to show that EGCG interacts directly with both the PPase and WW domains of Pin1, which inhibits its tumour-promoting activity. Therefore, Pin1 represent a possible target for anti-cancer therapies [83,213]. The dissociation constant of EGCG and Pin1 has been calculated as 21 μM, both by protease-coupled and isothermal titration calorimetric assays: this value is similar to the concentration of EGCG that was found to exert anti-cancer effects in experimental cancer models [40]. Since the Kd value that resulted was quite high, the interaction between EGCG and Pin1 was described as "not strong". Urusova and colleagues crystallized the Pin1-EGCG complex, resolving its structure at 1.9 Å resolution by X-ray diffraction. The crystal structure has revealed that a molecule of EGCG was bound to Pin1 WW domain (aminoacids 1–31), which is responsible for the interaction with the substrate, while another molecule of EGCG was bound to the Pin1 PPIase domain, necessary for the isomerization reaction. A recent study demonstrated that galloyl group in EGCG is required for Pin1 inhibition [214]. Binding between EGCG and Pin1 in solution has been studied recently by combining fluorescence spectrum, far-UV circular dichroism spectrum with molecular dynamics simulations. The analysis of the binding energy confirmed the strong inhibitory effect that is exerted by EGCG on Pin1 activity [215].

To analyze the functional consequence of Pin1-EGCG binding, Urusova and colleagues used mouse embryonal fibroblasts (MEF) collected from PIN1 KO and WT mice, and showed that Pin1 expression is required for EGCG (10–40 μM) inhibitory effect on MEFs growth. Furthermore, the formation of the EGCG-Pin1 complex prevented the binding of the Pin1 substrate c-Jun. Finally, EGCG effect on transcriptional regulation of AP-1 and NF-kB has been shown to be mediated by Pin1 [83].

Green tea catechins are mainly believed to prevent cancer. However, several epidemiological studies suggest that their activity also works against cancer progression; the interaction of EGCG with proteins that are involved in cancer progression and metastatic spread has been considered. One of the effects exerted by EGCG is the inhibition of TGF-β signaling transduction. TGF-β is a multifunctional cytokine that induces epithelial-mesenchymal transition (EMT) of cancer cells, and it is also responsible for the maintenance of EMT, a critical event during early metastatic growth. The mechanism by which EGCG modulates TGF-β pathway has not been completely elucidated. It has been shown that the binding between TGF-β and its receptor, TGFR-II, activates two different pathways leading to EMT: the canonical Smad-dependent pathway and the mitogen-activated protein kinase (MAPK) pathway. Tabuchi et al. used immunoprecipitation and affinity chromatography assays to demonstrate binding between EGCG and TGFR-II protein. This interaction may be responsible for the inhibitory effect of EGCG on the expression of alpha-SMA (considered a marker of the EMT) via the TGF-beta Smad2/3 pathway in human lung fibroblast cells [94].

EGCG has also been shown to bind to metalloproteinases (MMPs). MMPs are matrix degrading enzymes that are involved in tumor invasion and metastasis [50] whose expression is regulated by several growth factors, including TGF-β1 [216–219]. Sazuka et al. have demonstrated that EGCG inhibits the collagenase activity of MMP-2 and MMP-9 produced by lung carcinoma cells. The authors suggest that the mechanism of inhibition relies on direct binding between EGCG and MMP proteins, as proved by affinity gel chromatography experiments [50]. In 2017, Chowdhury et al. performed a preliminary in silico analysis and then showed a strong interaction of pro-/active MMP2 with the galloyl group of EGCG and ECG in pulmonary artery smooth muscle cell culture supernatant. They showed that EGCG and ECG were better inhibitors of proMMP2 when compared to MMP2, and they demonstrated that a strong interaction with MT1/MMP is involved in the conversion of proMMP2 to active MMP2 [220]. Further, investigating the interactions of pro-/active MMP-9 with green tea catechins by computational methods, they showed strong interactions between pro-/active MMP9 and EGCG/ECG [221].

4. EGCG Epigenetic Regulation

Another mechanism that can explain the pleiotropic effects exerted by green tea catechins in tumor cells is the epigenetic change in gene expression and chromatin organization. Mutations in oncogenes and tumor suppressor genes are often the cause of cancer development and alterations of gene expression count for cancer progression.

Many biologically active compounds, including EGCG, have been demonstrated to modulate DNA methylation and histone acetylation status [222].

DNA methyltransferases (DNMTs) and histone deacetylases (HDACs) are enzymes that are involved in transcriptional gene silencing and histone acetyl transferases (HATs) positively regulate gene expression regulation [223,224]. Several studies reported EGCG contribution in epigenetic control acting on DNMTs, HDACs and HATs expression and activity in different tumours. We will briefly mention different genes whose expression is enhanced or reduced by EGCG-dependent epigenetic control.

Fang et al. demonstrated that EGCG binds to DNMT and competitively inhibits the enzymatic activity (Ki of 6.89 μM), yielding the reactivation of methylation-silenced genes in prostate cancer PC3 cells [225]. Molecular modeling and docking studies supported the binding of EGCG to DNMT3B and HDAC1 [39].

In HeLa cell line, it has been observed that EGCG can direct bind to and inhibit DNMT1, DNMT3B, and HDAC1 activity, causing a reduction in DNA hypermethylation and restoring the expression of repressed genes as retinoic acid receptor β (RARβ), CDH1 (e-cadherine gene), and DAPK1 [29,39]. Furthermore, in the same the same cell line, EGCG combination with eugenol-amrogentin (active compounds of clove and Swertia Chirata, respectively) reduces DNMT1 expression with the consequent hypomethylation of the cell cycle inhibitors p16 and LimD1 promoters [226]. In acute promyelocytic leukemia cells, EGCG down-regulates DNMT1, HDAC1, HDAC2, G9a, and Polycomb repressive complex 2 (PRC2) core components expression and favours the binding of hyperacetylated H4 and acetylated H3K14 histones to promoter regions of p27, CAF, C/EBPα, and C/EBPε genes [63]. In the lung cell line PC-9, EGCG combination with Am80 (a synthetic retinoid used for acute promyelocytic leukemia therapy) causes a decrease of HDAC4, HDAC5, and HDAC6 protein levels and reduction of HDAC activity, leading to increased p53 and α-tubulin acetylation [227]. In in vitro and in vivo models of lung cancer, EGCG has been found to resensitize tumor cells to Cisplatin (DDP)-based combination chemotherapy through DNMT and HDAC activity inhibition, and the subsequent re-expression of GAS1, TIMP4, ICAM1, and WISP2 genes [228]. In in vivo model of lung cancer, EGCG epigenetic action in down-regulating DNMT1 is accompanied by phospho-histone H2AX (γ-H2AX) and p-AKT reduction [229]. In skin cancer cells, it has demonstrated EGCG capability in reducing DNMT1, DNMT3A, and DNMT3B activity and expression, and also in increasing histones H3 and H4 acetylation. As a consequence of the described epigenetic changes, a restored expression of the cell cycle inhibitors p16 and p21 has been observed [48]. In breast cancer cells, EGCG-dependent reduction of HDAC1 and zeste homolog 2 (EZH2) protein levels leads to tissue inhibitor of matrix metalloproteinase-3 (TIMP-3) gene transcriptional activation [72]. In prostate cancer cell lines, it has been observed that the EGCG-dependent reduction of the acetylated androgen receptor (AR) gene might be induced by EGCG reduction in HAT activity [65]. EGCG also acts on teleomerase, reducing its activity in different tumor types as esophageal carcinoma [230], glioma [231], cervical cancer [232], breast cancer [100], nasopharyngeal carcinoma [233], ovarian cancer [68], laryngeal squamous cell carcinoma [234], and lung cancer [235]. It has also been shown that EGCG can translocate from the cytoplasm to the nucleus where it can bind to DNA, suggesting a possible role in gene expression regulation also through the direct binding to nucleic acid [236,237]. However, the effects of EGCG/DNA direct interaction need to be clarified.

5. Conclusions

Because of their anti-proliferative, pro-apoptotic, and anti-oxidative properties, green tea catechins and especially EGCG are receiving much attention in cancer biology. Several in vitro, in vivo, and clinical studies, have demonstrated that EGCG exerts anti-cancer effects in different models through the activation/inhibition of several signalling pathways, most of which are triggered by the direct interaction between EGCG and specific protein targets. The array of EGCG interactors is wide and growing, and it includes intracellular molecules, membranes receptors, membrane microdomains, and the plasma membrane itself. One of the first EGCG direct target identified was 67LR, but in recent years, others interactors, such as Pin1 or TGFR-II, have been recognized. Appropriate identification and study of EGCG direct targets will allow a better understanding of its mechanisms of action and a better exploitation of its anti-cancer properties. From 2004, when the 67LR was first identified as direct target of EGCG by Tachibana et al., several research teams have investigated the pathways modulated by EGCG-67LR interaction. Today, we know that the anti-proliferative action of EGCG is mediated by the binding to 67LR, whose expression is increased in tumour cells. Convincing experimental data also showed that membrane composition is involved in the inhibitory activity of EGCG in some cancer cells lines. Since 67LR is generally located in lipid rafts, EGCG-mediated microdomains composition and the alteration of their functions triggers the downstream signalling cascades. In addition, new experimental data have brought to light novel EGCG signalling cascades leading to cell apoptosis, cell cycle arrest, reduction in CSC colony and spheroid formation, as well as regulation of miRNAs expression. EGCG binding to membrane receptors, such as TGFR-II, intracellular molecules, such as Pin1 and secreted enzymes, such as MMPs, provided noteworthy information about the mechanisms of EGCG-mediated tumour suppression. Another mechanism to explain the pleiotropic anti-cancer effects that are exerted by EGCG and green tea catechins that is gaining the attention of the researchers is the modulation of epigenetic processes. Long-term administration of green tea catechins leads to the re-activation of tumour suppressor genes that are silenced during carcinogenesis and downregulation of oncogenes through the inhibition of enzymes, such as DNMTs and HDACs involved in DNA methylation and chromatin remodelling. Further studies on the interaction of EGCG with protein targets will provide new insights enabling the development of more pharmacological treatments targeting EGCG-activated master regulators of key pathways.

Author Contributions: A.N., V.N., F.R. and S.B. critically reviewed the literature and wrote the manuscript.

Funding: This research received no external funding.

Acknowledgments: V.N. was supported by a fellowship by Fondazione Umberto Veronesi. We thank Paul Wegener for English editing support.

Conflicts of Interest: The authors declare no conflict of interest.

References

1. Graham, H.N. Green tea composition, consumption, and polyphenol chemistry. *Prev. Med.* **1992**, *21*, 334–350. [CrossRef]
2. Lowe, G.M.; Gana, K.; Rahman, K. Dietary supplementation with green tea extract promotes enhanced human leukocyte activity. *J. Complement. Integr. Med.* **2015**, *12*, 277–282. [CrossRef] [PubMed]
3. Boschmann, M.; Thielecke, F. The effects of epigallocatechin-3-gallate on thermogenesis and fat oxidation in obese men: A pilot study. *J. Am. Coll. Nutr.* **2007**, *26*, 389S–395S. [CrossRef] [PubMed]
4. Basu, A.; Sanchez, K.; Leyva, M.J.; Wu, M.; Betts, N.M.; Aston, C.E.; Lyons, T.J. Green tea supplementation affects body weight, lipids, and lipid peroxidation in obese subjects with metabolic syndrome. *J. Am. Coll. Nutr.* **2010**, *29*, 31–40. [CrossRef] [PubMed]
5. Ide, K.; Yamada, H.; Takuma, N.; Park, M.; Wakamiya, N.; Nakase, J.; Ukawa, Y.; Sagesaka, Y.M. Green tea consumption affects cognitive dysfunction in the elderly: A pilot study. *Nutrients* **2014**, *6*, 4032–4042. [CrossRef] [PubMed]

6.   Bettuzzi, S.; Brausi, M.; Rizzi, F.; Castagnetti, G.; Peracchia, G.; Corti, A. Chemoprevention of human prostate cancer by oral administration of green tea catechins in volunteers with high-grade prostate intraepithelial neoplasia: A preliminary report from a one-year proof-of-principle study. *Cancer Res.* **2006**, *66*, 1234–1240. [CrossRef]

7.   Khan, N.; Afaq, F.; Saleem, M.; Ahmad, N.; Mukhtar, H. Targeting multiple signaling pathways by green tea polyphenol (−)-epigallocatechin-3-gallate. *Cancer Res.* **2006**, *66*, 2500–2505. [CrossRef]

8.   Yang, C.S.; Sang, S.; Lambert, J.D.; Lee, M.J. Bioavailability issues in studying the health effects of plant polyphenolic compounds. *Mol. Nutr. Food Res.* **2008**, *52* (Suppl. 1), S139–S151. [CrossRef]

9.   Lee, M.J.; Wang, Z.Y.; Li, H.; Chen, L.; Sun, Y.; Gobbo, S.; Balentine, D.A.; Yang, C.S. Analysis of plasma and urinary tea polyphenols in human subjects. *Cancer Epidemiol. Biomarkers Prev.* **1995**, *4*, 393–399.

10.   Gan, R.Y.; Li, H.B.; Sui, Z.Q.; Corke, H. Absorption, metabolism, anti-cancer effect and molecular targets of epigallocatechin gallate (egcg): An updated review. *Crit. Rev. Food Sci. Nutr.* **2018**, *58*, 924–941. [CrossRef]

11.   Zubair, H.; Azim, S.; Ahmad, A.; Khan, M.A.; Patel, G.K.; Singh, S.; Singh, A.P. Cancer chemoprevention by phytochemicals: Nature's healing touch. *Molecules* **2017**, *22*, 395. [CrossRef] [PubMed]

12.   Jin, G.; Yang, Y.; Liu, K.; Zhao, J.; Chen, X.; Liu, H.; Bai, R.; Li, X.; Jiang, Y.; Zhang, X.; et al. Combination curcumin and (−)-epigallocatechin-3-gallate inhibits colorectal carcinoma microenvironment-induced angiogenesis by jak/stat3/il-8 pathway. *Oncogenesis* **2017**, *6*, e384. [PubMed]

13.   Chan, M.M.; Chen, R.; Fong, D. Targeting cancer stem cells with dietary phytochemical—Repositioned drug combinations. *Cancer Lett.* **2018**, *433*, 53–64. [CrossRef] [PubMed]

14.   Wang, W.; Chen, D.; Zhu, K. Sox2ot variant 7 contributes to the synergistic interaction between egcg and doxorubicin to kill osteosarcoma via autophagy and stemness inhibition. *J. Exp. Clin. Cancer Res.* **2018**, *37*, 37. [CrossRef] [PubMed]

15.   Mayr, C.; Wagner, A.; Neureiter, D.; Pichler, M.; Jakab, M.; Illig, R.; Berr, F.; Kiesslich, T. The green tea catechin epigallocatechin gallate induces cell cycle arrest and shows potential synergism with cisplatin in biliary tract cancer cells. *BMC Complement. Altern. Med.* **2015**, *15*, 194. [CrossRef]

16.   Zhou, Y.; Tang, J.; Du, Y.; Ding, J.; Liu, J.Y. The green tea polyphenol egcg potentiates the antiproliferative activity of sunitinib in human cancer cells. *Tumour. Biol.* **2016**, *37*, 8555–8566. [CrossRef]

17.   Yuan, X.; He, Y.; Zhou, G.; Li, X.; Feng, A.; Zheng, W. Target challenging-cancer drug delivery to gastric cancer tissues with a fucose graft epigallocatechin-3-gallate-gold particles nanocomposite approach. *J. Photochem. Photobiol. B* **2018**, *183*, 147–153. [CrossRef]

18.   Hajipour, H.; Hamishehkar, H.; Nazari Soltan Ahmad, S.; Barghi, S.; Maroufi, N.F.; Taheri, R.A. Improved anticancer effects of epigallocatechin gallate using rgd-containing nanostructured lipid carriers. *Artif. Cells Nanomed. Biotechnol.* **2018**. [CrossRef]

19.   Sanna, V.; Singh, C.K.; Jashari, R.; Adhami, V.M.; Chamcheu, J.C.; Rady, I.; Sechi, M.; Mukhtar, H.; Siddiqui, I.A. Targeted nanoparticles encapsulating (−)-epigallocatechin-3-gallate for prostate cancer prevention and therapy. *Sci. Rep.* **2017**, *7*, 41573. [CrossRef]

20.   Krupkova, O.; Ferguson, S.J.; Wuertz-Kozak, K. Stability of (−)-epigallocatechin gallate and its activity in liquid formulations and delivery systems. *J. Nutr. Biochem.* **2016**, *37*, 1–12. [CrossRef]

21.   Rizzi, F.; Naponelli, V.; Silva, A.; Modernelli, A.; Ramazzina, I.; Bonacini, M.; Tardito, S.; Gatti, R.; Uggeri, J.; Bettuzzi, S. Polyphenon e(r), a standardized green tea extract, induces endoplasmic reticulum stress, leading to death of immortalized pnt1a cells by anoikis and tumorigenic pc3 by necroptosis. *Carcinogenesis* **2014**, *35*, 828–839. [CrossRef] [PubMed]

22.   Modernelli, A.; Naponelli, V.; Giovanna Troglio, M.; Bonacini, M.; Ramazzina, I.; Bettuzzi, S.; Rizzi, F. Egcg antagonizes bortezomib cytotoxicity in prostate cancer cells by an autophagic mechanism. *Sci. Rep.* **2015**, *5*, 15270. [CrossRef] [PubMed]

23.   Thawonsuwan, J.; Kiron, V.; Satoh, S.; Panigrahi, A.; Verlhac, V. Epigallocatechin-3-gallate (egcg) affects the antioxidant and immune defense of the rainbow trout, oncorhynchus mykiss. *Fish. Physiol. Biochem.* **2010**, *36*, 687–697. [CrossRef] [PubMed]

24.   Lambert, J.D.; Elias, R.J. The antioxidant and pro-oxidant activities of green tea polyphenols: A role in cancer prevention. *Arch. Biochem. Biophys.* **2010**, *501*, 65–72. [CrossRef] [PubMed]

25.   Gupta, S.; Hastak, K.; Afaq, F.; Ahmad, N.; Mukhtar, H. Essential role of caspases in epigallocatechin-3-gallate-mediated inhibition of nuclear factor kappa b and induction of apoptosis. *Oncogene* **2004**, *23*, 2507–2522. [CrossRef] [PubMed]

26. Shimizu, M.; Adachi, S.; Masuda, M.; Kozawa, O.; Moriwaki, H. Cancer chemoprevention with green tea catechins by targeting receptor tyrosine kinases. *Mol. Nutr. Food Res.* **2011**, *55*, 832–843. [CrossRef]

27. Singh, B.N.; Shankar, S.; Srivastava, R.K. Green tea catechin, epigallocatechin-3-gallate (egcg): Mechanisms, perspectives and clinical applications. *Biochem. Pharmacol.* **2011**, *82*, 1807–1821. [CrossRef]

28. Lin, C.H.; Shen, Y.A.; Hung, P.H.; Yu, Y.B.; Chen, Y.J. Epigallocathechin gallate, polyphenol present in green tea, inhibits stem-like characteristics and epithelial-mesenchymal transition in nasopharyngeal cancer cell lines. *BMC Complement. Altern. Med.* **2012**, *12*, 201. [CrossRef] [PubMed]

29. Lee, W.J.; Shim, J.Y.; Zhu, B.T. Mechanisms for the inhibition of DNA methyltransferases by tea catechins and bioflavonoids. *Mol. Pharmacol.* **2005**, *68*, 1018–1030. [CrossRef]

30. Shirakami, Y.; Shimizu, M. Possible mechanisms of green tea and its constituents against cancer. *Molecules* **2018**, *23*, 2284. [CrossRef]

31. Rahmani, A.H.; Al Shabrmi, F.M.; Allemailem, K.S.; Aly, S.M.; Khan, M.A. Implications of green tea and its constituents in the prevention of cancer via the modulation of cell signalling pathway. *BioMed Res. Int.* **2015**, *2015*, 925640. [CrossRef] [PubMed]

32. Naponelli, V.; Ramazzina, I.; Lenzi, C.; Bettuzzi, S.; Rizzi, F. Green tea catechins for prostate cancer prevention: Present achievements and future challenges. *Antioxidants* **2017**, *6*, 26. [CrossRef] [PubMed]

33. Ellinger, S.; Muller, N.; Stehle, P.; Ulrich-Merzenich, G. Consumption of green tea or green tea products: Is there an evidence for antioxidant effects from controlled interventional studies? *Phytomedicine* **2011**, *18*, 903–915. [CrossRef] [PubMed]

34. Shankar, S.; Ganapathy, S.; Hingorani, S.R.; Srivastava, R.K. Egcg inhibits growth, invasion, angiogenesis and metastasis of pancreatic cancer. *Front. Biosci.* **2008**, *13*, 440–452. [CrossRef] [PubMed]

35. Gupta, S.; Hussain, T.; Mukhtar, H. Molecular pathway for (−)-epigallocatechin-3-gallate-induced cell cycle arrest and apoptosis of human prostate carcinoma cells. *Arch. Biochem. Biophys.* **2003**, *410*, 177–185. [CrossRef]

36. Shimizu, M.; Shirakami, Y.; Moriwaki, H. Targeting receptor tyrosine kinases for chemoprevention by green tea catechin, egcg. *Int. J. Mol. Sci.* **2008**, *9*, 1034–1049. [CrossRef]

37. Shimizu, M.; Weinstein, I.B. Modulation of signal transduction by tea catechins and related phytochemicals. *Mutat. Res.* **2005**, *591*, 147–160. [CrossRef] [PubMed]

38. Pandey, M.; Shukla, S.; Gupta, S. Promoter demethylation and chromatin remodeling by green tea polyphenols leads to re-expression of gstp1 in human prostate cancer cells. *Int. J. Cancer* **2010**, *126*, 2520–2533. [CrossRef] [PubMed]

39. Khan, M.A.; Hussain, A.; Sundaram, M.K.; Alalami, U.; Gunasekera, D.; Ramesh, L.; Hamza, A.; Quraishi, U. (−)-epigallocatechin-3-gallate reverses the expression of various tumor-suppressor genes by inhibiting DNA methyltransferases and histone deacetylases in human cervical cancer cells. *Oncol. Rep.* **2015**, *33*, 1976–1984. [CrossRef] [PubMed]

40. Rouzer, C.A.; Marnett, L.J. Green tea gets molecular. *Cancer Prev. Res.* **2011**, *4*, 1343–1345. [CrossRef]

41. Saeki, K.; Hayakawa, S.; Nakano, S.; Ito, S.; Oishi, Y.; Suzuki, Y.; Isemura, M. In vitro and in silico studies of the molecular interactions of epigallocatechin-3-o-gallate (egcg) with proteins that explain the health benefits of green tea. *Molecules* **2018**, *23*, 1295. [CrossRef] [PubMed]

42. Ermakova, S.; Choi, B.Y.; Choi, H.S.; Kang, B.S.; Bode, A.M.; Dong, Z. The intermediate filament protein vimentin is a new target for epigallocatechin gallate. *J. Biol. Chem.* **2005**, *280*, 16882–16890. [CrossRef]

43. He, Z.; Tang, F.; Ermakova, S.; Li, M.; Zhao, Q.; Cho, Y.Y.; Ma, W.Y.; Choi, H.S.; Bode, A.M.; Yang, C.S.; et al. Fyn is a novel target of (−)-epigallocatechin gallate in the inhibition of jb6 cl41 cell transformation. *Mol. Carcinog.* **2008**, *47*, 172–183. [CrossRef] [PubMed]

44. Shim, J.H.; Choi, H.S.; Pugliese, A.; Lee, S.Y.; Chae, J.I.; Choi, B.Y.; Bode, A.M.; Dong, Z. (−)-epigallocatechin gallate regulates cd3-mediated t cell receptor signaling in leukemia through the inhibition of zap-70 kinase. *J. Biol. Chem.* **2008**, *283*, 28370–28379. [CrossRef] [PubMed]

45. Li, M.; He, Z.; Ermakova, S.; Zheng, D.; Tang, F.; Cho, Y.Y.; Zhu, F.; Ma, W.Y.; Sham, Y.; Rogozin, E.A.; et al. Direct inhibition of insulin-like growth factor-i receptor kinase activity by (−)-epigallocatechin-3-gallate regulates cell transformation. *Cancer Epidemiol. Biomarkers Prev.* **2007**, *16*, 598–605. [CrossRef] [PubMed]

46. Ermakova, S.P.; Kang, B.S.; Choi, B.Y.; Choi, H.S.; Schuster, T.F.; Ma, W.Y.; Bode, A.M.; Dong, Z. (−)-epigallocatechin gallate overcomes resistance to etoposide-induced cell death by targeting the molecular chaperone glucose-regulated protein 78. *Cancer Res.* **2006**, *66*, 9260–9269. [CrossRef] [PubMed]

47. Fujimura, Y. Small molecule-sensing strategy and techniques for understanding the functionality of green tea. *Biosci. Biotechnol. Biochem.* **2015**, *79*, 687–699. [CrossRef]

48. Nandakumar, V.; Vaid, M.; Katiyar, S.K. (−)-epigallocatechin-3-gallate reactivates silenced tumor suppressor genes, cip1/p21 and p16ink4a, by reducing DNA methylation and increasing histones acetylation in human skin cancer cells. *Carcinogenesis* **2011**, *32*, 537–544. [CrossRef]

49. Hu, Q.; Chang, X.; Yan, R.; Rong, C.; Yang, C.; Cheng, S.; Gu, X.; Yao, H.; Hou, X.; Mo, Y.; et al. (−)-epigallocatechin-3-gallate induces cancer cell apoptosis via acetylation of amyloid precursor protein. *Med. Oncol.* **2015**, *32*, 390. [CrossRef]

50. Sazuka, M.; Imazawa, H.; Shoji, Y.; Mita, T.; Hara, Y.; Isemura, M. Inhibition of collagenases from mouse lung carcinoma cells by green tea catechins and black tea theaflavins. *Biosci. Biotechnol. Biochem.* **1997**, *61*, 1504–1506. [CrossRef]

51. Fujimura, Y.; Tachibana, H.; Yamada, K. Lipid raft-associated catechin suppresses the fcepsilonri expression by inhibiting phosphorylation of the extracellular signal-regulated kinase1/2. *FEBS Lett.* **2004**, *556*, 204–210. [CrossRef]

52. Tsukamoto, S.; Huang, Y.; Kumazoe, M.; Lesnick, C.; Yamada, S.; Ueda, N.; Suzuki, T.; Yamashita, S.; Kim, Y.H.; Fujimura, Y.; et al. Sphingosine kinase-1 protects multiple myeloma from apoptosis driven by cancer-specific inhibition of rtks. *Mol. Cancer Ther.* **2015**, *14*, 2303–2312. [CrossRef] [PubMed]

53. Wu, P.P.; Kuo, S.C.; Huang, W.W.; Yang, J.S.; Lai, K.C.; Chen, H.J.; Lin, K.L.; Chiu, Y.J.; Huang, L.J.; Chung, J.G. (−)-epigallocatechin gallate induced apoptosis in human adrenal cancer nci-h295 cells through caspase-dependent and caspase-independent pathway. *Anticancer Res.* **2009**, *29*, 1435–1442. [PubMed]

54. Zhu, J.; Jiang, Y.; Yang, X.; Wang, S.; Xie, C.; Li, X.; Li, Y.; Chen, Y.; Wang, X.; Meng, Y.; et al. Wnt/beta-catenin pathway mediates (−)-epigallocatechin-3-gallate (egcg) inhibition of lung cancer stem cells. *Biochem. Biophys. Res. Commun.* **2017**, *482*, 15–21. [CrossRef] [PubMed]

55. Umeda, D.; Tachibana, H.; Yamada, K. Epigallocatechin-3-o-gallate disrupts stress fibers and the contractile ring by reducing myosin regulatory light chain phosphorylation mediated through the target molecule 67 kda laminin receptor. *Biochem. Biophys. Res. Commun.* **2005**, *333*, 628–635. [CrossRef] [PubMed]

56. Shankar, S.; Suthakar, G.; Srivastava, R.K. Epigallocatechin-3-gallate inhibits cell cycle and induces apoptosis in pancreatic cancer. *Front. Biosci.* **2007**, *12*, 5039–5051. [CrossRef]

57. Hwang, Y.S.; Park, K.K.; Chung, W.Y. Epigallocatechin-3 gallate inhibits cancer invasion by repressing functional invadopodia formation in oral squamous cell carcinoma. *Eur. J. Pharmacol.* **2013**, *715*, 286–295. [CrossRef]

58. Olotu, F.A.; Agoni, C.; Adeniji, E.; Abdullahi, M.; Soliman, M.E. Probing gallate-mediated selectivity and high-affinity binding of epigallocatechin gallate: A way-forward in the design of selective inhibitors for anti-apoptotic bcl-2 proteins. *Appl. Biochem. Biotechnol.* **2018**, *29*, 1–20. [CrossRef]

59. Shin, S.; Kim, M.K.; Jung, W.; Chong, Y. (−)-epigallocatechin gallate derivatives reduce the expression of both urokinase plasminogen activator and plasminogen activator inhibitor-1 to inhibit migration, adhesion, and invasion of mda-mb-231 cells. *Phytother. Res.* **2018**, *32*, 2086–2096. [CrossRef]

60. Shi, J.; Liu, F.; Zhang, W.; Liu, X.; Lin, B.; Tang, X. Epigallocatechin-3-gallate inhibits nicotine-induced migration and invasion by the suppression of angiogenesis and epithelial-mesenchymal transition in non-small cell lung cancer cells. *Oncol. Rep.* **2015**, *33*, 2972–2980. [CrossRef]

61. Umeda, D.; Yano, S.; Yamada, K.; Tachibana, H. Green tea polyphenol epigallocatechin-3-gallate signaling pathway through 67-kda laminin receptor. *J. Biol. Chem.* **2008**, *283*, 3050–3058. [CrossRef] [PubMed]

62. Jang, J.Y.; Lee, J.K.; Jeon, Y.K.; Kim, C.W. Exosome derived from epigallocatechin gallate treated breast cancer cells suppresses tumor growth by inhibiting tumor-associated macrophage infiltration and m2 polarization. *BMC Cancer* **2013**, *13*, 421. [CrossRef] [PubMed]

63. Borutinskaite, V.; Virksaite, A.; Gudelyte, G.; Navakauskiene, R. Green tea polyphenol egcg causes anti-cancerous epigenetic modulations in acute promyelocytic leukemia cells. *Leuk. Lymphoma* **2018**, *59*, 469–478. [CrossRef] [PubMed]

64. Ma, J.; Shi, M.; Li, G.; Wang, N.; Wei, J.; Wang, T.; Wang, Y. Regulation of id1 expression by epigallocatechin3gallate and its effect on the proliferation and apoptosis of poorly differentiated ags gastric cancer cells. *Int. J. Oncol.* **2013**, *43*, 1052–1058. [CrossRef]

65. Lee, Y.H.; Kwak, J.; Choi, H.K.; Choi, K.C.; Kim, S.; Lee, J.; Jun, W.; Park, H.J.; Yoon, H.G. Egcg suppresses prostate cancer cell growth modulating acetylation of androgen receptor by anti-histone acetyltransferase activity. *Int. J. Mol. Med.* **2012**, *30*, 69–74. [PubMed]

66. Balasubramanian, S.; Adhikary, G.; Eckert, R.L. The bmi-1 polycomb protein antagonizes the (−)-epigallocatechin-3-gallate-dependent suppression of skin cancer cell survival. *Carcinogenesis* **2010**, *31*, 496–503. [CrossRef] [PubMed]

67. Takahashi, A.; Watanabe, T.; Mondal, A.; Suzuki, K.; Kurusu-Kanno, M.; Li, Z.; Yamazaki, T.; Fujiki, H.; Suganuma, M. Mechanism-based inhibition of cancer metastasis with (−)-epigallocatechin gallate. *Biochem. Biophys. Res. Commun.* **2014**, *443*, 1–6. [CrossRef]

68. Chen, H.; Landen, C.N.; Li, Y.; Alvarez, R.D.; Tollefsbol, T.O. Epigallocatechin gallate and sulforaphane combination treatment induce apoptosis in paclitaxel-resistant ovarian cancer cells through htert and bcl-2 down-regulation. *Exp. Cell Res.* **2013**, *319*, 697–706. [CrossRef]

69. Basu, A.; Haldar, S. Combinatorial effect of epigallocatechin-3-gallate and trail on pancreatic cancer cell death. *Int. J. Oncol.* **2009**, *34*, 281–286. [CrossRef]

70. Belguise, K.; Guo, S.; Sonenshein, G.E. Activation of foxo3a by the green tea polyphenol epigallocatechin-3-gallate induces estrogen receptor alpha expression reversing invasive phenotype of breast cancer cells. *Cancer Res.* **2007**, *67*, 5763–5770. [CrossRef]

71. Harper, C.E.; Patel, B.B.; Wang, J.; Eltoum, I.A.; Lamartiniere, C.A. Epigallocatechin-3-gallate suppresses early stage, but not late stage prostate cancer in tramp mice: Mechanisms of action. *Prostate* **2007**, *67*, 1576–1589. [CrossRef]

72. Deb, G.; Thakur, V.S.; Limaye, A.M.; Gupta, S. Epigenetic induction of tissue inhibitor of matrix metalloproteinase-3 by green tea polyphenols in breast cancer cells. *Mol. Carcinog.* **2015**, *54*, 485–499. [CrossRef]

73. Moses, M.A.; Henry, E.C.; Ricke, W.A.; Gasiewicz, T.A. The heat shock protein 90 inhibitor, (−)-epigallocatechin gallate, has anticancer activity in a novel human prostate cancer progression model. *Cancer Prev. Res.* **2015**, *8*, 249–257. [CrossRef] [PubMed]

74. Kumazoe, M.; Sugihara, K.; Tsukamoto, S.; Huang, Y.; Tsurudome, Y.; Suzuki, T.; Suemasu, Y.; Ueda, N.; Yamashita, S.; Kim, Y.; et al. 67-kda laminin receptor increases cgmp to induce cancer-selective apoptosis. *J. Clin. Investig.* **2013**, *123*, 787–799. [CrossRef]

75. Vahora, H.; Khan, M.A.; Alalami, U.; Hussain, A. The potential role of nitric oxide in halting cancer progression through chemoprevention. *J. Cancer Prev.* **2016**, *21*, 1–12. [CrossRef]

76. Surh, Y.J.; Chun, K.S.; Cha, H.H.; Han, S.S.; Keum, Y.S.; Park, K.K.; Lee, S.S. Molecular mechanisms underlying chemopreventive activities of anti-inflammatory phytochemicals: Down-regulation of cox-2 and inos through suppression of nf-kappa b activation. *Mutat. Res.* **2001**, *480–481*, 243–268. [CrossRef]

77. Hayakawa, S.; Saito, K.; Miyoshi, N.; Ohishi, T.; Oishi, Y.; Miyoshi, M.; Nakamura, Y. Anti-cancer effects of green tea by either anti- or pro- oxidative mechanisms. *Asian Pac. J. Cancer Prev.* **2016**, *17*, 1649–1654. [CrossRef]

78. Dhakshinamoorthy, S.; Porter, A.G. Nitric oxide-induced transcriptional up-regulation of protective genes by nrf2 via the antioxidant response element counteracts apoptosis of neuroblastoma cells. *J. Biol. Chem.* **2004**, *279*, 20096–20107. [CrossRef]

79. Li, Y.J.; Wu, S.L.; Lu, S.M.; Chen, F.; Guo, Y.; Gan, S.M.; Shi, Y.L.; Liu, S.; Li, S.L. (−)-epigallocatechin-3-gallate inhibits nasopharyngeal cancer stem cell self-renewal and migration and reverses the epithelial-mesenchymal transition via nf-kappab p65 inactivation. *Tumour. Biol.* **2015**, *36*, 2747–2761. [CrossRef]

80. He, L.; Zhang, E.; Shi, J.; Li, X.; Zhou, K.; Zhang, Q.; Le, A.D.; Tang, X. (−)-epigallocatechin-3-gallate inhibits human papillomavirus (hpv)-16 oncoprotein-induced angiogenesis in non-small cell lung cancer cells by targeting hif-1alpha. *Cancer Chemother. Pharmacol.* **2013**, *71*, 713–725. [CrossRef]

81. Yamada, S.; Tsukamoto, S.; Huang, Y.; Makio, A.; Kumazoe, M.; Yamashita, S.; Tachibana, H. Epigallocatechin-3-O-gallate up-regulates microrna-let-7b expression by activating 67-kda laminin receptor signaling in melanoma cells. *Sci. Rep.* **2016**, *6*, 19225. [CrossRef] [PubMed]

82. Wang, H.; Bian, S.; Yang, C.S. Green tea polyphenol egcg suppresses lung cancer cell growth through upregulating mir-210 expression caused by stabilizing hif-1alpha. *Carcinogenesis* **2011**, *32*, 1881–1889. [CrossRef] [PubMed]

83. Urusova, D.V.; Shim, J.H.; Kim, D.J.; Jung, S.K.; Zykova, T.A.; Carper, A.; Bode, A.M.; Dong, Z. Epigallocatechin-gallate suppresses tumorigenesis by directly targeting pin1. *Cancer Prev. Res.* **2011**, *4*, 1366–1377. [CrossRef] [PubMed]

84. Qin, J.; Chen, H.G.; Yan, Q.; Deng, M.; Liu, J.; Doerge, S.; Ma, W.; Dong, Z.; Li, D.W. Protein phosphatase-2a is a target of epigallocatechin-3-gallate and modulates p53-bak apoptotic pathway. *Cancer Res.* **2008**, *68*, 4150–4162. [CrossRef] [PubMed]

85. Toden, S.; Tran, H.M.; Tovar-Camargo, O.A.; Okugawa, Y.; Goel, A. Epigallocatechin-3-gallate targets cancer stem-like cells and enhances 5-fluorouracil chemosensitivity in colorectal cancer. *Oncotarget* **2016**, *7*, 16158–16171. [CrossRef] [PubMed]

86. Tsukamoto, S.; Huang, Y.; Umeda, D.; Yamada, S.; Yamashita, S.; Kumazoe, M.; Kim, Y.; Murata, M.; Yamada, K.; Tachibana, H. 67-kda laminin receptor-dependent protein phosphatase 2a (pp2a) activation elicits melanoma-specific antitumor activity overcoming drug resistance. *J. Biol. Chem.* **2014**, *289*, 32671–32681. [CrossRef] [PubMed]

87. Saldanha, S.N.; Kala, R.; Tollefsbol, T.O. Molecular mechanisms for inhibition of colon cancer cells by combined epigenetic-modulating epigallocatechin gallate and sodium butyrate. *Exp. Cell Res.* **2014**, *324*, 40–53. [CrossRef]

88. Zhang, Y.; Wang, S.X.; Ma, J.W.; Li, H.Y.; Ye, J.C.; Xie, S.M.; Du, B.; Zhong, X.Y. Egcg inhibits properties of glioma stem-like cells and synergizes with temozolomide through downregulation of p-glycoprotein inhibition. *J. Neurooncol.* **2015**, *121*, 41–52. [CrossRef]

89. Suzuki, Y.; Isemura, M. Binding interaction between (−)-epigallocatechin gallate causes impaired spreading of cancer cells on fibrinogen. *Biomed. Res.* **2013**, *34*, 301–308. [CrossRef]

90. Tachibana, H.; Koga, K.; Fujimura, Y.; Yamada, K. A receptor for green tea polyphenol egcg. *Nat. Struct. Mol. Biol.* **2004**, *11*, 380–381. [CrossRef]

91. Lee, S.H.; Nam, H.J.; Kang, H.J.; Kwon, H.W.; Lim, Y.C. Epigallocatechin-3-gallate attenuates head and neck cancer stem cell traits through suppression of notch pathway. *Eur. J. Cancer* **2013**, *49*, 3210–3218. [CrossRef] [PubMed]

92. Adachi, S.; Nagao, T.; Ingolfsson, H.I.; Maxfield, F.R.; Andersen, O.S.; Kopelovich, L.; Weinstein, I.B. The inhibitory effect of (−)-epigallocatechin gallate on activation of the epidermal growth factor receptor is associated with altered lipid order in ht29 colon cancer cells. *Cancer Res.* **2007**, *67*, 6493–6501. [CrossRef] [PubMed]

93. Duhon, D.; Bigelow, R.L.; Coleman, D.T.; Steffan, J.J.; Yu, C.; Langston, W.; Kevil, C.G.; Cardelli, J.A. The polyphenol epigallocatechin-3-gallate affects lipid rafts to block activation of the c-met receptor in prostate cancer cells. *Mol. Carcinog.* **2010**, *49*, 739–749. [CrossRef]

94. Tabuchi, M.; Hayakawa, S.; Honda, E.; Ooshima, K.; Itoh, T.; Yoshida, K.; Park, A.M.; Higashino, H.; Isemura, M.; Munakata, H. Epigallocatechin-3-gallate suppresses transforming growth factor-beta signaling by interacting with the transforming growth factor-beta type ii receptor. *World J. Exp. Med.* **2013**, *3*, 100–107. [CrossRef]

95. Wubetu, G.Y.; Shimada, M.; Morine, Y.; Ikemoto, T.; Ishikawa, D.; Iwahashi, S.; Yamada, S.; Saito, Y.; Arakawa, Y.; Imura, S. Epigallocatechin gallate hinders human hepatoma and colon cancer sphere formation. *J. Gastroenterol. Hepatol.* **2016**, *31*, 256–264. [CrossRef] [PubMed]

96. Punathil, T.; Tollefsbol, T.O.; Katiyar, S.K. Egcg inhibits mammary cancer cell migration through inhibition of nitric oxide synthase and guanylate cyclase. *Biochem. Biophys. Res. Commun.* **2008**, *375*, 162–167. [CrossRef]

97. Sen, T.; Dutta, A.; Chatterjee, A. Epigallocatechin-3-gallate (egcg) downregulates gelatinase-b (mmp-9) by involvement of fak/erk/nfkappab and ap-1 in the human breast cancer cell line mda-mb-231. *Anticancer Drugs* **2010**, *21*, 632–644. [CrossRef] [PubMed]

98. Singh, T.; Katiyar, S.K. Green tea polyphenol, (−)-epigallocatechin-3-gallate, induces toxicity in human skin cancer cells by targeting beta-catenin signaling. *Toxicol. Appl. Pharmacol.* **2013**, *273*, 418–424. [CrossRef] [PubMed]

99. Shankar, S.; Marsh, L.; Srivastava, R.K. Egcg inhibits growth of human pancreatic tumors orthotopically implanted in balb c nude mice through modulation of fkhrl1/foxo3a and neuropilin. *Mol. Cell. Biochem.* **2013**, *372*, 83–94. [CrossRef] [PubMed]

100. Moradzadeh, M.; Hosseini, A.; Erfanian, S.; Rezaei, H. Epigallocatechin-3-gallate promotes apoptosis in human breast cancer t47d cells through down-regulation of pi3k/akt and telomerase. *Pharmacol. Rep.* **2017**, *69*, 924–928. [CrossRef] [PubMed]

101. Ketchart, W.; Smith, K.M.; Krupka, T.; Wittmann, B.M.; Hu, Y.; Rayman, P.A.; Doughman, Y.Q.; Albert, J.M.; Bai, X.; Finke, J.H.; et al. Inhibition of metastasis by hexim1 through effects on cell invasion and angiogenesis. *Oncogene* **2013**, *32*, 3829–3839. [CrossRef] [PubMed]

102. Lu, C.L.; Xu, J.; Yao, H.J.; Luo, K.L.; Li, J.M.; Wu, T.; Wu, G.Z. Inhibition of human 67-kda laminin receptor sensitizes multidrug resistance colon cancer cell line sw480 for apoptosis induction. *Tumour. Biol.* **2016**, *37*, 1319–1325. [CrossRef] [PubMed]

103. Montuori, N.; Selleri, C.; Risitano, A.M.; Raiola, A.M.; Ragno, P.; Del Vecchio, L.; Rotoli, B.; Rossi, G. Expression of the 67-kda laminin receptor in acute myeloid leukemia cells mediates adhesion to laminin and is frequently associated with monocytic differentiation. *Clin. Cancer Res.* **1999**, *5*, 1465–1472. [PubMed]

104. Yu, H.N.; Zhang, L.C.; Yang, J.G.; Das, U.N.; Shen, S.R. Effect of laminin tyrosine-isoleucine-glycine-serine-arginine peptide on the growth of human prostate cancer (pc-3) cells in vitro. *Eur. J. Pharmacol.* **2009**, *616*, 251–255. [CrossRef] [PubMed]

105. Liu, L.; Sun, L.; Zhang, H.; Li, Z.; Ning, X.; Shi, Y.; Guo, C.; Han, S.; Wu, K.; Fan, D. Hypoxia-mediated up-regulation of mgr1-ag/37lrp in gastric cancers occurs via hypoxia-inducible-factor 1-dependent mechanism and contributes to drug resistance. *Int. J. Cancer* **2009**, *124*, 1707–1715. [CrossRef] [PubMed]

106. Pesapane, A.; Ragno, P.; Selleri, C.; Montuori, N. Recent advances in the function of the 67 kda laminin receptor and its targeting for personalized therapy in cancer. *Curr. Pharm. Des.* **2017**, *23*, 4745–4757.

107. Pesapane, A.; Di Giovanni, C.; Rossi, F.W.; Alfano, D.; Formisano, L.; Ragno, P.; Selleri, C.; Montuori, N.; Lavecchia, A. Discovery of new small molecules inhibiting 67 kda laminin receptor interaction with laminin and cancer cell invasion. *Oncotarget* **2015**, *6*, 18116–18133. [CrossRef]

108. Li, Y.; Li, D.; Chen, J.; Wang, S. A polysaccharide from pinellia ternata inhibits cell proliferation and metastasis in human cholangiocarcinoma cells by targeting of cdc42 and 67kda laminin receptor (lr). *Int. J. Biol. Macromol.* **2016**, *93*, 520–525. [CrossRef]

109. Fujimura, Y.; Sumida, M.; Sugihara, K.; Tsukamoto, S.; Yamada, K.; Tachibana, H. Green tea polyphenol egcg sensing motif on the 67-kda laminin receptor. *PLoS ONE* **2012**, *7*, e37942. [CrossRef]

110. Fujimura, Y.; Yamada, K.; Tachibana, H. A lipid raft-associated 67kda laminin receptor mediates suppressive effect of epigallocatechin-3-o-gallate on fcepsilonri expression. *Biochem. Biophys. Res. Commun.* **2005**, *336*, 674–681. [CrossRef]

111. Simons, K.; Ikonen, E. Functional rafts in cell membranes. *Nature* **1997**, *387*, 569–572. [CrossRef] [PubMed]

112. Xu, L.; Auzins, A.; Sun, X.; Xu, Y.; Harnischfeger, F.; Lu, Y.; Li, Z.; Chen, Y.H.; Zheng, W.; Liu, W. The synaptic recruitment of lipid rafts is dependent on cd19-pi3k module and cytoskeleton remodeling molecules. *J. Leukoc. Biol.* **2015**, *98*, 223–234. [CrossRef] [PubMed]

113. Varshney, P.; Yadav, V.; Saini, N. Lipid rafts in immune signalling: Current progress and future perspective. *Immunology* **2016**, *149*, 13–24. [CrossRef] [PubMed]

114. Simons, K.; Toomre, D. Lipid rafts and signal transduction. *Nat. Rev. Mol. Cell. Biol.* **2000**, *1*, 31–39. [CrossRef] [PubMed]

115. Pike, L.J. Growth factor receptors, lipid rafts and caveolae: An evolving story. *Biochim. Biophys. Acta* **2005**, *1746*, 260–273. [CrossRef] [PubMed]

116. Diluvio, G.; Del Gaudio, F.; Giuli, M.V.; Franciosa, G.; Giuliani, E.; Palermo, R.; Besharat, Z.M.; Pignataro, M.G.; Vacca, A.; d'Amati, G.; et al. Notch3 inactivation increases triple negative breast cancer sensitivity to gefitinib by promoting egfr tyrosine dephosphorylation and its intracellular arrest. *Oncogenesis* **2018**, *7*, 42. [CrossRef]

117. Pike, L.J.; Han, X.; Gross, R.W. Epidermal growth factor receptors are localized to lipid rafts that contain a balance of inner and outer leaflet lipids: A shotgun lipidomics study. *J. Biol. Chem.* **2005**, *280*, 26796–26804. [CrossRef] [PubMed]

118. Masuda, M.; Wakasaki, T.; Toh, S.; Shimizu, M.; Adachi, S. Chemoprevention of head and neck cancer by green tea extract: Egcg-the role of egfr signaling and "lipid raft". *J. Oncol.* **2011**, *2011*, 540148. [CrossRef]

119. Guo, T.; Xu, L.; Che, X.; Zhang, S.; Li, C.; Wang, J.; Gong, J.; Ma, R.; Fan, Y.; Hou, K.; et al. Formation of the igf1r/cav1/src tri-complex antagonizes trail-induced apoptosis in gastric cancer cells. *Cell. Biol. Int.* **2017**, *41*, 749–760. [CrossRef]

120. Alawin, O.A.; Ahmed, R.A.; Ibrahim, B.A.; Briski, K.P.; Sylvester, P.W. Antiproliferative effects of gamma-tocotrienol are associated with lipid raft disruption in her2-positive human breast cancer cells. *J. Nutr. Biochem.* **2016**, *27*, 266–277. [CrossRef]

121. Sur, S.; Pal, D.; Roy, R.; Barua, A.; Roy, A.; Saha, P.; Panda, C.K. Tea polyphenols egcg and tf restrict tongue and liver carcinogenesis simultaneously induced by n-nitrosodiethylamine in mice. *Toxicol. Appl. Pharmacol.* **2016**, *300*, 34–46. [CrossRef]

122. Ma, Y.C.; Li, C.; Gao, F.; Xu, Y.; Jiang, Z.B.; Liu, J.X.; Jin, L.Y. Epigallocatechin gallate inhibits the growth of human lung cancer by directly targeting the egfr signaling pathway. *Oncol. Rep.* **2014**, *31*, 1343–1349. [CrossRef] [PubMed]

123. Filippi, A.; Picot, T.; Aanei, C.M.; Nagy, P.; Szollosi, J.; Campos, L.; Ganea, C.; Mocanu, M.M. Epigallocatechin-3-o-gallate alleviates the malignant phenotype in a-431 epidermoid and sk-br-3 breast cancer cell lines. *Int. J. Food Sci. Nutr.* **2018**, *69*, 584–597. [CrossRef] [PubMed]

124. Pike, L.J. Rafts defined: A report on the keystone symposium on lipid rafts and cell function. *J. Lipid. Res.* **2006**, *47*, 1597–1598. [CrossRef]

125. Kim, J.Y.; Wang, L.; Lee, J.; Ou, J.J. Hepatitis c virus induces the localization of lipid rafts to autophagosomes for its rna replication. *J. Virol.* **2017**, *91*. [CrossRef]

126. Rosenberger, C.M.; Brumell, J.H.; Finlay, B.B. Microbial pathogenesis: Lipid rafts as pathogen portals. *Curr. Biol.* **2000**, *10*, R823–R825. [CrossRef]

127. Guimaraes, A.J.; de Cerqueira, M.D.; Zamith-Miranda, D.; Lopez, P.H.; Rodrigues, M.L.; Pontes, B.; Viana, N.B.; DeLeon-Rodriguez, C.M.; Rossi, D.C.P.; Casadevall, A.; et al. Host membrane glycosphingolipids and lipid microdomains facilitate histoplasma capsulatum internalization by macrophages. *Cell. Microbiol.* **2018**, e12976. [CrossRef] [PubMed]

128. Smart, E.J.; Graf, G.A.; McNiven, M.A.; Sessa, W.C.; Engelman, J.A.; Scherer, P.E.; Okamoto, T.; Lisanti, M.P. Caveolins, liquid-ordered domains, and signal transduction. *Mol. Cell. Biol.* **1999**, *19*, 7289–7304. [CrossRef]

129. Hwangbo, C.; Tae, N.; Lee, S.; Kim, O.; Park, O.K.; Kim, J.; Kwon, S.H.; Lee, J.H. Syntenin regulates tgf-beta1-induced smad activation and the epithelial-to-mesenchymal transition by inhibiting caveolin-mediated tgf-beta type i receptor internalization. *Oncogene* **2016**, *35*, 389–401. [CrossRef] [PubMed]

130. Laurenzana, A.; Fibbi, G.; Chilla, A.; Margheri, G.; Del Rosso, T.; Rovida, E.; Del Rosso, M.; Margheri, F. Lipid rafts: Integrated platforms for vascular organization offering therapeutic opportunities. *Cell. Mol. Life Sci.* **2015**, *72*, 1537–1557. [CrossRef]

131. Mollinedo, F.; Gajate, C. Lipid rafts as major platforms for signaling regulation in cancer. *Adv. Biol. Regul.* **2015**, *57*, 130–146. [CrossRef] [PubMed]

132. Tai, Y.T.; Podar, K.; Catley, L.; Tseng, Y.H.; Akiyama, M.; Shringarpure, R.; Burger, R.; Hideshima, T.; Chauhan, D.; Mitsiades, N.; et al. Insulin-like growth factor-1 induces adhesion and migration in human multiple myeloma cells via activation of beta1-integrin and phosphatidylinositol 3'-kinase/akt signaling. *Cancer Res.* **2003**, *63*, 5850–5858.

133. Raghu, H.; Sodadasu, P.K.; Malla, R.R.; Gondi, C.S.; Estes, N.; Rao, J.S. Localization of upar and mmp-9 in lipid rafts is critical for migration, invasion and angiogenesis in human breast cancer cells. *BMC Cancer* **2010**, *10*, 647. [CrossRef] [PubMed]

134. Lacour, S.; Hammann, A.; Grazide, S.; Lagadic-Gossmann, D.; Athias, A.; Sergent, O.; Laurent, G.; Gambert, P.; Solary, E.; Dimanche-Boitrel, M.T. Cisplatin-induced cd95 redistribution into membrane lipid rafts of ht29 human colon cancer cells. *Cancer Res.* **2004**, *64*, 3593–3598. [PubMed]

135. George, K.S.; Wu, S. Lipid raft: A floating island of death or survival. *Toxicol. Appl. Pharmacol.* **2012**, *259*, 311–319.

136. Alves, A.C.S.; Dias, R.A.; Kagami, L.P.; das Neves, G.M.; Torres, F.C.; Eifler-Lima, V.L.; Carvalho, I.; de Miranda Silva, C.; Kawano, D.F. Beyond the "lock and key" paradigm: Targeting lipid rafts to induce the selective apoptosis of cancer cells. *Curr. Med. Chem.* **2018**, *25*, 2082–2104. [CrossRef]

137. Tsukamoto, S.; Hirotsu, K.; Kumazoe, M.; Goto, Y.; Sugihara, K.; Suda, T.; Tsurudome, Y.; Suzuki, T.; Yamashita, S.; Kim, Y.; et al. Green tea polyphenol egcg induces lipid-raft clustering and apoptotic cell death by activating protein kinase cdelta and acid sphingomyelinase through a 67 kda laminin receptor in multiple myeloma cells. *Biochem. J.* **2012**, *443*, 525–534. [CrossRef]

138. Mocanu, M.M.; Ganea, C.; Georgescu, L.; Varadi, T.; Shrestha, D.; Baran, I.; Katona, E.; Nagy, P.; Szollosi, J. Epigallocatechin 3-o-gallate induces 67 kda laminin receptor-mediated cell death accompanied by downregulation of erbb proteins and altered lipid raft clustering in mammary and epidermoid carcinoma cells. *J. Nat. Prod.* **2014**, *77*, 250–257. [CrossRef]

139. Huang, Y.; Kumazoe, M.; Bae, J.; Yamada, S.; Takai, M.; Hidaka, S.; Yamashita, S.; Kim, Y.; Won, Y.; Murata, M.; et al. Green tea polyphenol epigallocatechin-o-gallate induces cell death by acid sphingomyelinase activation in chronic myeloid leukemia cells. *Oncol. Rep.* **2015**, *34*, 1162–1168. [CrossRef]

140. Yang, C.S.; Wang, H. Cancer preventive activities of tea catechins. *Molecules* **2016**, *21*, 1679. [CrossRef]

141. Luo, K.W.; Lung, W.Y.; Chun, X.; Luo, X.L.; Huang, W.R. Egcg inhibited bladder cancer t24 and 5637 cell proliferation and migration via pi3k/akt pathway. *Oncotarget* **2018**, *9*, 12261–12272. [CrossRef]

142. Velavan, B.; Divya, T.; Sureshkumar, A.; Sudhandiran, G. Nano-chemotherapeutic efficacy of (−)-epigallocatechin 3-gallate mediating apoptosis in a549cells: Involvement of reactive oxygen species mediated nrf2/keap1signaling. *Biochem. Biophys. Res. Commun.* **2018**, *503*, 1723–1731. [CrossRef] [PubMed]

143. Gu, J.J.; Qiao, K.S.; Sun, P.; Chen, P.; Li, Q. Study of egcg induced apoptosis in lung cancer cells by inhibiting pi3k/akt signaling pathway. *Eur. Rev. Med. Pharmacol. Sci.* **2018**, *22*, 4557–4563.

144. Wang, Y.Q.; Lu, J.L.; Liang, Y.R.; Li, Q.S. Suppressive effects of egcg on cervical cancer. *Molecules* **2018**, *23*, 2334. [CrossRef] [PubMed]

145. Britschgi, A.; Simon, H.U.; Tobler, A.; Fey, M.F.; Tschan, M.P. Epigallocatechin-3-gallate induces cell death in acute myeloid leukaemia cells and supports all-trans retinoic acid-induced neutrophil differentiation via death-associated protein kinase 2. *Br. J. Haematol.* **2010**, *149*, 55–64. [CrossRef] [PubMed]

146. Shammas, M.A.; Neri, P.; Koley, H.; Batchu, R.B.; Bertheau, R.C.; Munshi, V.; Prabhala, R.; Fulciniti, M.; Tai, Y.T.; Treon, S.P.; et al. Specific killing of multiple myeloma cells by (−)-epigallocatechin-3-gallate extracted from green tea: Biologic activity and therapeutic implications. *Blood* **2006**, *108*, 2804–2810. [CrossRef]

147. Kirschnek, S.; Paris, F.; Weller, M.; Grassme, H.; Ferlinz, K.; Riehle, A.; Fuks, Z.; Kolesnick, R.; Gulbins, E. Cd95-mediated apoptosis in vivo involves acid sphingomyelinase. *J. Biol. Chem.* **2000**, *275*, 27316–27323. [PubMed]

148. Garcia-Barros, M.; Paris, F.; Cordon-Cardo, C.; Lyden, D.; Rafii, S.; Haimovitz-Friedman, A.; Fuks, Z.; Kolesnick, R. Tumor response to radiotherapy regulated by endothelial cell apoptosis. *Science* **2003**, *300*, 1155–1159. [CrossRef]

149. Zhang, Y.; Mattjus, P.; Schmid, P.C.; Dong, Z.; Zhong, S.; Ma, W.Y.; Brown, R.E.; Bode, A.M.; Schmid, H.H. Involvement of the acid sphingomyelinase pathway in uva-induced apoptosis. *J. Biol. Chem.* **2001**, *276*, 11775–11782. [CrossRef]

150. Goni, F.M.; Alonso, A. Sphingomyelinases: Enzymology and membrane activity. *FEBS Lett.* **2002**, *531*, 38–46. [CrossRef]

151. Morita, Y.; Perez, G.I.; Paris, F.; Miranda, S.R.; Ehleiter, D.; Haimovitz-Friedman, A.; Fuks, Z.; Xie, Z.; Reed, J.C.; Schuchman, E.H.; et al. Oocyte apoptosis is suppressed by disruption of the acid sphingomyelinase gene or by sphingosine-1-phosphate therapy. *Nat. Med.* **2000**, *6*, 1109–1114. [CrossRef] [PubMed]

152. Gulbins, E. Regulation of death receptor signaling and apoptosis by ceramide. *Pharmacol. Res.* **2003**, *47*, 393–399. [CrossRef]

153. Hueber, A.O.; Bernard, A.M.; Herincs, Z.; Couzinet, A.; He, H.T. An essential role for membrane rafts in the initiation of fas/cd95-triggered cell death in mouse thymocytes. *EMBO Rep.* **2002**, *3*, 190–196. [CrossRef] [PubMed]

154. Kischkel, F.C.; Hellbardt, S.; Behrmann, I.; Germer, M.; Pawlita, M.; Krammer, P.H.; Peter, M.E. Cytotoxicity-dependent apo-1 (fas/cd95)-associated proteins form a death-inducing signaling complex (disc) with the receptor. *EMBO J.* **1995**, *14*, 5579–5588. [CrossRef] [PubMed]

155. Grassme, H.; Cremesti, A.; Kolesnick, R.; Gulbins, E. Ceramide-mediated clustering is required for cd95-disc formation. *Oncogene* **2003**, *22*, 5457–5470. [CrossRef] [PubMed]

156. Gajate, C.; Mollinedo, F. The antitumor ether lipid et-18-och(3) induces apoptosis through translocation and capping of fas/cd95 into membrane rafts in human leukemic cells. *Blood* **2001**, *98*, 3860–3863. [CrossRef] [PubMed]

157. London, E. Ceramide selectively displaces cholesterol from ordered lipid domains (rafts): Implications for lipid raft structure and function. *J. Biol. Chem.* **2004**, *279*, 9997–10004.

158. Cremesti, A.; Paris, F.; Grassme, H.; Holler, N.; Tschopp, J.; Fuks, Z.; Gulbins, E.; Kolesnick, R. Ceramide enables fas to cap and kill. *J. Biol. Chem.* **2001**, *276*, 23954–23961. [CrossRef]
159. Fanzo, J.C.; Lynch, M.P.; Phee, H.; Hyer, M.; Cremesti, A.; Grassme, H.; Norris, J.S.; Coggeshall, K.M.; Rueda, B.R.; Pernis, A.B.; et al. Cd95 rapidly clusters in cells of diverse origins. *Cancer Biol. Ther.* **2003**, *2*, 392–395. [CrossRef]
160. Wu, L.Y.; De Luca, T.; Watanabe, T.; Morre, D.M.; Morre, D.J. Metabolite modulation of hela cell response to enox2 inhibitors egcg and phenoxodiol. *Biochim. Biophys. Acta* **2011**, *1810*, 784–789. [CrossRef]
161. Kim, M.H.; Chung, J. Synergistic cell death by egcg and ibuprofen in du-145 prostate cancer cell line. *Anticancer Res.* **2007**, *27*, 3947–3956. [PubMed]
162. Tan, X.; Zhang, Y.; Jiang, B.; Zhou, D. Changes in ceramide levels upon catechins-induced apoptosis in lovo cells. *Life Sci.* **2002**, *70*, 2023–2029. [CrossRef]
163. Zhou, L.; Yang, F.; Li, G.; Huang, J.; Liu, Y.; Zhang, Q.; Tang, Q.; Hu, C.; Zhang, R. Coptisine induces apoptosis in human hepatoma cells through activating 67-kda laminin receptor/cgmp signaling. *Front. Pharmacol.* **2018**, *9*, 517. [CrossRef] [PubMed]
164. Kumazoe, M.; Kim, Y.; Bae, J.; Takai, M.; Murata, M.; Suemasu, Y.; Sugihara, K.; Yamashita, S.; Tsukamoto, S.; Huang, Y.; et al. Phosphodiesterase 5 inhibitor acts as a potent agent sensitizing acute myeloid leukemia cells to 67-kda laminin receptor-dependent apoptosis. *FEBS Lett.* **2013**, *587*, 3052–3057. [CrossRef] [PubMed]
165. Kumazoe, M.; Tsukamoto, S.; Lesnick, C.; Kay, N.E.; Yamada, K.; Shanafelt, T.D.; Tachibana, H. Vardenafil, a clinically available phosphodiesterase inhibitor, potentiates the killing effect of egcg on cll cells. *Br. J. Haematol.* **2015**, *168*, 610–613. [CrossRef] [PubMed]
166. Casaletto, J.B.; McClatchey, A.I. Spatial regulation of receptor tyrosine kinases in development and cancer. *Nat. Rev. Cancer* **2012**, *12*, 387–400. [CrossRef] [PubMed]
167. Brizuela, L.; Dayon, A.; Doumerc, N.; Ader, I.; Golzio, M.; Izard, J.C.; Hara, Y.; Malavaud, B.; Cuvillier, O. The sphingosine kinase-1 survival pathway is a molecular target for the tumor-suppressive tea and wine polyphenols in prostate cancer. *FASEB J.* **2010**, *24*, 3882–3894. [CrossRef] [PubMed]
168. Olivera, A.; Spiegel, S. Sphingosine-1-phosphate as second messenger in cell proliferation induced by pdgf and fcs mitogens. *Nature* **1993**, *365*, 557–560. [CrossRef] [PubMed]
169. Cuvillier, O.; Pirianov, G.; Kleuser, B.; Vanek, P.G.; Coso, O.A.; Gutkind, S.; Spiegel, S. Suppression of ceramide-mediated programmed cell death by sphingosine-1-phosphate. *Nature* **1996**, *381*, 800–803. [CrossRef] [PubMed]
170. Tsukamoto, S.; Kumazoe, M.; Huang, Y.; Lesnick, C.; Kay, N.E.; Shanafelt, T.D.; Tachibana, H. Sphk1 inhibitor potentiates the anti-cancer effect of egcg on leukaemia cells. *Br. J. Haematol.* **2017**, *178*, 155–158. [CrossRef] [PubMed]
171. Chakrabarty, S.; Ganguli, A.; Das, A.; Nag, D.; Chakrabarti, G. Epigallocatechin-3-gallate shows anti-proliferative activity in hela cells targeting tubulin-microtubule equilibrium. *Chem. Biol. Interact.* **2015**, *242*, 380–389. [CrossRef] [PubMed]
172. Shenouda, N.S.; Zhou, C.; Browning, J.D.; Ansell, P.J.; Sakla, M.S.; Lubahn, D.B.; Macdonald, R.S. Phytoestrogens in common herbs regulate prostate cancer cell growth in vitro. *Nutr. Cancer* **2004**, *49*, 200–208. [CrossRef] [PubMed]
173. Umeda, D.; Yano, S.; Yamada, K.; Tachibana, H. Involvement of 67-kda laminin receptor-mediated myosin phosphatase activation in antiproliferative effect of epigallocatechin-3-*O*-gallate at a physiological concentration on caco-2 colon cancer cells. *Biochem. Biophys. Res. Commun.* **2008**, *371*, 172–176. [CrossRef] [PubMed]
174. D'Avino, P.P.; Giansanti, M.G.; Petronczki, M. Cytokinesis in animal cells. *Cold Spring Harb. Perspect. Biol.* **2015**, *7*, a015834. [CrossRef] [PubMed]
175. Wang, Y.L. The mechanism of cortical ingression during early cytokinesis: Thinking beyond the contractile ring hypothesis. *Trends Cell. Biol.* **2005**, *15*, 581–588. [CrossRef]
176. Matsumura, F. Regulation of myosin ii during cytokinesis in higher eukaryotes. *Trends Cell. Biol.* **2005**, *15*, 371–377. [CrossRef]
177. Moussavi, R.S.; Kelley, C.A.; Adelstein, R.S. Phosphorylation of vertebrate nonmuscle and smooth muscle myosin heavy chains and light chains. *Mol. Cell. Biochem.* **1993**, *127–128*, 219–227. [CrossRef]
178. Scholey, J.M.; Taylor, K.A.; Kendrick-Jones, J. Regulation of non-muscle myosin assembly by calmodulin-dependent light chain kinase. *Nature* **1980**, *287*, 233–235. [CrossRef]

179. Ikebe, M.; Koretz, J.; Hartshorne, D.J. Effects of phosphorylation of light chain residues threonine 18 and serine 19 on the properties and conformation of smooth muscle myosin. *J. Biol. Chem.* **1988**, *263*, 6432–6437.

180. Kawano, Y.; Fukata, Y.; Oshiro, N.; Amano, M.; Nakamura, T.; Ito, M.; Matsumura, F.; Inagaki, M.; Kaibuchi, K. Phosphorylation of myosin-binding subunit (mbs) of myosin phosphatase by rho-kinase in vivo. *J. Cell. Biol.* **1999**, *147*, 1023–1038. [CrossRef]

181. Negrutskii, B.S.; El'skaya, A.V. Eukaryotic translation elongation factor 1 alpha: Structure, expression, functions, and possible role in aminoacyl-trna channeling. *Prog. Nucleic Acid Res. Mol. Biol.* **1998**, *60*, 47–78. [PubMed]

182. Gangwani, L.; Mikrut, M.; Galcheva-Gargova, Z.; Davis, R.J. Interaction of zpr1 with translation elongation factor-1alpha in proliferating cells. *J. Cell. Biol.* **1998**, *143*, 1471–1484. [CrossRef] [PubMed]

183. Lamberti, A.; Caraglia, M.; Longo, O.; Marra, M.; Abbruzzese, A.; Arcari, P. The translation elongation factor 1a in tumorigenesis, signal transduction and apoptosis: Review article. *Amino Acids* **2004**, *26*, 443–448. [CrossRef] [PubMed]

184. Izawa, T.; Fukata, Y.; Kimura, T.; Iwamatsu, A.; Dohi, K.; Kaibuchi, K. Elongation factor-1 alpha is a novel substrate of rho-associated kinase. *Biochem. Biophys. Res. Commun.* **2000**, *278*, 72–78. [CrossRef] [PubMed]

185. Peterson, R.T.; Desai, B.N.; Hardwick, J.S.; Schreiber, S.L. Protein phosphatase 2a interacts with the 70-kda s6 kinase and is activated by inhibition of fkbp12-rapamycinassociated protein. *Proc. Natl. Acad. Sci. USA* **1999**, *96*, 4438–4442. [CrossRef]

186. Zhang, Q.; Claret, F.X. Phosphatases: The new brakes for cancer development? *Enzym. Res.* **2012**, *2012*, 659649. [CrossRef] [PubMed]

187. Kiss, A.; Becsi, B.; Kolozsvari, B.; Komaromi, I.; Kover, K.E.; Erdodi, F. Epigallocatechin-3-gallate and penta-o-galloyl-beta-d-glucose inhibit protein phosphatase-1. *FEBS J.* **2013**, *280*, 612–626. [CrossRef]

188. Kitano, K.; Nam, K.Y.; Kimura, S.; Fujiki, H.; Imanishi, Y. Sealing effects of (−)-epigallocatechin gallate on protein kinase c and protein phosphatase 2a. *Biophys. Chem.* **1997**, *65*, 157–164. [CrossRef]

189. Janssens, V.; Goris, J.; Van Hoof, C. Pp2a: The expected tumor suppressor. *Curr. Opin. Genet. Dev.* **2005**, *15*, 34–41. [CrossRef]

190. Stamenkovic, I.; Yu, Q. Merlin, a "magic" linker between extracellular cues and intracellular signaling pathways that regulate cell motility, proliferation, and survival. *Curr. Protein Pept. Sci.* **2010**, *11*, 471–484. [CrossRef]

191. Horiguchi, A.; Zheng, R.; Shen, R.; Nanus, D.M. Inactivation of the nf2 tumor suppressor protein merlin in du145 prostate cancer cells. *Prostate* **2008**, *68*, 975–984. [CrossRef] [PubMed]

192. Malhotra, A.; Shibata, Y.; Hall, I.M.; Dutta, A. Chromosomal structural variations during progression of a prostate epithelial cell line to a malignant metastatic state inactivate the nf2, nipsnap1, ugt2b17, and lpin2 genes. *Cancer Biol. Ther.* **2013**, *14*, 840–852. [CrossRef] [PubMed]

193. Petrilli, A.M.; Fernandez-Valle, C. Role of merlin/nf2 inactivation in tumor biology. *Oncogene* **2016**, *35*, 537–548. [CrossRef] [PubMed]

194. Ambros, V. Micrornas: Tiny regulators with great potential. *Cell* **2001**, *107*, 823–826. [CrossRef]

195. Johnson, S.M.; Grosshans, H.; Shingara, J.; Byrom, M.; Jarvis, R.; Cheng, A.; Labourier, E.; Reinert, K.L.; Brown, D.; Slack, F.J. Ras is regulated by the let-7 microrna family. *Cell* **2005**, *120*, 635–647. [CrossRef] [PubMed]

196. Schultz, J.; Lorenz, P.; Gross, G.; Ibrahim, S.; Kunz, M. Microrna let-7b targets important cell cycle molecules in malignant melanoma cells and interferes with anchorage-independent growth. *Cell Res.* **2008**, *18*, 549–557. [CrossRef] [PubMed]

197. Zedan, A.H.; Hansen, T.F.; Assenholt, J.; Pleckaitis, M.; Madsen, J.S.; Osther, P.J.S. Microrna expression in tumour tissue and plasma in patients with newly diagnosed metastatic prostate cancer. *Tumour. Biol.* **2018**, *40*, 1010428318775864. [CrossRef]

198. Zhou, H.; Chen, J.X.; Yang, C.S.; Yang, M.Q.; Deng, Y.; Wang, H. Gene regulation mediated by micrornas in response to green tea polyphenol egcg in mouse lung cancer. *BMC Genom.* **2014**, *15* (Suppl. 11), S3. [CrossRef]

199. Pan, X.; Zhao, B.; Song, Z.; Han, S.; Wang, M. Estrogen receptor-alpha36 is involved in epigallocatechin-3-gallate induced growth inhibition of er-negative breast cancer stem/progenitor cells. *J. Pharmacol. Sci.* **2016**, *130*, 85–93. [CrossRef]

200. Jiang, P.; Xu, C.; Chen, L.; Chen, A.; Wu, X.; Zhou, M.; Haq, I.U.; Mariyam, Z.; Feng, Q. Egcg inhibits csc-like properties through targeting mir-485/cd44 axis in a549-cisplatin resistant cells. *Mol. Carcinog.* **2018**, *57*, 1835–1844. [CrossRef]

201. Nishimura, N.; Hartomo, T.B.; Pham, T.V.; Lee, M.J.; Yamamoto, T.; Morikawa, S.; Hasegawa, D.; Takeda, H.; Kawasaki, K.; Kosaka, Y.; et al. Epigallocatechin gallate inhibits sphere formation of neuroblastoma be(2)-c cells. *Environ. Health Prev. Med.* **2012**, *17*, 246–251. [CrossRef]

202. Kumazoe, M.; Takai, M.; Hiroi, S.; Takeuchi, C.; Yamanouchi, M.; Nojiri, T.; Onda, H.; Bae, J.; Huang, Y.; Takamatsu, K.; et al. Pde3 inhibitor and egcg combination treatment suppress cancer stem cell properties in pancreatic ductal adenocarcinoma. *Sci. Rep.* **2017**, *7*, 1917. [CrossRef] [PubMed]

203. Kumazoe, M.; Takai, M.; Bae, J.; Hiroi, S.; Huang, Y.; Takamatsu, K.; Won, Y.; Yamashita, M.; Hidaka, S.; Yamashita, S.; et al. Foxo3 is essential for cd44 expression in pancreatic cancer cells. *Oncogene* **2017**, *36*, 2643–2654. [CrossRef] [PubMed]

204. Eddy, S.F.; Kane, S.E.; Sonenshein, G.E. Trastuzumab-resistant her2-driven breast cancer cells are sensitive to epigallocatechin-3 gallate. *Cancer Res.* **2007**, *67*, 9018–9023. [CrossRef] [PubMed]

205. Farabegoli, F.; Govoni, M.; Ciavarella, C.; Orlandi, M.; Papi, A. A rxr ligand 6-oh-11-o-hydroxyphenanthrene with antitumour properties enhances (−)-epigallocatechin-3-gallate activity in three human breast carcinoma cell lines. *BioMed Res. Int.* **2014**, *2014*, 853086. [CrossRef]

206. Lugnier, C. Cyclic nucleotide phosphodiesterase (pde) superfamily: A new target for the development of specific therapeutic agents. *Pharmacol. Ther.* **2006**, *109*, 366–398. [CrossRef] [PubMed]

207. Lu, K.P.; Zhou, X.Z. The prolyl isomerase pin1: A pivotal new twist in phosphorylation signalling and disease. *Nat. Rev. Mol. Cell Biol.* **2007**, *8*, 904–916. [CrossRef] [PubMed]

208. Dominguez-Sola, D.; Dalla-Favera, R. Pinning down the c-myc oncoprotein. *Nat. Cell Biol.* **2004**, *6*, 288–289. [CrossRef] [PubMed]

209. Sears, R.C. The life cycle of c-myc: From synthesis to degradation. *Cell Cycle* **2004**, *3*, 1133–1137. [CrossRef] [PubMed]

210. Ryo, A.; Nakamura, M.; Wulf, G.; Liou, Y.C.; Lu, K.P. Pin1 regulates turnover and subcellular localization of beta-catenin by inhibiting its interaction with apc. *Nat. Cell Biol.* **2001**, *3*, 793–801. [CrossRef]

211. Bao, L.; Kimzey, A.; Sauter, G.; Sowadski, J.M.; Lu, K.P.; Wang, D.G. Prevalent overexpression of prolyl isomerase pin1 in human cancers. *Am. J. Pathol.* **2004**, *164*, 1727–1737. [CrossRef]

212. Ayala, G.; Wang, D.; Wulf, G.; Frolov, A.; Li, R.; Sowadski, J.; Wheeler, T.M.; Lu, K.P.; Bao, L. The prolyl isomerase pin1 is a novel prognostic marker in human prostate cancer. *Cancer Res.* **2003**, *63*, 6244–6251.

213. Moore, J.D.; Potter, A. Pin1 inhibitors: Pitfalls, progress and cellular pharmacology. *Bioorg. Med. Chem. Lett.* **2013**, *23*, 4283–4291. [CrossRef]

214. Hidaka, M.; Kosaka, K.; Tsushima, S.; Uchida, C.; Takahashi, K.; Takahashi, N.; Tsubuki, M.; Hara, Y.; Uchida, T. Food polyphenols targeting peptidyl prolyl cis/trans isomerase pin1. *Biochem. Biophys. Res. Commun.* **2018**, *499*, 681–687. [CrossRef]

215. Xi, L.; Wang, Y.; He, Q.; Zhang, Q.; Du, L. Interaction between pin1 and its natural product inhibitor epigallocatechin-3-gallate by spectroscopy and molecular dynamics simulations. *Spectrochim. Acta A Mol. Biomol. Spectrosc* **2016**, *169*, 134–143. [CrossRef]

216. Katsuno, Y.; Lamouille, S.; Derynck, R. Tgf-beta signaling and epithelial-mesenchymal transition in cancer progression. *Curr. Opin. Oncol.* **2013**, *25*, 76–84. [CrossRef] [PubMed]

217. Sun, L.; Diamond, M.E.; Ottaviano, A.J.; Joseph, M.J.; Ananthanarayan, V.; Munshi, H.G. Transforming growth factor-beta 1 promotes matrix metalloproteinase-9-mediated oral cancer invasion through snail expression. *Mol. Cancer Res.* **2008**, *6*, 10–20. [CrossRef]

218. Joseph, M.J.; Dangi-Garimella, S.; Shields, M.A.; Diamond, M.E.; Sun, L.; Koblinski, J.E.; Munshi, H.G. Slug is a downstream mediator of transforming growth factor-beta1-induced matrix metalloproteinase-9 expression and invasion of oral cancer cells. *J. Cell. Biochem.* **2009**, *108*, 726–736. [CrossRef]

219. Sinpitaksakul, S.N.; Pimkhaokham, A.; Sanchavanakit, N.; Pavasant, P. Tgf-beta1 induced mmp-9 expression in hnscc cell lines via smad/mlck pathway. *Biochem. Biophys. Res. Commun.* **2008**, *371*, 713–718. [CrossRef] [PubMed]

220. Chowdhury, A.; Nandy, S.K.; Sarkar, J.; Chakraborti, T.; Chakraborti, S. Inhibition of pro-/active mmp-2 by green tea catechins and prediction of their interaction by molecular docking studies. *Mol. Cell. Biochem.* **2017**, *427*, 111–122. [CrossRef] [PubMed]

221. Sarkar, J.; Nandy, S.K.; Chowdhury, A.; Chakraborti, T.; Chakraborti, S. Inhibition of mmp-9 by green tea catechins and prediction of their interaction by molecular docking analysis. *Biomed. Pharmacother.* **2016**, *84*, 340–347. [CrossRef]

222. Schramm, L. Going green: The role of the green tea component egcg in chemoprevention. *J. Carcinog. Mutagen.* **2013**, *4*, 1000142. [CrossRef] [PubMed]

223. Riley, P.A. Epimutation and cancer: Carcinogenesis viewed as error-prone inheritance of epigenetic information. *J. Oncol.* **2018**, *2018*, 2645095. [CrossRef] [PubMed]

224. Huang, Z.; Huang, Q.; Ji, L.; Wang, Y.; Qi, X.; Liu, L.; Liu, Z.; Lu, L. Epigenetic regulation of active Chinese herbal components for cancer prevention and treatment: A follow-up review. *Pharmacol. Res.* **2016**, *114*, 1–12. [CrossRef] [PubMed]

225. Fang, M.Z.; Wang, Y.; Ai, N.; Hou, Z.; Sun, Y.; Lu, H.; Welsh, W.; Yang, C.S. Tea polyphenol (−)-epigallocatechin-3-gallate inhibits DNA methyltransferase and reactivates methylation-silenced genes in cancer cell lines. *Cancer Res.* **2003**, *63*, 7563–7570.

226. Pal, D.; Sur, S.; Roy, R.; Mandal, S.; Kumar Panda, C. Epigallocatechin gallate in combination with eugenol or amarogentin shows synergistic chemotherapeutic potential in cervical cancer cell line. *J. Cell. Physiol.* **2018**, *234*, 825–836. [CrossRef]

227. Oya, Y.; Mondal, A.; Rawangkan, A.; Umsumarng, S.; Iida, K.; Watanabe, T.; Kanno, M.; Suzuki, K.; Li, Z.; Kagechika, H.; et al. Down-regulation of histone deacetylase 4, -5 and -6 as a mechanism of synergistic enhancement of apoptosis in human lung cancer cells treated with the combination of a synthetic retinoid, am80 and green tea catechin. *J. Nutr. Biochem.* **2017**, *42*, 7–16. [CrossRef]

228. Zhang, Y.; Wang, X.; Han, L.; Zhou, Y.; Sun, S. Green tea polyphenol egcg reverse cisplatin resistance of a549/ddp cell line through candidate genes demethylation. *Biomed. Pharmacother.* **2015**, *69*, 285–290. [CrossRef]

229. Jin, H.; Chen, J.X.; Wang, H.; Lu, G.; Liu, A.; Li, G.; Tu, S.; Lin, Y.; Yang, C.S. Nnk-induced DNA methyltransferase 1 in lung tumorigenesis in a/j mice and inhibitory effects of (−)-epigallocatechin-3-gallate. *Nutr. Cancer* **2015**, *67*, 167–176. [CrossRef]

230. Liu, L.; Zuo, J.; Wang, G. Epigallocatechin-3-gallate suppresses cell proliferation and promotes apoptosis in ec9706 and eca109 esophageal carcinoma cells. *Oncol. Lett.* **2017**, *14*, 4391–4395. [CrossRef]

231. Le, C.T.; Leenders, W.P.J.; Molenaar, R.J.; van Noorden, C.J.F. Effects of the green tea polyphenol epigallocatechin-3-gallate on glioma: A critical evaluation of the literature. *Nutr. Cancer* **2018**, *70*, 317–333. [CrossRef] [PubMed]

232. Li, W.G.; Li, Q.H.; Tan, Z. Epigallocatechin gallate induces telomere fragmentation in hela and 293 but not in mrc-5 cells. *Life Sci.* **2005**, *76*, 1735–1746. [CrossRef] [PubMed]

233. Zhang, W.; Yang, P.; Gao, F.; Yang, J.; Yao, K. Effects of epigallocatechin gallate on the proliferation and apoptosis of the nasopharyngeal carcinoma cell line cne2. *Exp. Ther. Med.* **2014**, *8*, 1783–1788. [CrossRef]

234. Wang, X.; Hao, M.W.; Dong, K.; Lin, F.; Ren, J.H.; Zhang, H.Z. Apoptosis induction effects of egcg in laryngeal squamous cell carcinoma cells through telomerase repression. *Arch. Pharm. Res.* **2009**, *32*, 1263–1269. [CrossRef] [PubMed]

235. Sadava, D.; Whitlock, E.; Kane, S.E. The green tea polyphenol, epigallocatechin-3-gallate inhibits telomerase and induces apoptosis in drug-resistant lung cancer cells. *Biochem. Biophys. Res. Commun.* **2007**, *360*, 233–237. [CrossRef]

236. Kuzuhara, T.; Sei, Y.; Yamaguchi, K.; Suganuma, M.; Fujiki, H. DNA and rna as new binding targets of green tea catechins. *J. Biol. Chem.* **2006**, *281*, 17446–17456. [CrossRef] [PubMed]

237. Kuzuhara, T.; Tanabe, A.; Sei, Y.; Yamaguchi, K.; Suganuma, M.; Fujiki, H. Synergistic effects of multiple treatments, and both DNA and rna direct bindings on, green tea catechins. *Mol. Carcinog.* **2007**, *46*, 640–645. [CrossRef]

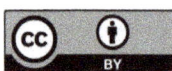

nutrients

MDPI

Review

Tea Polyphenols in Promotion of Human Health

Naghma Khan * and Hasan Mukhtar

4385 Medical Sciences Center, 1300 University Ave, Dept. of Dermatology, University of Wisconsin-Madison, Madison, WI 53706, USA; hmukhtar@dermatology.wisc.edu
* Correspondence: nkhan@dermatology.wisc.edu; Tel.: +1-608-263-5519

Received: 20 November 2018; Accepted: 21 December 2018; Published: 25 December 2018

Abstract: Tea is the most widely used beverage worldwide. Japanese and Chinese people have been drinking tea for centuries and in Asia, it is the most consumed beverage besides water. It is a rich source of pharmacologically active molecules which have been implicated to provide diverse health benefits. The three major forms of tea are green, black and oolong tea based on the degree of fermentation. The composition of tea differs with the species, season, leaves, climate, and horticultural practices. Polyphenols are the major active compounds present in teas. The catechins are the major polyphenolic compounds in green tea, which include epigallocatechin-3-gallate (EGCG), epigallocatechin, epicatechin-3-gallate and epicatechin, gallocatechins and gallocatechin gallate. EGCG is the predominant and most studied catechin in green tea. There are numerous evidences from cell culture and animal studies that tea polyphenols have beneficial effects against several pathological diseases including cancer, diabetes and cardiovascular diseases. The polyphenolic compounds present in black tea include theaflavins and thearubigins. In this review article, we will summarize recent studies documenting the role of tea polyphenols in the prevention of cancer, diabetes, cardiovascular and neurological diseases.

Keywords: cancer; EGCG; diseases; green tea; tea polyphenols

---

1. Introduction

The beverage tea is made from the infusion of the leaves of *Camellia sinensis*. The world's tea consumption is highest for black tea, followed by green tea, oolong tea, and white tea. Black tea is made by crushing and drying fresh tea leaves to effect fermentation prior to final processing and is consumed usually in the United States, Europe, Africa, and India. During fermentation, some of the catechins combine to form complex theaflavins and other flavonoids, which offer characteristic taste and color to black tea. To prevent fermentation, green tea is prepared when the fresh leaves are processed swiftly and the oolong tea is partially fermented.

Tea possesses antioxidant properties with traces of proteins, carbohydrates, amino acids, lipids, vitamins and minerals. It also contains an extensive range of chemical compounds, but mainly polyphenols account for the aroma and beneficial health effects of tea. The polyphenols in green tea are credited with its beneficial properties against several diseases in many reported studies [1]. These polyphenols are present in much higher concentrations in green tea than black or oolong tea and this accounts for their antioxidant properties. The distinctive polyphenolic compounds present in green tea are called as catechins, like (-)-epigallocatechin-3-gallate (EGCG), (-)-epigallocatechin (EGC), (-)-epicatechin-3-gallate (ECG) and (-)-epicatechin (EC). EGCG account for 50–70% of catechins. EGCG is the major catechin in tea and accounts for most of the research carried out with green tea. One cup of green tea contains up to 200 mg of EGCG, which has been shown to have chemopreventive/chemotherapeutic effects against several types of cancers [2,3]. Proper drinking of green tea is three to five cups per day, which accounts for a minimum of 250 mg of catechins per day [4]. Several in-vitro and in-vivo studies have reported the antioxidant effects of GTP. We have earlier discussed the anticarcinogenic effects of green tea, its effects on various receptor tyrosine kinases, signal transduction pathways and metastasis [1,5,6]. In this article, we present recent scientific evidences, for the anticarcinogenic effect of green tea and its role in diabetes, cardiovascular and neurological diseases. Anticarcinogenic effects of tea polyphenols and their mechanisms in different cancer types are shown in Table 1.

2. Green Tea Polyphenols and Lung Cancer

2.1. In-Vitro Studies

Lung cancer is the primary cause of cancer-related deaths worldwide, and non-small cell lung cancer (NSCLC) accounts for 80% of lung cancer cases. Recently, it was reported that EGCG inhibited programmed cell death ligand 1 (PD-L1) expression in NSCLC cells, induced by both interferon (IFN)-γ and epidermal growth factor (EGF) [7]. In NSCLC cells, pretreatment with EGCG and green tea extract (GTE) caused decrease in the mRNA and protein levels of IFN-γ-induced PD-L1, through inhibition of Janus kinase (JAK)/signal transducers and activators of transcription (STAT) signaling. Pre-treatment with EGCG also caused decrease in EGF-induced PD-L1 expression through inhibition of EGF receptor (EGFR)/Akt signaling [7].

ECG, a natural polyphenolic component of green tea, inhibited the invasion of NSCLC cells by suppressing the levels of matrix metalloproteinase (MMP)-2 and urokinase type plasminogen activator (uPA) [8]. It also reversed the transforming growth factor (TGF)-β1-induced epithelial-mesenchymal transition (EMT) and upregulated E-cadherin, while it caused the inhibition of mesenchymal markers, such as fibronectin and p-FAK. Subcutaneous inoculation of ECG also inhibited the tumor growth of NSCLC cells in xenograft model [8]. The clinical efficacy of tea polyphenols depends on efficient delivery and bioavailability [9–11]. Atomistic Molecular Dynamics simulations have shown that EGCG naturally binds to the hydrophilic regions of phospholipids, positioning mostly at the interface between water and lipid phases [12]. EGCG was encapsulated inside anionic liposomes made of 1-palmitoyl-2-oleoyl-sn-glycero-3-phosphocholine, 1,2-dioleoyl-sn-glycero-3-phosphoethanolamine and cholesteryl hemisuccinate to escalate its delivery. The ability of these liposomes to contrast H_2O_2-induced cell death was investigated in human retinal cells. Mitochondria were better preserved in cells treated with liposomes as compared to those treated with free EGCG. It was concluded that the produced formulation improved the efficacy of EGCG and could be used for diseases caused by oxidative damage [13].

Using nanochemoprevention, tea polyphenols, like theaflavin (TF) and EGCG were encapsulated in a biodegradable nanoparticulate formulation based on poly(lactide-co-glycolide) (PLGA) [14]. The ability of both bulk TF/EGCG and TF/EGCG-loaded PLGA-NPs to inhibit proliferation of lung carcinoma, cervical carcinoma and acute monocytic leukemia cells was determined. There was about three to seven fold reduction in IC_{50} doses on treatment with TF/EGCG-loaded NPs when compared with bulk doses of polyphenols. There was lack of toxicity of PLGA-NPs as evidenced by the treatment of cells. TF/EGCG-NPs were also more effective than bulk TF/EGCG in sensitizing lung cancer cells to cisplatin-induced apoptosis. The combination of TF/EGCG-NPs and cisplatin caused inhibition of NF-κB activation, cyclin D1, MMP-9 and vascular endothelial growth factor (VEGF). A proteomic-based approach was employed to identify proteins modulated by EGCG in A549 lung cancer cells [15]. Hepatoma-derived growth factor (HDGF) is considered as a therapeutic target in lung cancer. Treatment with EGCG caused three-fold suppression of HDGF and downregulation of HDGF by EGCG was confirmed using anti-HDGF antibodies in lung cancer cell lines. EGCG treatment also induced synergistic effect with cisplatin in causing lung cancer cell death and increased cytotoxicity was also noted in HDGF-silenced cells. Induction of apoptosis, disruption of the mitochondrial membrane potential, and activation of caspase-3 and -9 were linked to cell death. It was concluded that decreasing the levels of HDGF by treatment with EGCG may signify a novel approach in treatment of lung cancer. In addition, EGCG induced a marked synergistic effect with cisplatin in cell death. Consistently, an enhanced cytotoxicity in HDGF-silenced cells was also found. Cell death was associated to increased apoptosis, disruption of the mitochondrial membrane potential, and activation of caspase-3 and -9 [15]. Treatment of human lung cancer cells with EGCG caused inhibition of anchorage-independent growth and induction of G0/G1 phase cell-cycle arrest [16]. Suppression of EGFR pathway was found to be involved in the anticancer efficacy of EGCG. Short term exposure of human lung cancer cells with EGCG decreased EGF-induced EGFR, AKT and activation of ERK1/2. Chronic treatment with EGCG caused inhibition of total and membranous EGFR expression and decreased nuclear localization of EGFR with downregulation of cyclin D1. Also, sensitivity of lung cancer cells to EGCG was decreased on knockdown of EGFR, confirming that EGFR signaling may be involved in the anticancer activity of EGCG in human lung cancer cells [16]. The involvement of AP-1 in GTP-induced tumor inhibition was investigated in human NSCLC cell line H1299 and mouse SPON 10 cells [17]. These cell lines displayed high constitutive AP-1 activity and cell growth was inhibited when TAM67 expression was induced with doxycycline and connected with inhibited AP-1 activity. RNA-seq was used to define the global transcriptional effects of AP-1 inhibition and to elucidate the possible involvement of AP-1 in GTP-induced chemoprevention. AP-1 was identified as a key transcription regulator. In TAM67 expressing H1299 cells, 293 genes were downregulated on treatment with polyphenon E (PPE), and 10% of them had a direct AP-1 binding site, suggesting that AP-1 is the target of PPE. Regarding the inhibition of AP-1, chemopreventive properties of PPE were lost, signifying that AP-1 pathway is targeted by GTP [17].

2.2. In-Vivo Studies

In 4-(methylnitrosamino)-1-(3-pyridyl)-1-butanone (NNK)-induced lung cancer model, 0.3% GTE in drinking water decreased the tumor multiplicity and the percentage of PD-L1 positive cells. Thus, it was shown that EGCG acts as an alternative immune checkpoint inhibitor [7]. The PLGA-NPs in combination with cisplatin decreased tumor volume and increased longevity in mice bearing Ehrlich's ascites carcinoma cells. Thus, it was shown that EGCG and TF-NPs were more effective than bulk EGCG/TF [14]. Functional genomic approaches were used to explain the role of microRNA in the inhibition of tobacco carcinogen-induced lung tumors in A/J mice by EGCG [18]. Modest changes were noted in the expression levels of 21 microRNAs and by comparing these microRNAs with the mRNA expression profiles using the computation methods, 26 potential targeted genes of these microRNAs were identified. It was noted that Akt, NF-κB, MAP kinases and cell cycle pathways were modulated after treatment with EGCG, demonstrating that the miRNA-mediated regulation was involved in the anti-cancer activity of EGCG in-vivo [18].

2.3. Studies in Humans

A cross-sectional survey with the use of data from the Korean National Health and Nutritional Examination Survey collected between 2008 and 2015 reported an association between green tea intake and chronic obstructive lung disease (COPD) [19]. To examine the association between the frequency of green tea intake and risk of COPD, multiple linear and logistic regression models were used after adjusting for age, sex, body mass index, smoking status, alcohol consumption, physical activity, and socioeconomic status. It was reported that there was decrease in the incidence of COPD with an increase in the consumption of green tea from never to ≥2 times per day, highlighting that the intake of green tea is associated with a reduced risk of COPD in Korean populations [19].

3. Green Tea Polyphenols and Colorectal Cancer

3.1. In-Vitro Studies

Colorectal cancer (CRC) is regarded as one of the most prevalent form of cancer because of its predominant incidences in both males and females worldwide. Recently, it has been reported that treatment of CRC cells with EGCG and radiation augmented the sensitivity to radiation by inhibition of cell proliferation and induction of nuclear factor (erythroid-derived 2)-like 2 (Nrf2) nuclear translocation and autophagy. Treatment with combination of EGCG and radiation also induced the expression of LC3 and caspase-9 mRNA [20]. Increased expression of the enhancer of zeste homologue 2 (EZH2) is associated with disease progression and a poorer prognosis in several types of cancers. Ying et al., investigated whether EGCG could be a potential EZH2 inhibitor, with a mechanism similar to that of GSK343 (EZH2 inhibitor) in CRC cells [21]. Levels of the EZH2 were found to be significantly higher in CRC tissues compared to normal adjacent tissues and different human CRC cell lines displayed contradictory expression of the EZH2 protein levels. In RKO CRC cells, EGCG and GSK343 inhibited proliferation, invasion and migration and caused suppression of the protein expression of trimethylated lysine 27 on histone H3 (H3K27me3), which may be caused by the loss of the enzymatic function of EZH2. There was synergistic effect of EGCG and GSK343 on the growth of CRC cells at low doses. Both EGCG and GSK343 caused G0/G1 phase arrest in cell cycle, signifying that EGCG and GSK343 work through a common mechanism of action in CRC cells [21]. Cancer stem cells (CSCs) are an infrequent subpopulation of cancer cells that demonstrates the abilities of self-renewal and multipotent differentiation and have an important part in initiation and development of tumors [22,23]. Treatment with EGCG inhibited the spheroid formation competency of CRC cells, expression of colorectal CSC markers, inhibition of cell proliferation, induction of apoptosis accompanied by downregulation of the activation of Wnt/β-catenin pathway [24]. The platinum-based chemotherapy treatments are used extensively for the treatment of CRC, but they have various adverse cytotoxic effects. A combination of EGCG with cisplatin or oxaliplatin was used to minimize the side effects of platinum-based therapy [25]. Treatment of human CRC cells with EGCG plus cisplatin or oxaliplatin showed a synergistic effect on the inhibition of cell proliferation and induction of cell death. EGCG treatment also improved the effect of cisplatin and oxaliplatin-induced autophagy as shown by the accumulation of LC3-II protein, rise of acidic vesicular organelles and the formation of autophagosome. These findings recommend that combination of EGCG with cisplatin or oxaliplatin could decrease cytotoxicity in CRC cells through autophagy related pathways [25]. The chemosensitizing effects of EGCG in 5-fluorouracil (FU)-resistant (5-FUR) CRC cells and spheroid-derived CSCs (SDCSCs) were investigated in a recent study [26]. Treatment with EGCG boosted 5-FU induced cytotoxicity and suppressed proliferation in 5-FUR cell lines through enhancement of apoptosis and cell cycle arrest. The higher spheroid forming capacity was shown in 5-FUR cells as compared to parental cells, representing higher CSC population. Treatment with EGCG led to suppression of SDCSC formation and enhanced 5-FU sensitivity to SDCSCs. EGCG also inhibited pathways targeted in 5-FUR CRC cells such as Notch1, Bmi1, Suz12, and Ezh2, and upregulated self-renewal suppressive-miRNAs, miR-34a, miR-145, and miR-200c [26].

3.2. In-Vivo Studies

The inhibitory effects of orally administered PPE on colon carcinogenesis in azoxymethane-treated rats have been reported. PPE is a defined GTP preparation containing about 65% EGCG and less than 0.1% caffeine. Treatment with PPE in diet significantly increased the plasma and colonic levels of tea polyphenols, reduced tumor multiplicity, tumor size and decreased the incidence and multiplicity of adenocarcinoma. It also caused decrease in the levels of proinflammatory eicosanoids, prostaglandin E2 and leukotriene B4. PPE treatment also lowered β-catenin nuclear expression and caused induction of apoptosis and augmented expression levels of RXR α, β and γ in adenocarcinomas [27]. Treatment with EGCG caused inhibition of tumor growth in a SDCSC xenograft model. It was concluded from the study that EGCG may assist as an adjunctive treatment to conventional chemotherapeutic drugs in CRC patients [26].

3.3. Studies in Humans

In a randomized clinical trial, the effect of green tea extract (GTE) supplements on metachronous colorectal adenoma and cancer in the Korean population was determined [28]. Patients who had undergone complete removal of colorectal adenomas by endoscopic polypectomy were divided into two groups. One group was control and the other was given 0.9 g GTE/day for 12 months. It was found that the incidence of metachronous adenomas at the end-point colonoscopy was higher in control group (42.3%) than GTE-supplemented group (23.6%). Relapsed adenoma was also decreased in the GTE group as compared to the control group, although no differences were noted between two groups in regards to body mass index, dietary intakes, serum lipid profiles, fasting serum glucose and serum C-reactive protein levels. It was concluded that GTE supplements were promising for the chemoprevention of metachronous colorectal adenomas in Korean patients [28].

4. Green Tea Polyphenols and Skin Cancer

4.1. In-Vitro Studies

Skin cancer can be classified as basal cell carcinoma, squamous cell carcinoma, and melanoma, according to histological characteristics [29]. The effect of tea polyphenols on Toll-like receptor 4 (TLR4) in melanoma cell lines has been reported recently [30]. Treatment of melanoma cell lines (B16F10 and A375) with tea polyphenols inhibited the proliferation, migration and invasion ability of melanoma cells dose and time dependently. As compared with normal skin cells, TLR4 was greatly expressed in melanoma cells. Treatment with tea polyphenols inhibited TLR4 expression both in normal melanomas and in stimulated melanomas by TLR4 agonist lipopolysaccharides. The inhibition of TLR4 in melanoma cell lines inhibited cell proliferation, migration, and invasion, and blocking the expression of 67LR eliminated the effects of tea polyphenols on TLR4 [30]. It has been shown that the physiological doses of EGCG (0.1–1 µM) inhibited the proliferation of human metastatic melanoma cell lines [31]. Treatment with EGCG also inhibited NF-κB activity and IL-1β secretion, which was related with downregulation of NLRP1 and a decrease in the activation of caspase-1. The inhibitory effect of EGCG on tumor proliferation was eliminated by silencing NLRP1, signifying a key role of inflammasomes in the tumor-inhibitory effect of EGCG in human melanoma cells [31]. TRAF6, a member of the tumor necrosis factor receptor-associated factor (TRAF) family, has been identified as a novel target of EGCG [32]. They employed a structure-based virtual screening to identify TRAF6 as a potential target of EGCG, and a pull-down assay revealed that EGCG directly binds to TRAF6. EGCG was found to bind with TRAF6 at the residues of Gln54, Gly55, ILe72, Cys73, Asp57 and Lys96. EGCG also inhibited the E3 ubiquitin ligase activity of TRAF6 both in-vitro and in-vivo. EGCG treatment blocked the regulation of NF-κB pathway activation by TRAF6 and inhibits melanoma cell growth, invasion and migration. Therefore, this study suggests that EGCG is an E3 ubiquitin ligase inhibitor and inhibits melanoma cell growth and metastasis by targeting TRAF6 [32]. The 67-kDa laminin receptor (67LR) has been identified as a cell surface receptor of EGCG and has a role in its anticancer effects. EGCG inhibited melanoma tumor growth by activating 67-kDa laminin receptor (67LR) signaling [33]. Treatment of melanoma cells with EGCG up-regulated miRNA-let-7b expression through 67LR, which in turn, caused downregulation of high mobility group A2 (HMGA2), a target gene connected to tumor progression. It was demonstrated that the upregulation of let-7b expression by EGCG followed activation of 67LR-dependent cAMP/protein kinase A (PKA)/protein phosphatase 2A (PP2A) signaling pathway [33].

4.2. In-Vivo Studies

Oral gavage treatment with tea polyphenols inhibited B16F10 melanoma cells growth in-vivo. Treatment with tea polyphenols decreased the tumor size and tumor volume along with the inhibition of TLR4 protein expression as compared with the control group [30]. The effects of tea polyphenols against UVB-induced skin cancer has been reported [34]. GTP can be easily oxidized in the environment and slowly lose their activity. Preserving the activity of GTP for topical formulations is challenging as browning takes place during the storage of skin cream supplemented with green tea catechins. Therefore, Li et al., demonstrated the stabilizing effect of carboxymethyl cellulose sodium (CMC-Na) on GTP under aqueous conditions [35]. Topical application of GTP, emulsified in CMC-Na had a strong photoprotective effect against acute UVB induced photodamage in hairless mice skin. It was reported that 93% of GTP was preserved after 8 h of incubation at 50 °C with CMC-Na, whereas in the absence of CMC-Na, only 61% was preserved. There was also inhibition of acute UVB-induced infiltration of inflammatory cells, increase of skin thickness, depletion of antioxidant enzymes and lipid oxidation, and induction of nuclear accumulation of Nrf2 in mice skin on topical treatment of emulsified GTP [35].

4.3. Studies in Humans

In a case-control study, data from 767 non-Hispanic Whites under age 40 was evaluated to understand the effects of tea, coffee, and caffeine on the early-onset of basal cell carcinoma (BCC). Inverse relationship was found to be associated with combined regular consumption of caffeinated coffee plus hot tea with early-onset of BCC. There was 43% reduced risk of BCC in people consuming the highest category of caffeine from these sources as compared with non-consumers. This study concluded that there was a modest protective effect for caffeinated coffee plus tea in relation to early-onset BCC [36].

5. Green Tea Polyphenols and Prostate Cancer

5.1. In-Vitro Studies

Prostate cancer (PCa) is the most commonly diagnosed malignancy in males and we have earlier reported in detail the effects of GTP on various signaling pathways in PCa [37,38], and its preclinical and clinical effects [1,39]. Polymeric EGCG-encapsulated nanoparticles (NPs) targeted with small molecular entities that were able to bind to prostate specific membrane antigen (PSMA) were developed [40]. Increased anti-proliferative activity and induction of apoptosis in PCa cell lines was observed on treatment with EGCG encapsulating NPs compared to the free EGCG [40]. We have earlier reported the synthesis, characterization and efficacy assessment of a nanotechnology-based oral formulation of chitosan nanoparticles with a size in the range of 150–200 nm diameter encapsulating EGCG (Chit-nanoEGCG) for the treatment of PCa in a preclinical setting [41]. We synthesized nanoparticles made up of the natural biopolymer chitosan with encapsulated EGCG, which appeared to be stable in the acidic environment of the stomach and prevented release of EGCG in the stomach. These nanoparticles showed a slow release of EGCG in acidic pH (simulated gastric juice) and faster release in simulated intestinal fluid (neutral pH) [41]. It has been shown that there was decrease in PCa cell survival and induction of apoptosis with a low dose of 1 μM EGCG [42]. Treatment with EGCG also boosted the capacity of cisplatin to promote apoptosis, and EGCG, both alone and in combination with cisplatin, stimulated the expression of the pro-apoptotic splice isoform of caspase-9 in PCa cells [42]. In human PCa cells, GTP and EGCG activated p53 through acetylation at the Lys373 and Lys382 residues by inhibiting class I Histone deacetylases (HDACs) [43]. There was dose- and time-dependent inhibition of class I HDACs (HDAC1, 2, 3 and 8) on treatment of PCa cells with GTP (2.5–10 μg/mL) and EGCG (5–20 μM), while loss of p53 acetylation at both the sites was observed on withdrawal of treatment with GTP/EGCG. Increased expression of p21/WAF1 was also noted on treatment with GTP/EGCG in PCa cells. The increased GTP/EGCG-mediated p53 acetylation improved its binding on the promoters of p21/WAF1 and Bax. This in turn was connected with an increase in the accumulation of cells in the G0/G1 phase of the cell cycle and induction of apoptosis [43]. The effect of epicatechin (EC), epigallocatechin (EGC) and EGCG (EGCG) on the regulation of androgen receptor acetylation in androgen-dependent PCa cells was demonstrated by histone acetyl-transferase (HAT) activity [44]. Treatment with EC, EGC and EGCG caused PCa cell death, inhibited agonist-dependent androgen receptor (AR) activation and AR-regulated gene transcription. EGCG was the most potent HAT inhibitor among all other catechins and it downregulated AR acetylation. In the presence of the agonist, there was inhibition of AR protein translocation to the nucleus from cytoplasmic compartment [44].

Table 1. Anticarcinogenic effects of tea polyphenols, reported from 2011–2018.

Target Organ	Mechanism of Action	References
Lung cancer	Decrease in the mRNA and protein levels of IFN-γ-induced PD-L1, through inhibition of JAK/STAT signaling. Decrease in EGF-induced PD-L1expression through inhibition of EGFR/Akt signaling. Decreased tumor multiplicity in NNK-induced mice.	[7]
	In Korean population, decrease in the incidence of COPD with an increase in the consumption of green tea intake from never to ≥2 times/day	[8]
	Suppression of the levels of MMP-2 and uPA	[9]
	Upregulation of E-cadherin, inhibition of fibronectin and p-FAK. Inhibition of tumor growth in xenograft model	[10]
	Inhibition of NF-κB activation, cyclin D1, MMP-9 and VEGF on combination of EGCG and TF-nanoparticles with cisplatin	[11]
	Suppression of EGFR pathway	[13]
Colorectal Cancer	Inhibition of cell proliferation and induction of Nrf2 nuclear translocation and autophagy, expression of LC3 and caspase-9 mRNA	[15]
	Decrease in the expression of colorectal CSC markers, inhibition of cell proliferation, induction of apoptosis and downregulation of Wnt/β-catenin pathway	[19]
	Reduced tumor multiplicity, tumor size, decrease in the incidence and multiplicity of adenocarcinoma in rats. Decrease in PGE2, leukotriene B4, β-catenin nuclear expression and increase in RXR α, β and γ	[20]
Skin Cancer	Inhibition of the proliferation, migration and invasion of melanoma cells, inhibition of TLR4 expression	[25]
	Inhibition of NF-κB activity, IL-1β secretion related with downregulation of NLRP1	[28]
	Inhibition of melanoma tumor growth by activation of 67-kDa laminin receptor (67LR) signaling	[30]
Prostate Cancer	Inverse association of PCa risk among Chinese men in Hong Kong with green tea consumption and EGCG intake	[34]
	In mouse xenograft model of prostatic tumor, nanoformulated EGCG had better efficacy than native EGCG	[35]
	In xenograft study, Chit-nanoEGCG caused inhibition of tumor growth and PSA levels, induction of PARP cleavage, increase in Bax with decrease in Bcl-2, activation of caspases and decrease in Ki-67, PCNA, CD-31 and VEGF	[37]
	Inhibition of class I HDACs (HDAC1, 2, 3 and 8), arrest of cells in G0/G01 phase of cell cycle and induction of apoptosis	[39]
	Inhibition of agonist-dependent AR activation and AR-regulated gene transcription	[40]
Breast Cancer	Inhibition of cell growth, activation of caspases-3, -8 -9, promotion of mitochondrial depolarization, inhibition of the activity of the enzymes hexokinase, phosphofructokinase and lactic dehydrogenase	[41]
	Decrease in cell-viability, β-catenin, p-AKT and cyclin D1	[43]
	Increase in PTEN, caspases-3 and -9, decreased AKT and increased Bax/Bcl-2 ratio, comparable to tamoxifen	[44]

This list provides selected examples.

5.2. In-Vivo Studies

In mouse xenograft model of prostatic tumor, nanoformulated EGCG displayed better efficacy than native EGCG and there was 30% tumor growth inhibition in EGCG-treated groups whereas 55 and 60% tumor growth inhibition on treatment with non-targeted- and targeted-NPs, respectively, at the end of the study [40]. It has been reported that certain stages are more or less sensitive to EGCG and that sensitivity is related to heat shock protein 90 (HSP90) inhibition in non-tumorigenic (BPH-1), tumorigenic (BCaPT1, BCaPT10) and metastatic (BCaPM-T10) cancer cells from a human PCa progression model [45]. Further strong cytotoxic effects were observed on the treatment of tumorigenic and metastatic cells with EGCG, novobiocin, or N-terminal inhibitor, 17-AAG. Animals given 0.06% EGCG in drinking water developed significantly smaller tumors than untreated mice when tumorigenic or metastatic cells were grown in-vivo. EGCG-Sepharose was found to bind more HSP90 from metastatic cells compared with non-tumorigenic cells and binding occurred through the HSP90 C-terminus, as determined by binding assays with EGCG-Sepharose, a C-terminal HSP90 antibody, and HSP90 mutants. EGCG, novobiocin, and 17-AAG also led to induction of changes in HSP90-client proteins in non-tumorigenic cells and larger differences in metastatic cells, suggesting that EGCG preferentially targets cancer cells and prevents a molecular chaperone supportive of the malignant phenotype [45].

Chit-nanoEGCG treatment of athymic nude mice subcutaneously implanted with PCa cells caused significant inhibition of tumor growth and secreted prostate-specific antigen (PSA) levels compared with EGCG and control groups. There was also induction of poly (ADP-ribose) polymerases (PARP) cleavage, increase in the protein expression of Bax with decrease in Bcl-2, activation of caspases and decrease in Ki-67, proliferating cell nuclear antigen (PCNA), CD-31 and vascular endothelial growth factor (VEGF) in tumor tissues of mice treated with Chit-nanoEGCG, as compared with groups treated with EGCG and control group [41]. This study addressed concerns related to bioavailability of EGCG and suggested that this nanoformulation also has the potential to be used as a carrier system for many of the bioactive compounds that have sensitivity to acidic pH [41].

5.3. Studies in Humans

The relationship between prostate cancer (PCa) risk and habitual green tea intake was investigated among Chinese men in Hong Kong [46]. The 404 PCa patients and 395 controls were recruited in the study from the same hospital that had complete data on habitual tea consumption of green, oolong, black and pu'er tea. Habitual green tea drinking was reported in a total of 32 cases and 50 controls, while a modest excess risk was detected among the habitual pu'er tea drinkers. An inverse gradient of PCa risk with the increasing consumption of EGCG was observed due to lower intake of EGCG among PCa patients than the controls. It was concluded that there is an inverse association of PCa risk among Chinese men in Hong Kong with green tea consumption and EGCG intake [46]. In a double-blind, placebo-controlled study, sixty volunteers with high-grade prostate intraepithelial neoplasia (HGPIN), without any given therapy was enrolled to determine whether the administration of green tea catechins (GTCs) could stop malignancy in men at high-risk [47]. Volunteers were given daily treatment of three GTCs capsules, 200 mg each. It was noted that only one tumor was diagnosed among the 30 GTCs-treated men after 1 year, as compared with nine cancers among the 30 placebo-treated men. There was not much effect on total prostate-specific antigen between the two arms, but lower values were recorded in GTCs-treated men with respect to placebo-treated ones. There was improvement in International Prostate Symptom Score and quality of life scores of GTCs-treated men with coexistent benign prostate hyperplasia with no significant side effects. Lower urinary tract symptoms also decreased on administration of GTCs, signifying that green tea could also be beneficial for benign prostate hyperplasia [47]. The role of GTCs for prostate cancer chemoprevention was further investigated in a randomized, double-blind, placebo controlled trial. PPE, as a standardized formulation of GTCs containing 400 mg EGCG/day was given to men with HGPIN and/or atypical small acinar proliferation (ASAP) [48]. The primary endpoint of the study was a comparison of the cumulative one-year PCa rates on the two study arms and there were no differences in the number of PCa cases. In a pre-specified secondary analysis performed in men with HGPIN without ASAP at baseline, a decrease in the composite endpoint of PCa plus ASAP was observed for the PPE arm. In addition, fewer men with HGPIN without ASAP at baseline were subsequently diagnosed with ASAP on the PPE than on the placebo arm. It was concluded that daily consumption of a standardized, decaffeinated catechins mixture containing 400 mg EGCG/day for 1 year accumulated in plasma and was well tolerated but did not lessen the likelihood of PCa in men with baseline HGPIN or ASAP [48].

6. Green Tea Polyphenols and Breast Cancer

6.1. In-Vitro Studies

Breast cancer is the most commonly diagnosed cancer and the main reason of cancer-related deaths among women globally. The anticancer effects of EGCG in breast cancer were investigated both in-vitro and in-vivo, based on its effect on tumor glucose metabolism [49]. Treatment of breast cancer 4T1 cells with EGCG inhibited cell growth and induced apoptosis as shown by activation of caspases-3, -8 -9, modulation of apoptotic related genes and promotion of mitochondrial depolarization. EGCG treatment also inhibited the activity of the enzymes hexokinase, phosphofructokinase and lactic dehydrogenase, enzymes related to the glycolytic pathway, specifying that modulating glucose metabolism plays an important part in the anticancer effects of EGCG [49]. Treatment with EGCG inhibited the MDA-MB-231 cell-viability, expression of β-catenin, phosphorylated Akt and cyclin D1. This study suggested that EGCG inhibits the growth of breast cancer cells through the inactivation of the β-catenin signaling pathway [50]. The effects of EGCG on proliferation and apoptosis of T47D estrogen receptor α-positive breast cancer cells, and compared with tamoxifen were reported recently. Treatment of cells with EGCG decreased cell viability in a dose and time-dependent manner. EGCG treatment of cells significantly increased PTEN, caspases-3 and -9, decreased AKT and increased Bax/Bcl-2 ratio, almost similar to tamoxifen [51]. The stability of EGCG in solutions of different pH was investigated to define the pH range of stability of EGCG under room temperature conditions. Very low stability profile of EGCG at physiological pH was observed with rapid degradation under alkaline conditions. Hence, EGCG was encapsulated in solid lipid nanoparticles (SLN) for enhancing the stability and anticancer activity. SLN control the release of encapsulated drug and consequently, prevent the premature degradation of encapsulated drug in the biological system. EGCG and EGCG loaded nanoparticles (EGCG-SLN) were compared by cellular proliferation assay in MDA-MB-231 human breast cancer and DU-145 PCa cell lines. The cytotoxicity of EGCG-SLN was found to be 8.1 times higher against human breast cancer cells and 3.8 times higher against human PCa cells, as compared with pure EGCG [52].

6.2. In-Vivo Studies

The effects of a nutrient mixture containing ascorbic acid, lysine, proline and green tea extract were investigated in a model of metastatic breast cancer. Treatment with nutrient mixture inhibited tumor weight and burden of metastatic breast tumors and also decreased lung metastasis, as compared to control mice. There was also decrease in the metastasis to liver, spleen, kidney and heart with NM treatment, suggesting that nutrient mixture may be explored further for the treatment of breast cancer [53].

6.3. Studies in Humans

Among patients who underwent surgery at Chonbuk National University Hospital, Jeonju, Korea, for primary breast cancers, 74 breast cancer patients were identified and admitted in the study to investigate the expression profiles of the β-catenin signaling pathway in breast cancer patients. The β-catenin expression was analyzed according to the clinicopathological factors of female breast cancer patients diagnosed with invasive ductal carcinoma. It was found that β-catenin was expressed at higher levels in breast cancer tissue than in normal tissue. β-catenin expression was related with lymph node metastasis, tumor-node-metastasis stage and estrogen receptor status. [50]. In a randomized phase II controlled trial, the effects of daily consumption of GTE containing 800 mg EGCG for 12 months were evaluated on changes in mammographic density (MD) measures in healthy postmenopausal women at high risk of breast cancer due to dense breast tissue. It was observed that supplementation of GTE did not significantly change percent MD (PMD) or absolute MD in all women. In younger women, GTE supplementation significantly reduced PMD as compared with the placebo, but had no effect in older women. Administration of GTE also did not prompt MD change in other subgroups of women stratified by catechol-*O*-methyltransferase genotype or level of body mass index. This study concluded that 12 months administration of a high dose of EGCG did not have a significant effect on MD measures in all women, but reduced PMD in younger women, an age-dependent effect comparable to those of tamoxifen [54].

6.4. Green Tea Polyphenols and Diabetes

Diabetes is one of the major health problems worldwide. Type-1 diabetes is not preventable and is treated by insulin supplementation. However. Type-2 diabetes can be prevented or reversed by altering diet and management of lifestyle factors. EGCG has been reported to inhibit starch hydrolysis and acted as an inhibitor by binding to the active site of α-amylase and α-glucosidase. The anti-diabetic action of EGCG was explored in high fat diet and streptozotocin (STZ)-induced type-2 diabetes. Treatment with EGCG enhanced glucose homeostasis and repressed the process of gluconeogenesis and lipogenesis in the liver. It also activated PXR/CAR, accompanied by upgrading PXR/CAR-mediated phase II drug metabolism enzyme expression in small intestine and liver, relating SULT1A1, UGT1A1 and SULT2B1b [55]. Diabetes mellitus (DM) can cause compromised wound healing by disturbing the biological mechanisms of the process. It was shown that the late wound healing in STZ-induced DM mice could be enhanced by EGCG. In the skin wounds of DM mice, EGCG treatment inhibited macrophage accumulation, inflammation response, and Notch signaling and directly bind with mouse Notch-1. Diabetic wound healing was improved on treatment with EGCG before or after the inflammation period by targeting the Notch signaling pathway, signifying that the pre-existing diabetic wound healing was enhanced by EGCG [56]. The mechanisms by which EGCG alleviates insulin resistance (IR) were explored in human hepatoma HepG2 cells. Treatment of cells with EGCG increased glucose uptake and decreased glucose content. It also reduced the intracellular levels of tumor necrosis factor-α, reactive oxygen species, malondialdehyde, with increase in antioxidant enzymes like superoxide dismutases (SOD) and glutathione peroxidase. There was also increase in the glucose transporter 2 (GLUT2) protein and its downstream proteins peroxisome proliferator-activated receptor coactivator (PGC)-1β, when cells were treated with EGCG [57]. In 3T3-L1 pre-adipocytes, EGCG has been reported to increase the activity of browning in inguinal white adipose tissue (iWAT), inhibited adipocyte differentiation and relieved TNF-α-triggered insulin resistance through the suppression of oxidative stress and regulation of mitochondrial function [58].

7. Green Tea Polyphenols and Cardiovascular Diseases

Cardiovascular disease is the leading cause of deaths worldwide and includes coronary heart disease (CHD), congenital heart disease, rheumatic heart disease, cerebrovascular disease and peripheral arterial disease. The relationship between plasma tea catechin and risk of stroke and CHD was investigated in a nested case-control study in men and women aged 40–69 years without history of heart disease, stroke or cancer. Participants completed a survey and donated blood samples between 1990 and 1994, and were followed-up through 2008. No significant association between plasma tea catechin and the incidence of stroke or CHD in either men or women was observed, although high plasma levels of EGCG were associated with decreased risk of stroke in non-smoking men. It was concluded that plasma tea catechin was not connected with decreased risks of either stroke or CHD, though, for male non-smokers, a protective effect of tea catechin on stroke risk was proposed [59]. The protective effect of EGCG in a mouse model of heart failure and the underlying mechanisms were investigated recently [60]. Echocardiography was employed to measure alterations in ejection fraction, left ventricular internal diastolic diameter (LVIDd) and left ventricular internal systolic diameter (LVIDs). The experiments revealed that EGCG reversed the changes in LVIDd and LVIDs, induced by establishment of the model of heart failure. There was also inhibition of myocardial fibrosis, oxidative stress, inflammatory and cardiomyocyte apoptosis, and decrease in the expression levels of collagen I and collagen III. The effect of EGCG against heart failure was diminished on treatment with TGF-β1 inhibitor, showing that EGCG inhibited the progression and development of heart failure in mice via inhibition of myocardial fibrosis and decrease of ventricular collagen remodeling, through inhibition of TGF-β1/smad3 signaling pathway [60].

The effects of EGCG on cardiac function by desensitization of 1-AR and GRK2 in heart failure (HF) rats were studied. Left ventricular end diastolic pressure, mean blood pressure, heart/body weight and posterior wall thickness were significantly increased in the HF group as compared to control group. Left ventricular systolic pressure, maximum rate of left ventricular pressure rise and maximum rate of left ventricular pressure fall were also lowered, whereas, treatment with EGCG recovered cardiac function by regulation of these parameters. There was decrease in the expression of 1-AR in the left ventricle tissue of HF rats and increase in expression of GRK2. Treatment with EGCG downregulated the membrane expression of GRK2 and upregulated the expression of 1-AR, suggesting it has therapeutic effects on the heart function of HF rats [61]. The protective effect of EGCG against Doxorubicin (DOX)-induced cardiotoxicity via effects on oxidative stress, inflammatory and apoptotic markers was investigated in Male Wistar rats. Treatment with EGCG was found to protect against DOX-induced ECG changes, leakage of cardiac enzymes and histopathological changes. Treatment with EGCG decreased glutathione depletion and lipid peroxidation and promotion of antioxidant enzyme activities. ErbB2 expression was reduced on treatment with DOX and it improved on treatment with EGCG. Treatment with DOX reduced expression of ErbB2, NF-κB, p53, caspases-3, -12 and basal level of Hsp70, while EGCG pretreatment significantly reversed these effects [62].

8. Green Tea Polyphenols and Neurological Diseases

Neurological diseases account for principal causes of disability and have high impact on the quality of life of patients and their caregivers. The effect of EGCG was investigated against neuronal injury in rat models of middle cerebral artery occlusion (MCAO). Treatment with EGCG reduced neurological function score, protected nerve cells, repressed neuronal apoptosis, and inhibited oxidative stress injury and brain injury markers level after MCAO. There was also decrease in the apoptotic rate of neurons expression, caspase-3, Bax with increase in the expression of Bcl-2. The protective effect of EGCG was decreased after administration of LY294002, a phosphoinositide 3-kinase (PI3K) inhibitor [63]. Subarachnoid hemorrhage (SAH), an exceptional subtype of stroke, has a high mortality rate. EGCG has been reported to regulate the Ca^{2+}-mitochondrial dynamic axis to protect mitochondrial function after SAH. It was shown that EGCG antagonized the overloaded Ca^{2+}-induced damage of mitochondrial dynamics and mitochondrial dysfunction, finally displaying neuroprotective effects after SAH. EGCG treatment improved the neurological score by reducing cell death through the Cytochrome *c*-mediated intrinsic apoptotic pathway [64]. Parkinson's disease (PD) is a movement disorder categorized by degeneration of dopaminergic neurons and generation of intracellular deposits known as Lewy bodies and dystrophic neurites, composed primarily of alpha-synuclein (SNCA) and phosphorylated SNCA [65]. Xu et al., investigated whether EGCG inhibit the SNCA aggregation using biochemical, and tissue biological methods. They also utilized the human brain tissue for the experiment. EGCG inhibited the SNCA aggregation in a concentration dependent manner. The SNCA amino acid sites, which possibly interacted with EGCG, were detected on peptide membranes and it was suggested that EGCG inhibited the SNCA aggregation by instable intermolecular hydrophobic interactions [66].

9. Conclusions and Future Prospects

Tea polyphenols, especially EGCG has been the focus of research owing to it multiple protective effects against cancer and other diseases such as diabetes, neurological and cardiovascular diseases. Large amount of epidemiological and clinical studies have indicated that supplementation of green tea has significant protective effects against chronic diseases.

Natural products with various pharmacological effects may cause drug or food interactions when administered simultaneously with narrow therapeutic index drugs. There are still many challenges for clinical application of EGCG. It has low bioavailability when given orally and it is very perplexing to derive ways to deliver EGCG effectively to target sites. The consumers should be made aware of its potential interactions with conventional medications. The tannin content of green tea interferes with intestinal absorption of some nutrients and drugs and it has inhibitory effects on CYP450 isozymes such as CYP3A4, 1A1, and 1A2. There is very restricted data on the drug and nutrient interaction of green tea in humans [67].

We have earlier reported in detail that EGCG modulates several signal transduction pathways and has robust cancer chemopreventive/chemotherapeutic effects [5,37,38]. It is important to recognize molecules in the cell signaling pathways which are affected on treatment with EGCG as deregulation of the network cause several chronic diseases such as cancer. The effect of EGCG on cell signaling network is evidenced by activation of cell death and induction of apoptosis in cancer cells which leads to the development of cancer progression. Tea catechins act through multiple mechanisms and these act synergistically to elicit cancer preventive and therapeutic effects. Also, tea polyphenols in combination with other drugs for chemotherapy displayed synergistic effects. Although many clinical studies have reported the beneficial effects of tea in humans [19,46,47], we are lacking in the defined evidences about the mechanisms of cancer prevention by tea in humans. To obtain more definite information, well-designed large cohort studies and human intervention trials are necessary.

Author Contributions: N.K. and H.M. developed the contents of the manuscript. N.K. wrote the manuscript and H.M. contributed to the conceptualization and editing of the manuscript. Both authors approve the submitted version.

Funding: Naghma Khan is thankful for support from the American Cancer Society (Research Scholar Grant RSG-15-013-01-CNE) and University of Wisconsin Carbone Cancer Center (Support Grant P30 CA014520).

Acknowledgments: N.K. would like to thank American Cancer Society and University of Wisconsin Carbone Cancer Center for their funding support.

Conflicts of Interest: The authors declare no conflict of interest.

References

1. Khan, N.; Afaq, F.; Mukhtar, H. Cancer chemoprevention through dietary antioxidants: Progress and promise. *Antioxid. Redox Signal.* **2008**, *10*, 475–510. [CrossRef] [PubMed]
2. Yang, C.S.; Maliakal, P.; Meng, X. Inhibition of carcinogenesis by tea. *Annu. Rev. Pharmacol. Toxicol.* **2002**, *42*, 25–54. [CrossRef] [PubMed]
3. Yang, C.S.; Wang, X.; Lu, G.; Picinich, S.C. Cancer prevention by tea: Animal studies, molecular mechanisms and human relevance. *Nat. Rev. Cancer* **2009**, *9*, 429–439. [CrossRef] [PubMed]
4. Boehm, K.; Borrelli, F.; Ernst, E.; Habacher, G.; Hung, S.K.; Milazzo, S.; Horneber, M. Green tea (camellia sinensis) for the prevention of cancer. *Cochrane Database Syst. Rev.* **2009**, *8*, CD005004. [CrossRef] [PubMed]
5. Khan, N.; Afaq, F.; Saleem, M.; Ahmad, N.; Mukhtar, H. Targeting multiple signaling pathways by green tea polyphenol (-)-epigallocatechin-3-gallate. *Cancer Res.* **2006**, *66*, 2500–2505. [CrossRef] [PubMed]
6. Khan, N.; Mukhtar, H. Cancer and metastasis: Prevention and treatment by green tea. *Cancer Metastasis. Rev.* **2010**, *29*, 435–445. [CrossRef] [PubMed]
7. Rawangkan, A.; Wongsirisin, P.; Namiki, K.; Iida, K.; Kobayashi, Y.; Shimizu, Y.; Fujiki, H.; Suganuma, M. Green tea catechin is an alternative immune checkpoint inhibitor that inhibits pd-l1 expression and lung tumor growth. *Molecules* **2018**, *23*, 2071. [CrossRef]
8. Huang, S.F.; Horng, C.T.; Hsieh, Y.S.; Hsieh, Y.H.; Chu, S.C.; Chen, P.N. Epicatechin-3-gallate reverses tgf-beta1-induced epithelial-to-mesenchymal transition and inhibits cell invasion and protease activities in human lung cancer cells. *Food Chem. Toxicol.* **2016**, *94*, 1–10. [CrossRef]
9. Yang, C.S.; Sang, S.; Lambert, J.D.; Lee, M.J. Bioavailability issues in studying the health effects of plant polyphenolic compounds. *Mol. Nutr. Food Res.* **2008**, *52* (Suppl. 1), S139–S151. [CrossRef]
10. Yang, C.S.; Lambert, J.D.; Sang, S. Antioxidative and anti-carcinogenic activities of tea polyphenols. *Arch. Toxicol.* **2009**, *83*, 11–21. [CrossRef]
11. Shi, M.; Shi, Y.L.; Li, X.M.; Yang, R.; Cai, Z.Y.; Li, Q.S.; Ma, S.C.; Ye, J.H.; Lu, J.L.; Liang, Y.R.; et al. Food-grade encapsulation systems for (-)-epigallocatechin gallate. *Molecules* **2018**, *23*, 445. [CrossRef] [PubMed]
12. Laudadio, E.; Mobbili, G.; Minnelli, C.; Massaccesi, L.; Galeazzi, R. Salts influence cathechins and flavonoids encapsulation in liposomes: A molecular dynamics investigation. *Mol. Inform.* **2017**, *36*. [CrossRef] [PubMed]
13. Minnelli, C.; Moretti, P.; Fulgenzi, G.; Mariani, P.; Laudadio, E.; Armeni, T.; Galeazzi, R.; Mobbili, G. A poloxamer-407 modified liposome encapsulating epigallocatechin-3-gallate in the presence of magnesium: Characterization and protective effect against oxidative damage. *Int. J. Pharm.* **2018**, *552*, 225–234. [CrossRef] [PubMed]

14. Singh, M.; Bhatnagar, P.; Mishra, S.; Kumar, P.; Shukla, Y.; Gupta, K.C. Plga-encapsulated tea polyphenols enhance the chemotherapeutic efficacy of cisplatin against human cancer cells and mice bearing ehrlich ascites carcinoma. *Int. J. Nanomed.* **2015**, *10*, 6789–6809. [CrossRef] [PubMed]

15. Flores-Perez, A.; Marchat, L.A.; Sanchez, L.L.; Romero-Zamora, D.; Arechaga-Ocampo, E.; Ramirez-Torres, N.; Chavez, J.D.; Carlos-Reyes, A.; Astudillo-de la Vega, H.; Ruiz-Garcia, E.; et al. Differential proteomic analysis reveals that egcg inhibits hdgf and activates apoptosis to increase the sensitivity of non-small cells lung cancer to chemotherapy. *Proteom. Clin. Appl.* **2016**, *10*, 172–182. [CrossRef] [PubMed]

16. Ma, Y.C.; Li, C.; Gao, F.; Xu, Y.; Jiang, Z.B.; Liu, J.X.; Jin, L.Y. Epigallocatechin gallate inhibits the growth of human lung cancer by directly targeting the egfr signaling pathway. *Oncol. Rep.* **2014**, *31*, 1343–1349. [CrossRef] [PubMed]

17. Pan, J.; Zhang, Q.; Xiong, D.; Vedell, P.; Yan, Y.; Jiang, H.; Cui, P.; Ding, F.; Tichelaar, J.W.; Wang, Y.; et al. Transcriptomic analysis by rna-seq reveals ap-1 pathway as key regulator that green tea may rely on to inhibit lung tumorigenesis. *Mol. Carcinog.* **2014**, *53*, 19–29. [CrossRef] [PubMed]

18. Zhou, H.; Chen, J.X.; Yang, C.S.; Yang, M.Q.; Deng, Y.; Wang, H. Gene regulation mediated by micrornas in response to green tea polyphenol egcg in mouse lung cancer. *BMC Genom.* **2014**, *15* (Suppl. 11), S3. [CrossRef] [PubMed]

19. Oh, C.M.; Oh, I.H.; Choe, B.K.; Yoon, T.Y.; Choi, J.M.; Hwang, J. Consuming green tea at least twice each day is associated with reduced odds of chronic obstructive lung disease in middle-aged and older korean adults. *J. Nutr.* **2018**, *148*, 70–76. [CrossRef] [PubMed]

20. Enkhbat, T.; Nishi, M.; Yoshikawa, K.; Jun, H.; Tokunaga, T.; Takasu, C.; Kashihara, H.; Ishikawa, D.; Tominaga, M.; Shimada, M. Epigallocatechin-3-gallate enhances radiation sensitivity in colorectal cancer cells through nrf2 activation and autophagy. *Anticancer Res.* **2018**, *38*, 6247–6252. [CrossRef] [PubMed]

21. Ying, L.; Yan, F.; Williams, B.R.; Xu, P.; Li, X.; Zhao, Y.; Hu, Y.; Wang, Y.; Xu, D.; Dai, J. (-)-epigallocatechin-3-gallate and ezh2 inhibitor gsk343 have similar inhibitory effects and mechanisms of action on colorectal cancer cells. *Clin. Exp. Pharmacol. Physiol.* **2018**, *45*, 58–67. [CrossRef] [PubMed]

22. Ricci-Vitiani, L.; Lombardi, D.G.; Pilozzi, E.; Biffoni, M.; Todaro, M.; Peschle, C.; De Maria, R. Identification and expansion of human colon-cancer-initiating cells. *Nature* **2007**, *445*, 111–115. [CrossRef] [PubMed]

23. Todaro, M.; Francipane, M.G.; Medema, J.P.; Stassi, G. Colon cancer stem cells: Promise of targeted therapy. *Gastroenterology* **2010**, *138*, 2151–2162. [CrossRef] [PubMed]

24. Chen, Y.; Wang, X.Q.; Zhang, Q.; Zhu, J.Y.; Li, Y.; Xie, C.F.; Li, X.T.; Wu, J.S.; Geng, S.S.; Zhong, C.Y.; et al. (-)-epigallocatechin-3-gallate inhibits colorectal cancer stem cells by suppressing wnt/beta-catenin pathway. *Nutrients* **2017**, *9*, 572. [CrossRef] [PubMed]

25. Hu, F.; Wei, F.; Wang, Y.; Wu, B.; Fang, Y.; Xiong, B. Egcg synergizes the therapeutic effect of cisplatin and oxaliplatin through autophagic pathway in human colorectal cancer cells. *J. pharmacol. Sci.* **2015**, *128*, 27–34. [CrossRef] [PubMed]

26. Toden, S.; Tran, H.M.; Tovar-Camargo, O.A.; Okugawa, Y.; Goel, A. Epigallocatechin-3-gallate targets cancer stem-like cells and enhances 5-fluorouracil chemosensitivity in colorectal cancer. *Oncotarget* **2016**, *7*, 16158–16171. [CrossRef]

27. Hao, X.; Xiao, H.; Ju, J.; Lee, M.J.; Lambert, J.D.; Yang, C.S. Green tea polyphenols inhibit colorectal tumorigenesis in azoxymethane-treated f344 rats. *Nutr. Cancer* **2017**, *69*, 623–631. [CrossRef]

28. Shin, C.M.; Lee, D.H.; Seo, A.Y.; Lee, H.J.; Kim, S.B.; Son, W.C.; Kim, Y.K.; Lee, S.J.; Park, S.H.; Kim, N.; et al. Green tea extracts for the prevention of metachronous colorectal polyps among patients who underwent endoscopic removal of colorectal adenomas: A randomized clinical trial. *Clin. Nutr.* **2018**, *37*, 452–458. [CrossRef]

29. Sacco, A.G.; Daniels, G.A. Adjuvant and neoadjuvant treatment of skin cancer. *Facial Plast. Surg. Clin. N. Am.* **2019**, *27*, 139–150. [CrossRef]

30. Chen, X.; Chang, L.; Qu, Y.; Liang, J.; Jin, W.; Xia, X. Tea polyphenols inhibit the proliferation, migration, and invasion of melanoma cells through the down-regulation of tlr4. *Int. J. Immunopathol. Pharmacol.* **2018**, *32*. [CrossRef]

31. Ellis, L.Z.; Liu, W.; Luo, Y.; Okamoto, M.; Qu, D.; Dunn, J.H.; Fujita, M. Green tea polyphenol epigallocatechin-3-gallate suppresses melanoma growth by inhibiting inflammasome and il-1beta secretion. *Biochem. Biophys. Res. Commun.* **2011**, *414*, 551–556. [CrossRef] [PubMed]

32. Zhang, J.; Lei, Z.; Huang, Z.; Zhang, X.; Zhou, Y.; Luo, Z.; Zeng, W.; Su, J.; Peng, C.; Chen, X. Epigallocatechin-3-gallate(egcg) suppresses melanoma cell growth and metastasis by targeting traf6 activity. *Oncotarget* **2016**, *7*, 79557–79571. [CrossRef] [PubMed]

33. Yamada, S.; Tsukamoto, S.; Huang, Y.; Makio, A.; Kumazoe, M.; Yamashita, S.; Tachibana, H. Epigallocatechin-3-o-gallate up-regulates microrna-let-7b expression by activating 67-kda laminin receptor signaling in melanoma cells. *Sci. Rep.* **2016**, *6*, 19225. [CrossRef] [PubMed]

34. Sharma, P.; Montes de Oca, M.K.; Alkeswani, A.R.; McClees, S.F.; Das, T.; Elmets, C.A.; Afaq, F. Tea polyphenols for the prevention of uvb-induced skin cancer. *Photodermatol. Photoimmunol. Photomed.* **2018**, *34*, 50–59. [CrossRef] [PubMed]

35. Li, H.; Jiang, N.; Liu, Q.; Gao, A.; Zhou, X.; Liang, B.; Li, R.; Li, Z.; Zhu, H. Topical treatment of green tea polyphenols emulsified in carboxymethyl cellulose protects against acute ultraviolet light b-induced photodamage in hairless mice. *Photochem. Photobiol. Sci.* **2016**, *15*, 1264–1271. [CrossRef] [PubMed]

36. Ferrucci, L.M.; Cartmel, B.; Molinaro, A.M.; Leffell, D.J.; Bale, A.E.; Mayne, S.T. Tea, coffee, and caffeine and early-onset basal cell carcinoma in a case-control study. *Eur. J. Cancer Prev.* **2014**, *23*, 296–302. [CrossRef] [PubMed]

37. Khan, N.; Mukhtar, H. Modulation of signaling pathways in prostate cancer by green tea polyphenols. *Biochem. Pharmacol.* **2013**, *85*, 667–672. [CrossRef] [PubMed]

38. Khan, N.; Mukhtar, H. Multitargeted therapy of cancer by green tea polyphenols. *Cancer Lett.* **2008**, *269*, 269–280. [CrossRef] [PubMed]

39. Khan, N.; Adhami, V.M.; Mukhtar, H. Review: Green tea polyphenols in chemoprevention of prostate cancer: Preclinical and clinical studies. *Nutr. Cancer* **2009**, *61*, 836–841. [CrossRef]

40. Sanna, V.; Singh, C.K.; Jashari, R.; Adhami, V.M.; Chamcheu, J.C.; Rady, I.; Sechi, M.; Mukhtar, H.; Siddiqui, I.A. Targeted nanoparticles encapsulating (-)-epigallocatechin-3-gallate for prostate cancer prevention and therapy. *Sci. Rep.* **2017**, *7*, 41573. [CrossRef]

41. Khan, N.; Bharali, D.J.; Adhami, V.M.; Siddiqui, I.A.; Cui, H.; Shabana, S.M.; Mousa, S.A.; Mukhtar, H. Oral administration of naturally occurring chitosan-based nanoformulated green tea polyphenol egcg effectively inhibits prostate cancer cell growth in a xenograft model. *Carcinogenesis* **2014**, *35*, 415–423. [CrossRef] [PubMed]

42. Hagen, R.M.; Chedea, V.S.; Mintoff, C.P.; Bowler, E.; Morse, H.R.; Ladomery, M.R. Epigallocatechin-3-gallate promotes apoptosis and expression of the caspase 9a splice variant in pc3 prostate cancer cells. *Int. J. Oncol.* **2013**, *43*, 194–200. [CrossRef] [PubMed]

43. Thakur, V.S.; Gupta, K.; Gupta, S. Green tea polyphenols increase p53 transcriptional activity and acetylation by suppressing class i histone deacetylases. *Int. J. Oncol.* **2012**, *41*, 353–361. [PubMed]

44. Lee, Y.H.; Kwak, J.; Choi, H.K.; Choi, K.C.; Kim, S.; Lee, J.; Jun, W.; Park, H.J.; Yoon, H.G. Egcg suppresses prostate cancer cell growth modulating acetylation of androgen receptor by anti-histone acetyltransferase activity. *Int. J. Mol. Med.* **2012**, *30*, 69–74. [PubMed]

45. Moses, M.A.; Henry, E.C.; Ricke, W.A.; Gasiewicz, T.A. The heat shock protein 90 inhibitor, (-)-epigallocatechin gallate, has anticancer activity in a novel human prostate cancer progression model. *Cancer Prev. Res. (Phila)* **2015**, *8*, 249–257. [CrossRef] [PubMed]

46. Lee, P.M.Y.; Ng, C.F.; Liu, Z.M.; Ho, W.M.; Lee, M.K.; Wang, F.; Kan, H.D.; He, Y.H.; Ng, S.S.M.; Wong, S.Y.S.; et al. Reduced prostate cancer risk with green tea and epigallocatechin 3-gallate intake among hong kong chinese men. *Prostate Cancer Prostatic Dis.* **2017**, *20*, 318–322. [CrossRef]

47. Bettuzzi, S.; Brausi, M.; Rizzi, F.; Castagnetti, G.; Peracchia, G.; Corti, A. Chemoprevention of human prostate cancer by oral administration of green tea catechins in volunteers with high-grade prostate intraepithelial neoplasia: A preliminary report from a one-year proof-of-principle study. *Cancer Res.* **2006**, *66*, 1234–1240. [CrossRef]

48. Kumar, N.B.; Pow-Sang, J.; Egan, K.M.; Spiess, P.E.; Dickinson, S.; Salup, R.; Helal, M.; McLarty, J.; Williams, C.R.; Schreiber, F.; et al. Randomized, placebo-controlled trial of green tea catechins for prostate cancer prevention. *Cancer Prev. Res. (Phila)* **2015**, *8*, 879–887. [CrossRef]

49. Wei, R.; Mao, L.; Xu, P.; Zheng, X.; Hackman, R.M.; Mackenzie, G.G.; Wang, Y. Suppressing glucose metabolism with epigallocatechin-3-gallate (egcg) reduces breast cancer cell growth in preclinical models. *Food Funct.* **2018**, *9*, 5682–5696. [CrossRef]

50. Hong, O.Y.; Noh, E.M.; Jang, H.Y.; Lee, Y.R.; Lee, B.K.; Jung, S.H.; Kim, J.S.; Youn, H.J. Epigallocatechin gallate inhibits the growth of mda-mb-231 breast cancer cells via inactivation of the beta-catenin signaling pathway. *Oncol. Lett.* **2017**, *14*, 441–446. [CrossRef]

51. Moradzadeh, M.; Hosseini, A.; Erfanian, S.; Rezaei, H. Epigallocatechin-3-gallate promotes apoptosis in human breast cancer t47d cells through down-regulation of pi3k/akt and telomerase. *Pharmacol. Rep.* **2017**, *69*, 924–928. [CrossRef]

52. Radhakrishnan, R.; Kulhari, H.; Pooja, D.; Gudem, S.; Bhargava, S.; Shukla, R.; Sistla, R. Encapsulation of biophenolic phytochemical egcg within lipid nanoparticles enhances its stability and cytotoxicity against cancer. *Chem. Phys. Lipids* **2016**, *198*, 51–60. [CrossRef] [PubMed]

53. Roomi, M.W.; Kalinovsky, T.; Roomi, N.M.; Cha, J.; Rath, M.; Niedzwiecki, A. In vitro and in vivo effects of a nutrient mixture on breast cancer progression. *Int. J. Oncol.* **2014**, *44*, 1933–1944. [CrossRef] [PubMed]

54. Samavat, H.; Ursin, G.; Emory, T.H.; Lee, E.; Wang, R.; Torkelson, C.J.; Dostal, A.M.; Swenson, K.; Le, C.T.; Yang, C.S.; et al. A randomized controlled trial of green tea extract supplementation and mammographic density in postmenopausal women at increased risk of breast cancer. *Cancer Prev. Res. (Phila)* **2017**, *10*, 710–718. [CrossRef] [PubMed]

55. Li, X.; Li, S.; Chen, M.; Wang, J.; Xie, B.; Sun, Z. (-)-epigallocatechin-3-gallate (egcg) inhibits starch digestion and improves glucose homeostasis through direct or indirect activation of pxr/car-mediated phase ii metabolism in diabetic mice. *Food Funct.* **2018**, *9*, 4651–4663. [CrossRef] [PubMed]

56. Huang, Y.W.; Zhu, Q.Q.; Yang, X.Y.; Xu, H.H.; Sun, B.; Wang, X.J.; Sheng, J. Wound healing can be improved by (-)-epigallocatechin gallate through targeting notch in streptozotocin-induced diabetic mice. *FASEB J.* **2018**. [CrossRef]

57. Zhang, Q.; Yuan, H.; Zhang, C.; Guan, Y.; Wu, Y.; Ling, F.; Niu, Y.; Li, Y. Epigallocatechin gallate improves insulin resistance in hepg2 cells through alleviating inflammation and lipotoxicity. *Diabetes Res. Clin. Pract.* **2018**, *142*, 363–373. [CrossRef]

58. Mi, Y.; Liu, X.; Tian, H.; Liu, H.; Li, J.; Qi, G.; Liu, X. Egcg stimulates the recruitment of brite adipocytes, suppresses adipogenesis and counteracts tnf-alpha-triggered insulin resistance in adipocytes. *Food Funct.* **2018**, *9*, 3374–3386. [CrossRef]

59. Ikeda, A.; Iso, H.; Yamagishi, K.; Iwasaki, M.; Yamaji, T.; Miura, T.; Sawada, N.; Inoue, M.; Tsugane, S.; Group, J.S. Plasma tea catechins and risk of cardiovascular disease in middle-aged japanese subjects: The jphc study. *Atherosclerosis* **2018**, *277*, 90–97. [CrossRef]

60. Chen, K.; Chen, W.; Liu, S.L.; Wu, T.S.; Yu, K.F.; Qi, J.; Wang, Y.; Yao, H.; Huang, X.Y.; Han, Y.; et al. Epigallocatechingallate attenuates myocardial injury in a mouse model of heart failure through tgfbeta1/smad3 signaling pathway. *Mol. Med. Rep.* **2018**, *17*, 7652–7660.

61. Zhang, Q.; Hu, L.; Chen, L.; Li, H.; Wu, J.; Liu, W.; Zhang, M.; Yan, G. (-)-epigallocatechin-3-gallate, the major green tea catechin, regulates the desensitization of beta1 adrenoceptor via grk2 in experimental heart failure. *Inflammopharmacology* **2018**, *26*, 1081–1091. [CrossRef] [PubMed]

62. Saeed, N.M.; El-Naga, R.N.; El-Bakly, W.M.; Abdel-Rahman, H.M.; Salah ElDin, R.A.; El-Demerdash, E. Epigallocatechin-3-gallate pretreatment attenuates doxorubicin-induced cardiotoxicity in rats: A mechanistic study. *Biochem. Pharmacol.* **2015**, *95*, 145–155. [CrossRef] [PubMed]

63. Nan, W.; Zhonghang, X.; Keyan, C.; Tongtong, L.; Wanshu, G.; Zhongxin, X. Epigallocatechin-3-gallate reduces neuronal apoptosis in rats after middle cerebral artery occlusion injury via pi3k/akt/enos signaling pathway. *BioMed. Res. Int.* **2018**, *2018*, 6473580. [CrossRef] [PubMed]

64. Chen, Y.; Chen, J.; Sun, X.; Shi, X.; Wang, L.; Huang, L.; Zhou, W. Evaluation of the neuroprotective effect of egcg: A potential mechanism of mitochondrial dysfunction and mitochondrial dynamics after subarachnoid hemorrhage. *Food Funct.* **2018**, *9*, 6349–6359. [CrossRef] [PubMed]

65. Olanow, C.W.; Perl, D.P.; DeMartino, G.N.; McNaught, K.S. Lewy-body formation is an aggresome-related process: A hypothesis. *Lancet Neurol.* **2004**, *3*, 496–503. [CrossRef]

Nutrients **2019**, *11*, 39

66. Xu, Y.; Zhang, Y.; Quan, Z.; Wong, W.; Guo, J.; Zhang, R.; Yang, Q.; Dai, R.; McGeer, P.L.; Qing, H. Epigallocatechin gallate (egcg) inhibits alpha-synuclein aggregation: A potential agent for parkinson's disease. *Neurochem. Res.* **2016**, *41*, 2788–2796. [CrossRef]
67. Bedrood, Z.; Rameshrad, M.; Hosseinzadeh, H. Toxicological effects of camellia sinensis (green tea): A review. *Phytother. Res.* **2018**, *32*, 1163–1180. [CrossRef]

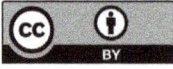

nutrients

MDPI

Article

Protection of UVB-Induced Photoaging by Fuzhuan-Brick Tea Aqueous Extract via MAPKs/*Nrf2*-Mediated Down-Regulation of MMP-1

Peijun Zhao [1,†], Md Badrul Alam [1,2,†] and Sang-Han Lee [1,2,*]

[1] Department of Food Science and Biotechnology, Graduate School, Kyungpook National University, Daegu 41566, Korea; laputaily@hotmail.com (P.Z.); mbalam@knu.ac.kr (M.B.A.)

[2] Food and Bio-Industry Research Institute, Inner Beauty/Antiaging Center, Kyungpook National University, Daegu 41566, Korea

* Correspondence: sang@knu.ac.kr; Tel.: +82-53-950-7754

† These authors contributed equally to this work.

Received: 1 November 2018; Accepted: 21 December 2018; Published: 28 December 2018

Abstract: Ultraviolet B (UVB) irradiation is viewed as the principal inducer of skin photo-aging, associated with acceleration of collagen degradation and upregulation of matrix metalloproteinases (MMPs). The ethnic groups of southern/western China use Fuzhuan brick-tea (FBT) as a beverage and as a nutritional supplement. In this study, we scrutinized the antagonistic effects of aqueous extract of Fuzhuan-brick tea (FBTA) on skin photo-aging in UVB-exposed human keratinocyte (HaCaT) cells. FBTA exhibited strong antioxidant activity and quenched UVB-induced generation of cellular reactive oxygen species (ROS) without showing any toxicity. FBTA was capable of combating oxidative stress by augmenting messenger RNA (mRNA) and protein levels of both phase I and phase II detoxifying enzymes, especially heme oxygenase 1 (HO-1), by upregulating the nuclear factor erythroid 2-related factor 2 (*Nrf2*)-mediated pathway in HaCaT cells via the phosphorylation of p38 and extracellular signal-regulated kinase (ERK). FBTA also downregulated the expression of matrix metalloproteinase-1 (MMP-1) while upregulating type I procollagen by modulating *Nrf2* signaling in UVB-irradiated HaCaT cells. Collectively, our results show that FBTA might be useful as a functional food while being a good candidate in the development of cosmetic products and medicines for the remedy of UVB-induced skin photo-aging.

Keywords: anti-oxidant; anti-photoaging; heme oxygenase-1; nuclear factor erythroid 2-related factor 2 (*Nrf2*); matrix metalloproteinase-1 (MMP-1)

1. Introduction

Ultraviolet (UV) irradiation is viewed as one of the main factors causing structural and functional alterations in the skin, triggering skin aging [1]. Accumulating evidences show that skin photo-aging induced by UV-irradiation is associated with either excessive production of reactive oxygen species (ROS) or inflammatory mediators and disturbance of extracellular matrix (ECM) proteins [2,3]. In particular, UVB-stimulated redundant formation of intracellular ROS can cause an imbalance of cellular oxygen levels, triggering oxidative stress and impairing the antioxidant defense system, causing of photo-aging [4]. ROS also boost the production of matrix metalloproteinases (MMPs) which can enhance the degradation of ECM proteins such as collagen and elastin, which are the foremost structural proteins in skin connective tissue, thereby leading to skin photo-aging [5,6]. Therefore, stimulation of the endogenous antioxidant system and/or suppression of ROS regeneration might be an effectual approach to lessening UVB-stimulated photo-aging or skin damage.

Various phase I and phase II detoxifying enzymes are readily abundant in skin cells and are capable of quenching ROS, thereby sustaining cellular redox homeostasis [7,8]. Heme oxygenase 1 (HO-1), among these antioxidant proteins, plays a pivotal role in protecting ROS-induced oxidative stress-mediated skin damage. [9]. It is noteworthy that the activation of nuclear factor E2-related factor 2 (*Nrf2*) is crucial for the upregulation of HO-1. Under quiescence, *Nrf2* is dormant in the cytoplasm due to the Kelch-like ECH-associated protein 1 (Keap1). However, responses to oxidative stress or conformational changes of Keap1 by inducers facilitate the nuclear translocation of *Nrf2* and binding to antioxidant response elements (ARE), modulating the expression of various antioxidant enzymes and mitigating ROS generation [10–12]. Furthermore, UV-induced oxidative stress has been shown to modulate the phosphorylation of mitogen-activated protein kinases (MAPKs) and induce MMP secretion and collagen destruction [13]. It is well known that enhanced MMP-1 secretion as well as suppression of type I procollagen by UV-irradiation are the most distinguished features of photoaged skin [14]. Thus, agents with potential antioxidant properties that lessen MMP-1 production and accelerate procollagen type I synthesis are deemed as potential nominees for prevention of skin photoaging.

Tea (*Camellia sinensis*) is one of the most extensively consumed beverages worldwide and is comprehensively associated with numerous biological functions. Teas such as unfermented (green tea), semifermented (oolong tea), and fermented tea or black tea (Fuzhuan-brick tea, pu-erh tea, or liubao tea) are extensively dependent on the degree of fermentation and the production process. Among them, Fuzhuan-brick tea (FBT), native to the Hunan province of China, is a popular beverage within ethnic groups in the border regions of southern/western China [15]. A unique fungal fermentation process with a mixture of several microorganisms (predominantly *Eurotium* spp.) controls the aroma, flavor, and the degree of quality of FBT, with a golden "fungal flora" appearing within the tea (Figure 1A) [16]. Mounting evidence has shown that the fermentation process results in FBT having a unique phytochemical profile, with teapolyphenol, theaflavins, and caffeine being dominant (Figure 1B, Supplementary Figure S1) compared to other types of tea [15,17–19]. Moreover, the aroma and taste of FBT are dependent on the presence of nitrogenous, carbonaceous, and volatile compounds [20]. Cumulative studies have reported that black teas possess various pharmacological activities such as lipid-lowering and anti-obesity [21], antioxidant [22], and anti-bacterial and anti-mutagenic [23] activities. However, no studies to date have been conducted to protect skin photoaging by black teas. We asked whether FBT is functionally affiliated with *Nrf2* and induces antioxidant enzymes, thereby hindering oxidative stress-mediated photo-aging. In the present study, emphasis was given to confirm the regulatory role of aqueous extract of FBT (FBTA) in the antioxidant capacity of HaCaT cells. We also elucidated the mechanism underlying oxidative stress-induced skin photo-aging by assessing the activation of *Nrf2* induced by FBTA.

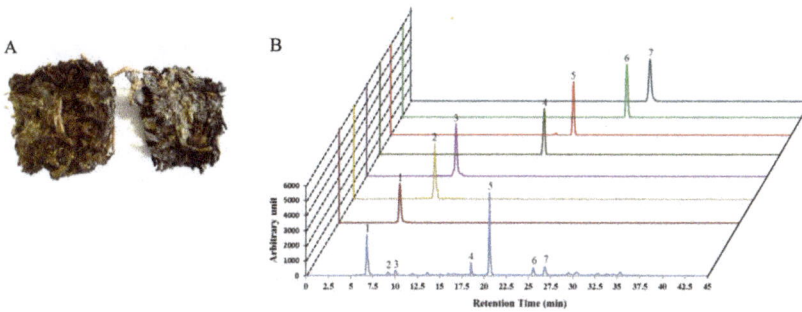

Figure 1. Fuzhuan-brick tea (FBT) (**A**) with the "golden flora" (the yellow dots) in its leaves. (**B**) High pressure liquid chromatography (HPLC) profile of Fuzhuan-brick tea aqueous extract (FBTA) with standards, including gallic acid (peak 1), theaflavins (peak 2), theobromine (peak 3), epigallocatechin (EGC) (peak 4), caffeine (peak 5), epicatechin (EC) (peak 6), and epigallocatechingallate (EGCG) (peak 7). A serving of 100 µg/mL of FBTA solution contains ~10 µM gallic acid, ~2 µM theoflavins, ~2 µM theobromine, ~4 µM EGC, ~15 µM caffiene, ~2 µM EC, and ~2 µM EGCG.

2. Materials and Methods

2.1. Plant Materials and Extraction

The Fuzhuan brick tea (FBT) was purchased from the Hunan Yiyang Tea Factory (Hunan, Yiyang, China). The voucher specimens of the plant and extracts have been deposited in the Laboratory of Enzyme Biotechnology, Kyungpook National University, Daegu, Republic of Korea. After air dying, 100 g tea powder were mixed with 15-folds of distilled water (DW) and placed in a shaking incubator at 60 °C for 24 h. Then, the supernatant was collected with filter paper (No. 1 Whatman Schleicher Schuell, Keene, NH, USA), and dried using a rotary vacuum evaporator (Tokyo Rikakikai Co. Ltd., Tokyo, Japan). Finally, the aqueous extracts of FBT (FBTA) were subjected to lyophilization and dissolved in deionized water at a concentration of 30 mg/mL as a stock solution.

2.2. Radical-Scavenging Activity Assays

2,2-diphenyl-1-picrylhydrazyl (DPPH-) and 2,20-azino-bis(3-ethylbenzothiazoline-6-sulphonic acid (ABTS-) radical scavenging assays, a ferric reducing antioxidant power (FRAP) assay, a cupric-reducing antioxidant capacity (CUPRAC) assay, and an oxygen radical absorbance capacity (ORAC) assay were carried out to evaluate the hydrogen and electron-donating capacity of FBTA, by which we confirmed the cell-free antioxidant potentiality of FBTA using previously described methods [24].

2.3. Cell Culture, UVB-Irradiation and Cell Viability Assay

HaCaT cells (1×10^5 cells/mL) were cultured in DMEM medium supplemented with fetal bovine serum (FBS) and penicillin/streptomycin at 37 °C in 5% CO_2 incubator. Then, sub-confluent cells were treated with indicated concentration (f.c. (final concentration) 3, 10, 30, or 100 µg/mL) of FBTA for 24 h. Subsequently, the cells was exposed to UVB at a dose of 60 mJ/cm² using a UVB source (Bio-Link Crosslinker, Vilber Lourmat, Cedex, France) set at a spectral peak of 312-nm for 20 s. After UVB irradiation, the cells were cultured in serum-free medium for 24 h. Cell viability was determined using the 3-(4,5-dimethylthiazol-2-yl)-2,5-diphenyltetrazolium bromide (MTT) colorimetric assay as described previously [11].

2.4. Measurement of Cellular ROS Generation

HaCaT cells (1×10^5 cells/mL) were cultured with indicated concentration of FBTA (f.c. 10, 30, or 100 µg/mL) in 96-well black plates for 24 h and then exposed to UVB-irradiation (60 mJ/cm²), followed by a change in the media and further incubation for 24 h. After that, the cells were washed with PBS twice and treated with 25 μM 2′,7′-dichlorofluorescin diacetate (DCF-DA) for 30 min at 37 °C in a CO_2 incubator. Finally, fluorescence intensity was measured at excitation and emission wavelengths of 485 and 528 nm, respectively, by a fluorescence microplate reader (Victor3, PerkinElmer, Waltham, MA, USA).

2.5. Reverse Transcription-Polymerase Chain Reaction (RT-PCR)

HaCaT cells (1×10^5 cells/mL) were cultured with indicated concentration of FBTA (f.c. 10, 30, or 100 μg/mL) in 6-well plates for 24 h. TRIzol reagent (Life Technologies, Gaithersburg, MD, USA) was used for the extraction of total RNA and complementary DNA (cDNA) was prepared using RT & GO Mastermix (MP Biomedicals, Seoul, Republic of Korea) and served as the PCR template. A PCR Thermal Cycler Dice TP600 (Takara Bio Inc., Otsu, Japan) was used to carry out RT-PCR using the various primer sequences (Supplementary Data Table S1) [24,25]. After electrophoresis, ethidium bromide staining was performed to visualize the PCR products.

2.6. Cell Lysates and Western Blotting

The lysates of HaCaT cells were prepared using radioimmunoprecipitation assay (RIPA) buffer with a phosphatase and protease inhibitor cocktail (Sigma-Aldrich, St. Louis, MO, USA) and the bicinchoninic acid (BCA) method was applied to quantify the protein content. A nuclear/cytosolic fractionation kit (Sigma-Aldrich, St. Louis, MO, USA) was used for the extraction of nuclear proteins. Aliquots of 50 μg of total proteins were used to carry out the Western blot analysis using various antibody (Supplementary Data Table S2) according to our previously described methods [24,25].

2.7. Statistical Analysis

The data were expressed as the mean ± standard deviation (SD; $n = 3$) and analyzed using the GraphPad Prism Software (GraphPad Software, Inc., San Diego, CA, USA). Statistical analysis was performed using one-way analysis of variance (ANOVA), followed by Dennett's test. A value of $p < 0.05$ was considered as significant.

3. Results

3.1. Radical Scavenging Abilities

Various cell free antioxidant assay systems such as DPPH-, and ABTS-radical scavenging as well as FRAP, CUPRAC, and ORAC assays were carried out to determine the antioxidant ability of FBTA along with other commercially available dark teas such as pu-erh tea and liubao tea. As described in results, FBTA markedly scavenged DPPH-radicals by 79.85 ± 3.38% followed by pu-erh tea (79.25 ± 1.38%) and liubao tea (74.56 ± 3.08%) at a dose of 300 μg/mL (Figure 2A; Supplementary Figure S2). In ABTS-radical scavenging activity, FBTA showed the highest ABTS-radical scavenging activity (75.78 ± 2.25%), followed by liubao tea (71.35 ± 1.56%) and pu-erh tea (68.98 ± 2.45%) (Figure 2B, Supplementary Figure S2). Furthermore, in Figure 2C, FBTA expressed a strong reducing power ability with respect to CUPRAC and FRAP assays with ascorbic acid equivalent antioxidant value at 80.98 ± 1.25 μM and 162.52 ± 1.86 μM, respectively, at a dose of 300 μg/mL. On the other hand, pu-erh tea and liubao tea had 65.78 ± 0.95 μM and 81.53 ± 2.15 μM ascorbic acid equivalent antioxidant value, respectively, in the CUPRAC assay, as well as 125.64 ± 2.19 μM and 164.25 ± 3.21 μM ascorbic acid equivalent antioxidant value, respectively, in the FRAP assay (Supplementary Figure S3). FBTA also meaningfully and concentration-dependently raised the net area under the curve (AUC) value in ORAC assay, confirming its strong reducing power activity (Figure 2D). We also further evaluated the radical scavenging ability of the identified polyphenolics of FBTA, at their presumed concentration in FBTA. Interestingly, all the identified constituents exhibited potent radical scavenging activity in the order of gallic acid > caffeine > (EGCG) > (EGC); > (EC) ≅ theaflavins > theobromine (Supplementary Figure S4).

3.2. Assay of Cell Viability in UVB-Irradiated HaCaT Cells

To examine the cytotoxic effects of UVB and FBTA on HaCaT cells, an MTT assay was performed. Since gallic acid at its putative concentration (9~10 µM) in FBTA has shown the highest antioxidant effects in cell free in vitro antioxidant assays, we used gallic acid as a positive control for cell-based assays. Gallic acid (f.c. 10 µM) and FBTA (f.c. 3 to 300 µg/mL) treatment did not show any significant cytotoxicity for 24 h (Figure 3A). Thus we fixed the concentration of FBTA as 3–100 µg/mL for further cell-based experiments. As shown in Figure 3B, UVB-irradiation significantly suppresses the cell growth in a concentration-dependent fashion. Interestingly, FBTA and gallic acid treatment substantially protected the cells from the toxic effect of UVB-irradiation at dose of 100 µg/mL and 10 µM, respectively (Figure 3C).

3.3. Effects of FBTA on ROS Generation

Spectrofluorometric analysis disclosed that UVB exposure significantly increased the intracellular ROS production in HaCaT cells (Figure 3D, column 2), whereas FBTA treatment significantly and dose-dependently repressed this trend (Figure 3D, column 6 to 9). In addition, to investigate the major constituents among the identified molecules in FBTA, which plays the crucial role in anti-photoaging effects of FBTA, we also examined the antagonist effect of all identified molecules, at their putative concentration in FBTA, on UVB-induced cellular ROS production. Our results revealed that gallic acid exhibited the highest quenching effects on cellular ROS generation, suggesting that gallic acid might be a principal constituent of FBTA for exhibiting anti-photoaging effects (Data Supplementary Data Figure S5) through lessening oxidative stress.

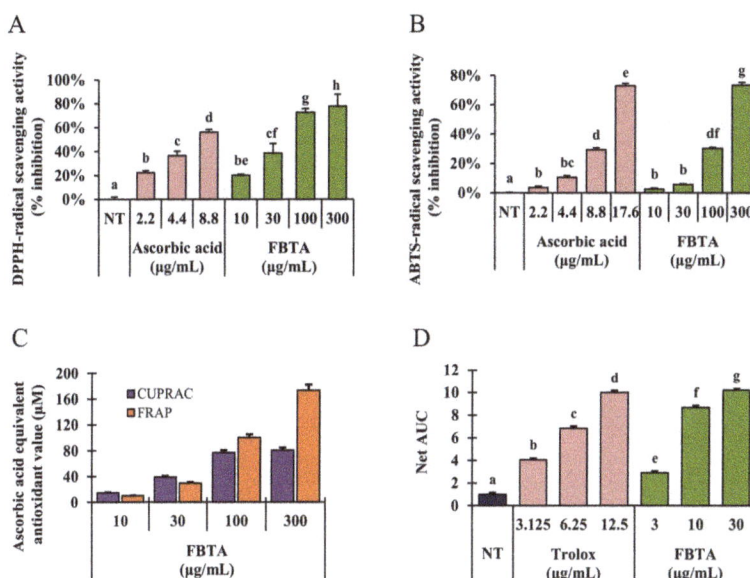

Figure 2. Cell free antioxidant activity of FBTA. (**A**) 2,2-diphenyl-1-picrylhydrazyl (DPPH-) and (**B**) 2,20-azino-bis(3-ethylbenzothiazoline-6-sulphonic acid) (ABTS)-radical scavenging activities. (**C**) Ferric- and (**D**) cupric-reducing activity was examined with different concentrations of FBTA in which ascorbic acid was used as standard. (**D**) The oxygen radical absorbance capacity (ORAC) activity of the samples was calculated by net area under the curve (net AUC). The different letters in each column are significant ($p < 0.05$). Different letters (a, b, c, d, e, f, g, be, cf, bc, df) are denoted as the statistical significance.

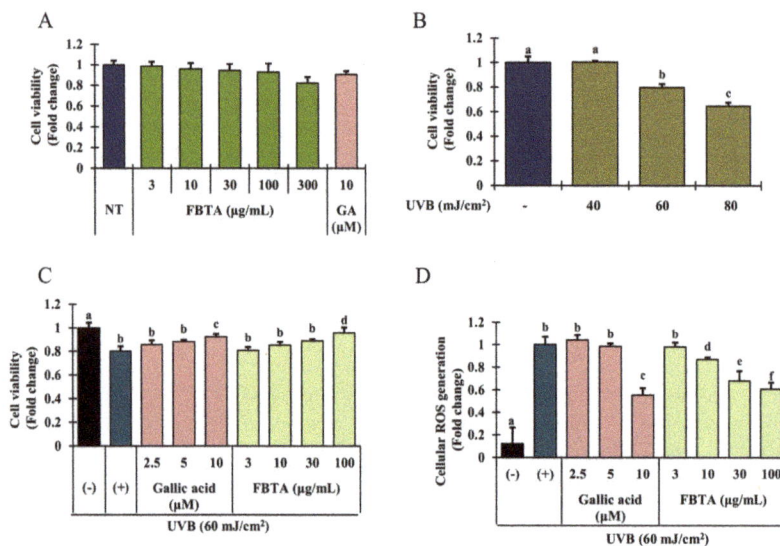

Figure 3. Cell viability activity of FBTA was evaluated by 3-(4,5-dimethylthiazol-2-yl)-2,5-diphenyl tetrazolium bromide (MTT) assay. (**A**) HaCaT cells (1×10^5) were treated with FBTA (f.c. (final concentration) 3–300 μg/mL) and gallic acid (10 μM) for 24 h; (**B**) HaCaT cells were seeded (1×10^5 cells/mL) in 96-well plates for 24 h, and then irradiated with UVB (40, 60 and 80 mJ/cm^2) followed by incubation for 24 h; (**C**) Cells (1×10^5) were pretreated with FBTA (10, 30 and 100 μg/mL) and gallic acid (GA) (2.5, 5, and 10 μM) for 24 h and then irradiated with UVB (60 mJ/cm^2). The cell viability was measured by MTT assay as described in materials and methods. The different letters of each column show significance ($p < 0.05$). (**D**) Pretreated HaCaT cells by FBTA and gallic acid were exposed to UVB irradiation (60 mJ/cm^2). Reactive oxygen species (ROS) levels were determined according to the Materials and Methods section. The different letters of each column show significance ($p < 0.05$). Different letters (a, b, c, d, e, f) are denoted as the statistical significance.

3.4. Effects of FBTA on Phase I and Phase II Antioxidant Enzyme Expression in HaCaT Cells

Results of immunoblotting analysis revealed that UVB-irradiation dramatically lessened the protein expression of phase I antioxidant enzymes such as superoxide dismutase 1 (SOD1), catalase (CAT), and glutathione peroxidase 1 (GPx-1). Interestingly, FBTA and gallic acid treatment expressively upregulated the protein levels in a dose-dependent manner (Figure 4A). Likewise, the transcriptional and translational level of HO-1, one of the phase II detoxifying enzymes, was also boosted by FBTA in concentration-dependent fashions (Figure 4B,C, Supplementary Figure S6). The information advocates an antioxidant role of FBTA through acceleration of the expression of antioxidant enzymes.

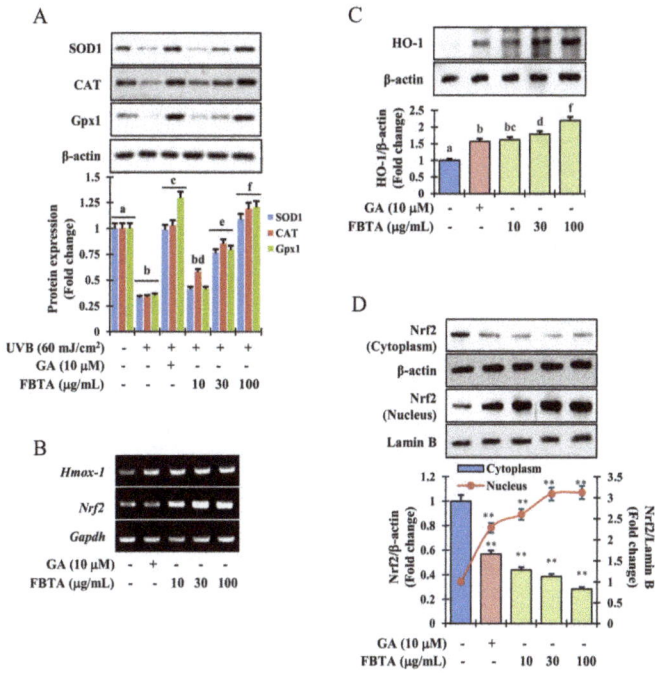

Figure 4. Effects of FBTA on the antioxidant enzyme expression through the nuclear factor erythroid 2-related factor 2 (*Nrf2*) signaling pathway. (**A**) FBTA pretreated HaCaT cells were exposed with UVB (60 mJ/cm^2), and the protein expression of superoxide dismutase 1 (SOD1), catalase (CAT), and glutathione peroxidase 1 (GPx-1) was detected by immunoblotting. The different letters of each column indicate significance ($p < 0.05$); (**B**) After treatment of HaCaT cells by FBTA, messenger RNA (mRNA) expressions of *Hmox-1* and *Nrf2* were detected by RT-PCR. (**C,D**) Heme oxygenase 1 (HO-1) and *Nrf2* expressions were detected by immunoblotting. Densitometric analysis was carried out to quantify the band intensity by β-actin normalization. ** $p < 0.01$ compared to the normal cells. GA: gallic acid. Different letters (a, b, c, d, e, f, g, bc, bd) are denoted as the statistical significance.

3.5. Acceleration of HO-1 Enzymes via Nrf2 Nuclear Translocation in HaCaT Cells

Mounting evidence suggests that the redox sensitive transcription factor *Nrf2* inevitably harmonizes the cellular antioxidant function by the triggering of a series of antioxidant genes, thereby acting against photo-aging in the skin [8]. We hypothesized that the effects FBTA against photo-aging could be due to its persuasive antioxidant capacity. To validate this, we determined the profile of mRNA and nuclear translocation of *Nrf2* in FBTA-treated HaCaT cells. As shown in Figure 4B, the transcriptional level of *Nrf2* was steadily raised in FBTA- and gallic acid-treated HaCaTs. Likewise, immunoblotting analysis revealed that FBTA and gallic acid enhanced the nuclear translocation of *Nrf2*, while simultaneously lessening the cytosolic *Nrf2* level (Figure 4D). Next, to authenticate the *Nrf2*-induced HO-1 expression by FBTA, we treated the cells by brusatol (f.c. 5 μM), a specific inhibitor of *Nrf2*, before FBTA and gallic acid treatment. As expected, brusatol significantly suppressed *Nrf2* expression, and reserved the FBTA as well as gallic acid effects (Figure 5A). In addition, the induction of HO-1 protein by FBTA and gallic acid was also effectively terminated at brusatol-treated cells (Figure 5A). These findings proposed that FBTA can improve the antioxidant defense system via upregulation of *Nrf2*-mediated HO-1 expression. Then, we sought to define whether FBTA could suppress oxidative cell death through the activation of *Nrf2* signaling. Remarkably, the cell proliferation and scavenging of ROS by FBTA was partially reduced in the presence of *Nrf2* inhibitors (Figure 5B,C), signifying that the activation of *Nrf2* signaling by FBTA is involved in the protection of UVB-stimulated oxidative stress-induced cell death.

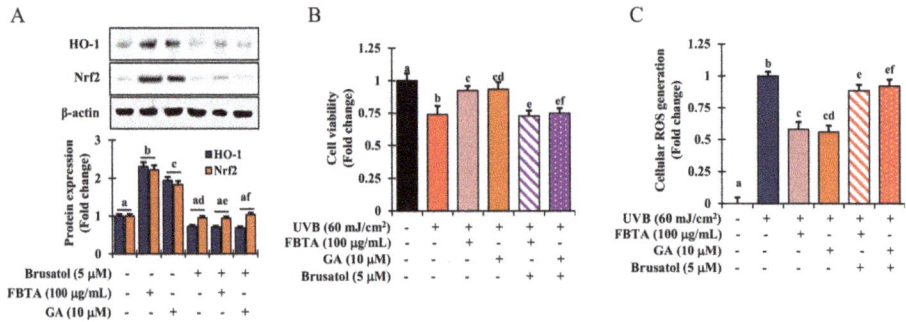

Figure 5. FBTA protects cell death by quenching cellular ROS through activation of *Nrf2*. Brusatol (f.c 5 μM) was added to the HaCaT cells and incubated for 30 min prior FBTA and gallic acid treatment. (**A**) HO-1 and *Nrf2* protein expression was detected by immunoblotting. Densitometric analysis was carried out to quantify the band intensity by β-actin normalization. The different letters of each column is significant ($p < 0.05$). GA: gallic acid; (**B**) Cells (1×10^5) were treated with brusatol for 30 min, followed by treatment with FBTA (f.c 100 μg/mL) and gallic acid (10 μM) for 24 h and were then subjected to UVB (60 mJ/cm^2) insult; (**B**) Cell viability was measured by MTT assay; (**C**) Cellular ROS generation was determined. The different letters of each column is significant ($p < 0.05$). Different letters (a, b, ad, ae, af, cd, ef) are denoted as the statistical significance.

3.6. Effects of FBTA on the MAPK Signaling Pathway

It has been reported that activation of MAPKs act as a crucial upstream signaling in modulating the activation of *Nrf2* [24]. Thus, to reveal the mechanics responsible for *Nrf2* activation, cells were pretreated with FBTA for indicated time interval and immunoblotting assay was performed to assess the phosphorylation of p38 mitogen-activated protein kinase, and extracellular signal-regulated kinase 1 and 2 (ERK1/2). Interestingly, FBTA treatment substantially augmented the phosphorylation of p38 and ERK1/2 after 30 min (Figure 6A). However, there was no detectable c-Jun N-terminal kinase (JNK) phosphorylation in FBTA-treated HaCaT cells (Supplementary Figure S7). Thus, to confirm whether FBTA-modulated *Nrf2*-induced HO-1 upregulation is associated with the MAPK signaling cascade, cells were treated with specific p38 and ERK1/2 inhibitors, such as SB239063 and U0126, respectively, before being treated with FBTA. FBTA exhibited the potential to accrue the protein expression of *Nrf2* and HO-1, while p38 and ERK1/2 inhibition intensely reversed this trend (Figure 6B). These data acknowledge that ERK and p38 are required in FBTA-induced triggering of *Nrf2*-mediated HO-1 expression in in HaCaT cells.

A

B

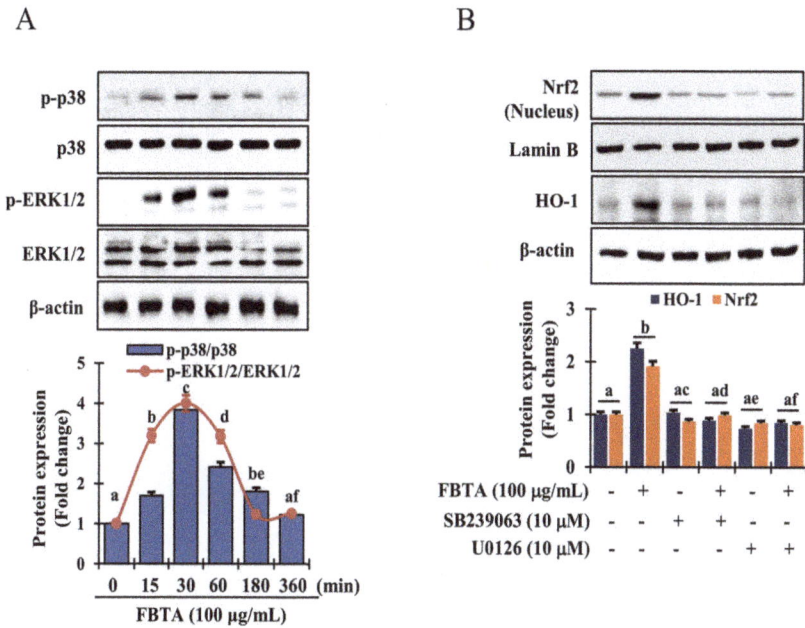

Figure 6. FBTA activates the mitogen-activated protein kinases (MAPKs) signaling pathway. (**A**) HaCaTs were treated with FBTA (100 μg/mL) at the indicated time point and the activated and non-activated forms of extracellular signal-regulated kinase 1 and 2 (ERK 1/2), and p38 were identified by immunoblotting assay. The different letters of each column indicate significance ($p < 0.05$). (**B**) Cells were treated with specific inhibitor U0126 and SB239063 in the presence and absence of FBTA (f.c. 100 μg/mL). *Nrf2* and HO-1 expressions were analyzed by immunoblotting. Densitometric analysis was carried out to quantify the band intensity by β-actin normalization. The different letters of each column indicate significance ($p < 0.05$). Different letters (a, b, c, d, ac, ad, ae, af, be) are denoted as the statistical significance.

3.7. Effects of FBTA on the Expressions of MMP-1 and Procollagen Type I

Accumulating research addressed that profound generation of MMPs and debasement of type I procollagen by UVB-irradiation predominantly leads to the pathogenesis of skin photoaging [14,26]. Thus to examine whether FBTA protects skin photoaging, UVB-exposed HaCaT cells were treated with FBTA and gallic acid and the expression of MMP-1 and type I procollagen was measured by Western blotting. Results displayed that FBTA treatment significantly downregulated the UVB-induced overexpression of MMP-1, as does gallic acid (Figure 7A). UVB alone induced a salient debasement of type I procollagen in HaCaT cells, while FBTA and gallic acid amended this trend. Nevertheless, FBTA and gallic acid remarkably elevated type 1 procollagen levels in UVB-stimulated cells (Figure 7A). These findings suggest that FBTA could prevent UVB-induced photoaging by lessening the MMP-1 upregulation and type I procollagen downregulation in skin keratinocytes, probably due to the presence of gallic acid, because during the permeation process, galloyl-catechins are metabolized by skin esterase and produce more gallic acid in the skin [27]. It is noteworthy that *Nrf2* plays a favorable role in delaying skin photoaging via the regulation of MMPs and type I procollagen [28,29]. There is a furthering pharmacological approach to delay skin photoaging by natural products via modulating *Nrf2*-induced antioxidant defense to combat oxidative stress. Thus, we examined *Nrf2* inhibition studies using brusatol in order to confirm the role of *Nrf2* activation in FBTA-mediated anti-photoaging effects against UVB exposure. Our results demonstrated that UVB-induced upregulation of MMP-1 in brusatol-treated cells remained high even after FBTA treatment, while FBTA extensively inhibited the MMP-1 expression (Figure 7B). Furthermore, FBTA treatment did not restore the UVB-induced degradation of type I procollagen in *Nrf2* inhibited cells (Figure 7B). These finding clarify that FBTA failed to hinder the UVB-induced MMP-1 overexpression and downregulation of type I procollagen in the absence of *Nrf2*.

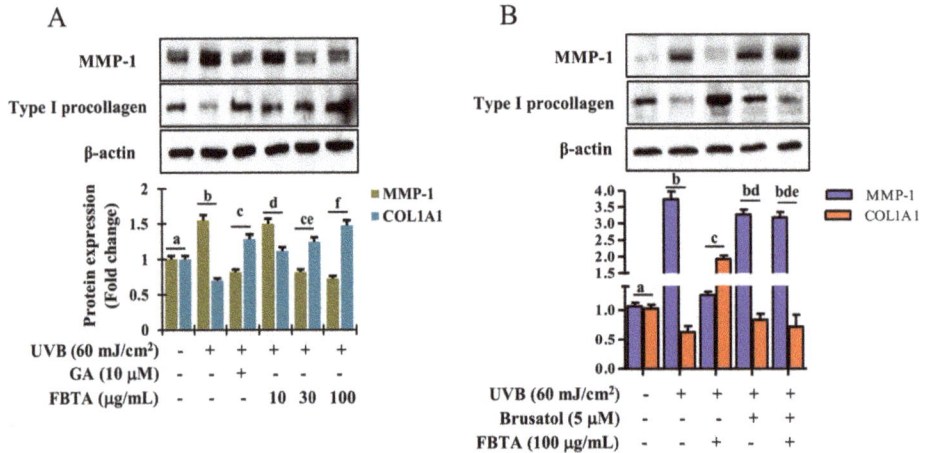

Figure 7. Effects of FBTA on matrix metalloproteinases (MMP)-1 and type I procollagen expression in UVB-stimulated HaCaT cells. The cells were pretreated with FBTA for 24 h, followed by UVB-irradiation. (**A**) MMP-1 and type I procollagen proteins were quantified by immunoblotting. The different letters of each column indicate significance ($p < 0.05$); (**B**) Cells were treated with brusatol for 30 min, followed by FBTA treatment (f.c. 100 µg/mL) for 24 h and were then subjected to UVB insult; the expressions of MMP-1 and type I procollagen were then analyzed by immunoblotting. Densitometric analysis was carried out to quantify the band intensity by β-actin normalization. The different letters of each column indicate significance ($p < 0.05$). Different letters (a, b, c, d, f, ce, bd, bde) are denoted as the statistical significance.

4. Discussion

Epidemiological studies addressed the number of photoaged skin patients are increasing due to overexposure of solar UV-irradiation. Chronic exposure of skin to solar UV radiation causes oxidative stress, ROS-mediated DNA damage, and modulation of extracellular matrix (ECM) components such as MMPs and collagen, thereby hastening skin photo-aging [4]. Among the cells of epidermis, keratinocytes are dominate and can absorb UVB radiation. UVB-induced photo-toxicity (photo-aging) to keratinocyte was characterized by a decline of cell viability (Figure 3A). Pretreatment of FBTA and gallic acid lessened the photo-toxicity triggered by UVB exposure, thereby protecting keratinocyte cells against UVB irradiation. Various concentrations of FBT (50–200 µg/mL) did not exhibit cytotoxicity towards Caco-2 cells and also protected the cells against H_2O_2-induced oxidative stress [30]. Our results are supported by previous findings that, FBTA had dermato-protective properties against UVB irradiation.

It is well known that elderly people have lower endogenous antioxidants activity resulting in more vulnerable to UV-irradiated skin damage, thus the improved strategies for skin photoprotection are needed. Botanicals with antioxidant properties are viewed as potential therapeutic agents to treat skin disorders such as photo-aging [31]. FBTA showed strong hydrogen- as well as electron-donating capacity in various in vitro cell free antioxidant assay systems (Figure 2), thereby confirming that FBTA has very strong antioxidant activity. In addition, we compared total phenol and flavonoid content (Supplementary Figure S1) as well as antioxidant activity with other commercially available dark teas including pu-erh tea and liubao tea (Supplementary Figures S2–S4). FBTA had strong ABTS-radical scavenging potential as compared to pu-erh tea and liubao tea, while in the DPPH-radical scavenging assay, FBTA and pu-erh tea showed similar effects. In contrast, liubao tea showed highest reducing power activity as compared to FBTA and pu-erh tea in both the CUPRAC and FRAP assay system. Our results are also supported by a previous study which stated that the polyphenolics and antioxidant activities of dark tea are dependent on the degree of fermentation. Excessive pile-fermentation reduced the antioxidant activities of dark tea [32,33].

The UVB irradiation of the epidermis causes ROS generation, resulting in attenuation of SOD, CAT, and GPx1 activity and hastening of oxidative damage [34]. Here, we found that FBTA treatment was markedly reserved the UVB-induced ROS generation (Figure 3D). In addition, among the identified bioactive molecules of FBTA, gallic acid showed the highest cellular ROS quenching activity (Supplementary Figure S5), suggesting that gallic acid could play the major role in attenuating the oxidative stress by FBTA. Moreover, FBTA treatment also restored the endogenous antioxidant enzymes such as SOD1, CAT, and GPx-1 in UVB-exposed HaCaT cells (Figure 4A). Our results also supported by the previous studies which reported the FBT significantly protected high fat diet-induced oxidative stress in liver by ameliorating the levels of SOD, CAT, and GSH-Px [35].

Heme oxygenase-1 (HO-1), a phase II-detoxifying enzymes, can convert heme into bilirubin, which acts as a strong antioxidant capable of protecting against cell death from oxidative insult [24]. Besides, a consistent increase in oxidative stress mediated by ROS results in a lowering the cellular HO-1 levels [36]. Upon treatment, FBTA showed a substantial enhance in both transcriptional and translational levles of HO-1 in HaCaT cells (Figure 4B,C, Supplementary Figure S2). Mounting evidence shows various polyphenols, such as gallic acid, EGC, and EGCG attenuate ROS-mediated oxidative stress-induced cell death through upregulation of HO-1 levels [37,38]. To validate this phenomenon, the transcriptional and translational level of *Nrf2*, the key regulator of HO-1 activation, was studied. Furthermore, Hirota et al. [39] discovered that knockdown of the *Nrf2* gene in mice exhibited the acceleration of UVB-induced photoaging process. Thus, *Nrf2*, a well-known redox-sensitive transcription factor, plays a critical role to protect cells against UVB-stimulated photoaging. The pharmacological approach for the activation of *Nrf2* has drawn substantial attention as a tactic for skin photoprotection [40]. Upon electrophilic and/or oxidative stress, *Nrf2* enters into the nucleus and triggers phase II-detoxifying enzymes such as HO-1, thereby indirectly ameliorating the cellular antioxidant defense system, and can protect skin against oxidative damage [41]. In our study, we found pretreatment of FBTA prompted *Nrf2* translocation of the nucleus, while inhibition of *Nrf2* strongly alleviated the upregulation of HO-1 (Figures 4D and 5A), confirming that *Nrf2* regulates the expression of phase II antioxidant enzymes such as HO-1. Gallic acid activates the *Nrf2*-mediated induction of HO-1 and glutathione-s-transferase alpha 3, preventing liver injury [42]. The apocarotenoid bixin, a natural food additive, was revealed to activate *Nrf2* and prevent skin damage by solar UV irradiation [40]. FBTA causes the activation of *Nrf2* and boosts antioxidant capacity, subsequently lessening UVB-induced oxidative stress by suppressing ROS generation. This suggests that FBTA acts as an *Nrf2* activator and has protective properties against photooxidative stress through the activation of *Nrf2*. Cumulating evidence has shown that the activation of *Nrf2* by various cytoprotective phytochemicals are involved in the modulation of various signaling molecules such as MAPKs including ERK1/2, p38, and JNK [8,43]. Our results demonstrated that FBTA-mediated *Nrf2* activation is accomplished through ERK1/2 and p38 MAPK signaling in HaCaT cells (Figure 6A). Pharmacological inhibition of these signaling cascades abolished FBTA-induced *Nrf2* nuclear accumulation and subsequently inhibited HO-1 amplification (Figure 6B). A current study disclosed that p38 and ERK1/2 are crucial for *Nrf2*-mediated HO-1 augmentation in HSC-3 cells [43]. Gallic acid activated the p38 pathway, enhancing the accumulation of *Nrf2* into nucleus and modulation of phase II P-form of phenol sulfotransferase, resulting in protecting oxidative stress induced HepG2 cell death [44]. Based on our findings, we speculated that p38 and ERK1/2 signaling molecules plays a pivotal role in *Nrf2* activation and demonstrate the dermato-protective properties of FBTA.

UVB-induced ROS were reported to be associated with MMP production and modulation of collagen and elastin components of ECM, thereby causing photo-aging and skin damage [7]. Therefore, natural products and/or nutrients with antioxidative properties which can suppress ROS production mitigate the upregulation of MMPs while enhancing type I procollagen synthesis are thought to be novel approaches to protecting against photo-aging. Dietary *Foeniculum vulgare* Mill extract attenuated UVB-induced skin photo-aging by suppression of ROS production and expression of MMP-1, while increasing the type I procollagen level in hairless mice [45]. Likewise, pretreatment with youngiasides A and C, from *Youngia denticulatum*, taken as a wild vegetables, has been reported to act as an antioxidant, abolishing UVB-induced upregulation of MMP-1 and degradation of procollagen I in HaCaT cells [46]. Gallic acid exhibited protection of skin from UVB-induced photo-aging via negative modulation of MMP-1 secretion and positive regulation of type I procollagen in hairless mice [47]. Topical administration of spent coffee ground extracts downregulate of MMPs, thereby protecting skin from UVB-induced photo-aging in hairless mice [48]. Our results demonstrated that FBTA pretreatment mitigated UVB-induced MMP-1 upregulation in a dose-dependent fashion, and renovated type I procollagen in HaCaT cells (Figure 7A). Interestingly, this trend was blocked by the inhibition of *Nrf2* (Figure 7B). It is of note that type I procollagen biosynthesis is considerably diminished in photo-aged skin, causing a loss in dermal elasticity, while restoration of type I procollagen with FBTA is evidence of its dermato-protective effect. This anti photo-aging effect appears to be arbitrated via activation of *Nrf2*-mediated downregulation of MMP-1 in UVB-exposed HaCaT cells.

Unfermented (green tea), semifermented (oolong tea), and fermented (Fuzhuan-brick tea, pu-erh tea or liubao) teas are some of the most widely consumed beverages in the world. The major chemical constituents of teas are polyphenols. Among them, flavan-3-ol such as EGCG and ECG are dominant. Flavonoids, gallic acid, caffeine, and amino acid are also present. Interestingly, during the production of black tea, catechins such as EC, ECG, EGC, and EGCG are oxidized by polyphenol oxidase (PPO) and peroxidase (POD) and consequently dimerized to theaflavins and polymers (thearubigins). There are some studies reporting on the pharmacokinetics profile of tea polyphenols, while the pharmacokinetics profiles of black tea polyphenols, theaflavins, and thearubigins have not been studied extensively [49]. However, gallic acid metabolites such as 3-*O*-methylgallic acid and 4-*O*-methylgallic acid found in the urine of humans who took black tea and are considered as an index of black tea consumption [50]. Mounting evidence has revealed that the half-lives of tea polyphenols are 2–4 h in humans. After oral administration, the peak plasma concentration is in the low µM range, which can be achieved within 1–3 h. Generally, it is known that 2~4 cups/day of Fuzhuan brick tea are consumed by healthy Chinese people (70 kg). The plasma concentration of gallic acid was found to be 2.09 µmol/L after oral consumption of 200 mL (equivalent to 1 cup) of Assam black tea [51]. Thus, it may assumed that in a healthy volunteer who drinks 2~4 cup of black tea per day, the plasma concentration of gallic acid could equivalent be to 5~9 µmol/L; a gallic acid concentration of 10 µmol/L is physiologically effective for exhibiting anti-skin aging effects. A number of studies have stated the low µM concentrations of tea polyphenol have diverse biological effects such as anti-inflammatory, antioxidant, anti-proliferative, and photoprotective effects in vitro [49]. This is also supported in our current study, where the used concentrations of FBTA and gallic acid were in the µM range.

Further studies should be focused on (1) finding active ingredients contributing anti-skin aging potential by investigating synergistic effects of polyphenolics, small molecules, and/or undetected compounds in FBTA, and (2) the pharmacokinetic parameters of tea polyphenols after oral administration of FBTA in a mice model. These are rewarding in that the future data will be beneficial to consumers for better skin and inner beauty care.

5. Conclusions

Our findings revealed for the first time that FBTA pretreatment mitigated UVB-induced photoaging in human keratinocyte HaCaT cells (Figure 8). FBTA stimulated the nuclear translocation of *Nrf2* via induction of p38 and ERK1/2 phosphorylation and subsequently induced HO-1, thereby successively quenching UVB-induced ROS production. Most prominently, significant stimulation of MMP-1 and downregulation of type I procollagen by UVB was restored by FBTA in HaCaT cells, probably through the activation of *Nrf2*. Collectively, our results demonstrated molecular evidence that FBTA could inhibit UVB-induced photoaging via quenching of ROS and triggering of *Nrf2* signaling cascades.

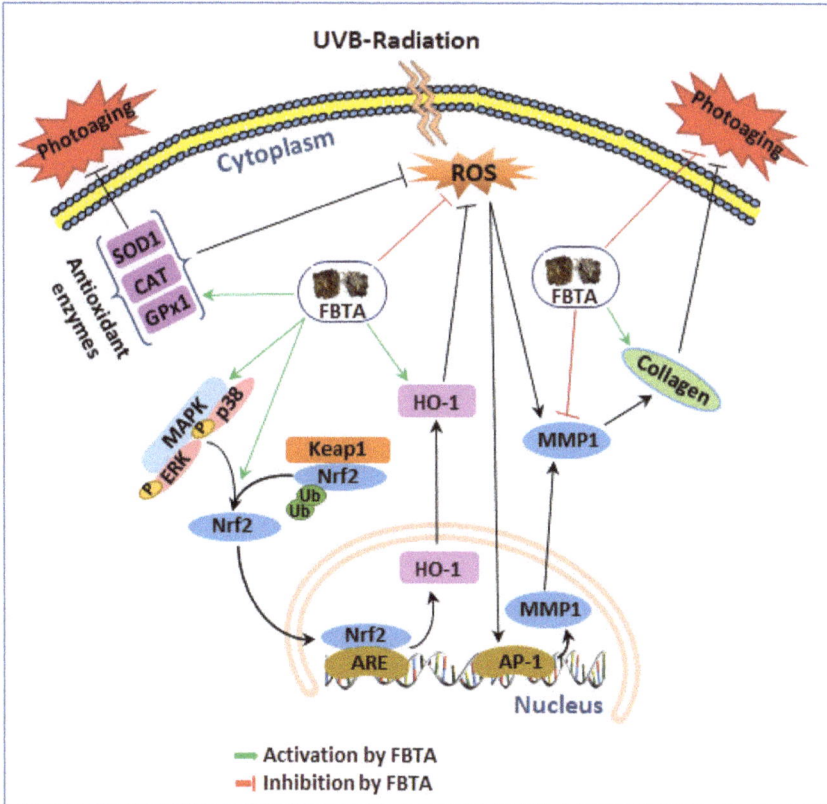

Figure 8. A proposed anti-aging mechanism of FBTA in the UVB-induced photoaging human keratinocytes. Ub, ubiquitin; ARE, antioxidant response element. Green arrows, activation by FBTA; red bars, inhibition by FBTA, black arrows, activation; black bar, inhibition.

Supplementary Materials: Supplementary Table S1: List of the primers used in the study; Supplementary Table S2: List of the antibodies used in the study; Supplementary Figure S1: Total phenolic and flavonoid contents of the aqueous extract of Fuzhuan-brick tea, pu-erh tea, and libao tea; Supplementary Figure S2: DPPH- and ABTS-radical scavenging activities of the aqueous extract of Fuzhuan-brick tea, pu-erh tea, and libao tea; Supplementary Figure S3: Reducing power activities of the aqueous extract of Fuzhuan-brick tea, pu-erh tea, and libao tea in CUPRAC and FRAP assays; Supplementary Figure S4: DPPH-radical scavenging activities of the aqueous extract of Fuzhuan-brick tea (FBTA) and the identified constituents at their putative concentrations in FBTA; Supplementary Figure S5: Cellular ROS quenching effects of the aqueous extract of Fuzhuan-brick tea (FBTA) and the identified constituents at their putative concentration in FBTA; Supplementary Figure S6: Effect of FBTA on HO-1 and *Nrf2* expression in UVB-exposed HaCaT cells; Supplementary Figure S7: Effects of Fuzhuan-brick tea aqueous extract on the activation of JNK.

Author Contributions: P.Z. and M.B.A. performed the research. P.Z., M.B.A. and S.H.L. designed the research study and analyzed the data. P.Z., M.B.A. and S.H.L. wrote the paper. M.B.A. and S.H.L. revised the paper.

Funding: This research received no external funding.

Conflicts of Interest: The authors declare no conflicts of interest.

References

1. Rittie, L.; Fisher, G.J. Uv-light-induced signal cascades and skin aging. *Ageing Res. Rev.* **2002**, *1*, 705–720. [CrossRef]
2. Hwang, B.M.; Noh, E.M.; Kim, J.S.; Kim, J.M.; Hwang, J.K.; Kim, H.K.; Kang, J.S.; Kim, D.S.; Chae, H.J.; You, Y.O.; et al. Decursin inhibits uvb-induced mmp expression in human dermal fibroblasts via regulation of nuclear factor-kappab. *Int. J. Mol. Med.* **2013**, *31*, 477–483. [CrossRef] [PubMed]
3. Kim, S.R.; Jung, Y.R.; An, H.J.; Kim, D.H.; Jang, E.J.; Choi, Y.J.; Moon, K.M.; Park, M.H.; Park, C.H.; Chung, K.W.; et al. Anti-wrinkle and anti-inflammatory effects of active garlic components and the inhibition of mmps via nf-kappab signaling. *PLoS ONE* **2013**, *8*, e73877.
4. Afaq, F.; Adhami, V.M.; Mukhtar, H. Photochemoprevention of ultraviolet b signaling and photocarcinogenesis. *Mutat. Res.* **2005**, *571*, 153–173. [CrossRef] [PubMed]
5. Ho, J.N.; Lee, Y.H.; Park, J.S.; Jun, W.J.; Kim, H.K.; Hong, B.S.; Shin, D.H.; Cho, H.Y. Protective effects of aucubin isolated from eucommia ulmoides against uvb-induced oxidative stress in human skin fibroblasts. *Biol. Pharm. Bull.* **2005**, *28*, 1244–1248. [CrossRef] [PubMed]
6. Sun, Z.; Park, S.Y.; Hwang, E.; Zhang, M.; Jin, F.; Zhang, B.; Yi, T.H. Salvianolic acid b protects normal human dermal fibroblasts against ultraviolet b irradiation-induced photoaging through mitogen-activated protein kinase and activator protein-1 pathways. *Photochem. Photobiol.* **2015**, *91*, 879–886. [CrossRef] [PubMed]
7. Chen, L.; Hu, J.Y.; Wang, S.Q. The role of antioxidants in photoprotection: A critical review. *J. Am. Acad. Dermatol.* **2012**, *67*, 1013–1024. [CrossRef] [PubMed]
8. Hseu, Y.C.; Lo, H.W.; Korivi, M.; Tsai, Y.C.; Tang, M.J.; Yang, H.L. Dermato-protective properties of ergothioneine through induction of nrf2/are-mediated antioxidant genes in uva-irradiated human keratinocytes. *Free Radic. Biol. Med.* **2015**, *86*, 102–117. [CrossRef]
9. Marrot, L.; Jones, C.; Perez, P.; Meunier, J.R. The significance of nrf2 pathway in (photo)-oxidative stress response in melanocytes and keratinocytes of the human epidermis. *Pigment Cell Melanoma Res.* **2008**, *21*, 79–88. [CrossRef]
10. Ben-Yehuda Greenwald, M.; Frusic-Zlotkin, M.; Soroka, Y.; Ben-Sasson, S.; Bianco-Peled, H.; Kohen, R. A novel role of topical iodine in skin: Activation of the nrf2 pathway. *Free Radic. Biol. Med.* **2017**, *104*, 238–248. [CrossRef]
11. Sun, Z.; Park, S.Y.; Hwang, E.; Zhang, M.; Seo, S.A.; Lin, P.; Yi, T.H. Thymus vulgaris alleviates uvb irradiation induced skin damage via inhibition of mapk/ap-1 and activation of nrf2-are antioxidant system. *J. Cell. Mol. Med.* **2017**, *21*, 336–348. [CrossRef] [PubMed]
12. Taguchi, K.; Motohashi, H.; Yamamoto, M. Molecular mechanisms of the keap1–nrf2 pathway in stress response and cancer evolution. *Genes Cells* **2011**, *16*, 123–140. [CrossRef]
13. Bae, J.Y.; Choi, J.S.; Choi, Y.J.; Shin, S.Y.; Kang, S.W.; Han, S.J.; Kang, Y.H. (-)epigallocatechin gallate hampers collagen destruction and collagenase activation in ultraviolet-b-irradiated human dermal fibroblasts: Involvement of mitogen-activated protein kinase. *Food Chem. Toxicol.* **2008**, *46*, 1298–1307. [CrossRef] [PubMed]
14. Pittayapruek, P.; Meephansan, J.; Prapapan, O.; Komine, M.; Ohtsuki, M. Role of matrix metalloproteinases in photoaging and photocarcinogenesis. *Int. J. Mol. Sci.* **2016**, *17*, 868. [CrossRef]
15. Wang, Y.; Xu, A.; Liu, P.; Li, Z. Effects of fuzhuan brick-tea water extract on mice infected with e. Coli o157:H7. *Nutrients* **2015**, *7*, 5309–5326. [CrossRef] [PubMed]
16. Mo, H.; Zhu, Y.; Chen, Z. Microbial fermented tea–a potential source of natural food preservatives. *Trends Food Sci. Technol.* **2008**, *19*, 124–130. [CrossRef]
17. Keller, A.C.; Weir, T.L.; Broeckling, C.D.; Ryan, E.P. Antibacterial activity and phytochemical profile of fermented camellia sinensis (fuzhuan tea). *Food Res. Int.* **2013**, *53*, 945–949. [CrossRef]
18. Luo, Z.M.; Ling, T.J.; Li, L.X.; Zhang, Z.Z.; Zhu, H.T.; Zhang, Y.J.; Wan, X.C. A new norisoprenoid and other compounds from fuzhuan brick tea. *Molecules* **2012**, *17*, 3539–3546. [CrossRef]
19. Ling, T.J.; Wan, X.C.; Ling, W.W.; Zhang, Z.Z.; Xia, T.; Li, D.X.; Hou, R.Y. New triterpenoids and other constituents from a special microbial-fermented tea-fuzhuan brick tea. *J. Agric. Food Chem.* **2010**, *58*, 4945–4950. [CrossRef]
20. Xu, X.; Mo, H.; Yan, M.; Zhu, Y. Analysis of characteristic aroma of fungal fermented fuzhuan brick-tea by gas chromatography/mass spectrophotometry. *J. Sci. Food Agric.* **2007**, *87*, 1502–1504. [CrossRef]

21. Li, Q.; Liu, Z.; Huang, J.; Luo, G.; Liang, Q.; Wang, D.; Ye, X.; Wu, C.; Wang, L.; Hu, J. Anti-obesity and hypolipidemic effects of fuzhuan brick tea water extract in high-fat diet-induced obese rats. *J. Sci. Food Agric.* **2013**, *93*, 1310–1316. [CrossRef] [PubMed]

22. Jie, G.; Lin, Z.; Zhang, L.; Lv, H.; He, P.; Zhao, B. Free radical scavenging effect of pu-erh tea extracts and their protective effect on oxidative damage in human fibroblast cells. *J. Agric. Food Chem.* **2006**, *54*, 8058–8064. [CrossRef] [PubMed]

23. Wu, S.-C.; Yen, G.-C.; Wang, B.-S.; Chiu, C.-K.; Yen, W.-J.; Chang, L.-W.; Duh, P.-D. Antimutagenic and antimicrobial activities of pu-erh tea. *LWT Food Sci. Technol.* **2007**, *40*, 506–512. [CrossRef]

24. Alam, M.B.; Ju, M.K.; Lee, S.H. DNA protecting activities of nymphaea nouchali (burm. F) flower extract attenuate t-bhp-induced oxidative stress cell death through nrf2-mediated induction of heme oxygenase-1 expression by activating map-kinases. *Int. J. Mol. Sci.* **2017**, *18*, 2069. [CrossRef] [PubMed]

25. Alam, M.B.; Kwon, K.R.; Lee, S.H.; Lee, S.H. Lannea coromandelica (houtt.) merr. Induces heme oxygenase 1 (ho-1) expression and reduces oxidative stress via the p38/c-jun n-terminal kinase-nuclear factor erythroid 2-related factor 2 (p38/jnk-nrf2)-mediated antioxidant pathway. *Int. J. Mol. Sci.* **2017**, *18*, 266. [CrossRef] [PubMed]

26. Buechner, N.; Schroeder, P.; Jakob, S.; Kunze, K.; Maresch, T.; Calles, C.; Krutmann, J.; Haendeler, J. Changes of mmp-1 and collagen type ialpha1 by uva, uvb and ira are differentially regulated by trx-1. *Exp. Gerontol.* **2008**, *43*, 633–637. [CrossRef] [PubMed]

27. Batchelder, R.J.; Calder, R.J.; Thomas, C.P.; Heard, C.M. In vitro transdermal delivery of the major catechins and caffeine from extract of camellia sinensis. *Int. J. Pharm.* **2004**, *283*, 45–51. [CrossRef]

28. Chaiprasongsuk, A.; Lohakul, J.; Soontrapa, K.; Sampattavanich, S.; Akarasereenont, P.; Panich, U. Activation of nrf2 reduces uva-mediated mmp-1 upregulation via mapk/ap-1 signaling cascades: The photoprotective effects of sulforaphane and hispidulin. *J. Pharmacol. Exp. Ther.* **2017**, *360*, 388–398. [CrossRef]

29. Hseu, Y.C.; Korivi, M.; Lin, F.Y.; Li, M.L.; Lin, R.W.; Wu, J.J.; Yang, H.L. Trans-cinnamic acid attenuates uva-induced photoaging through inhibition of ap-1 activation and induction of nrf2-mediated antioxidant genes in human skin fibroblasts. *J. Dermatol. Sci.* **2018**, *90*, 123–134. [CrossRef]

30. Song, J.L.; Gao, Y. Effects of methanolic extract form fuzhuan brick-tea on hydrogen peroxide-induced oxidative stress in human intestinal epithelial adenocarcinoma caco-2 cells. *Mol. Med. Rep.* **2014**, *9*, 1061–1067. [CrossRef]

31. Seo, S.A.; Park, B.; Hwang, E.; Park, S.Y.; Yi, T.H. Borago officinalis l. Attenuates uvb-induced skin photodamage via regulation of ap-1 and nrf2/are pathway in normal human dermal fibroblasts and promotion of collagen synthesis in hairless mice. *Exp. Gerontol.* **2018**, *107*, 178–186. [CrossRef] [PubMed]

32. Lv, H.P.; Zhang, Y.; Shi, J.; Lin, Z. Phytochemical profiles and antioxidant activities of chinese dark teas obtained by different processing technologies. *Food Res. Int.* **2017**, *100*, 486–493. [CrossRef] [PubMed]

33. Zhang, L.; Wang, D.; Chen, W.; Tan, X.; Wang, P. Impact of fermentation degree on the antioxidant activity of pu-erh tea in vitro. *J. Food Biochem.* **2012**, *36*, 262–267. [CrossRef]

34. Shin, D.; Lee, S.; Huang, Y.H.; Lim, H.W.; Lee, Y.; Jang, K.; Cho, Y.; Park, S.J.; Kim, D.D.; Lim, C.J. Protective properties of geniposide against uv-b-induced photooxidative stress in human dermal fibroblasts. *Pharm. Biol.* **2018**, *56*, 176–182. [CrossRef] [PubMed]

35. Chen, G.; Wang, M.; Xie, M.; Wan, P.; Chen, D.; Hu, B.; Ye, H.; Zeng, X.; Liu, Z. Evaluation of chemical property, cytotoxicity and antioxidant activity in vitro and in vivo of polysaccharides from fuzhuan brick teas. *Int. J. Biol. Macromol.* **2018**, *116*, 120–127. [CrossRef] [PubMed]

36. Mishra, M.; Fomusi Ndisang, J. A critical and comprehensive insight on heme oxygenase and related products including carbon monoxide, bilirubin, biliverdin and ferritin in type-1 and type-2 diabetes. *Curr. Pharm. Des.* **2014**, *20*, 1370–1391. [CrossRef] [PubMed]

37. Pullikotil, P.; Chen, H.; Muniyappa, R.; Greenberg, C.C.; Yang, S.; Reiter, C.E.; Lee, J.-W.; Chung, J.H.; Quon, M.J. Epigallocatechin gallate induces expression of heme oxygenase-1 in endothelial cells via p38 mapk and nrf-2 that suppresses proinflammatory actions of tnf-α. *J. Nutr. Biochem.* **2012**, *23*, 1134–1145. [CrossRef]

38. Martín, M.Á.; Serrano, A.B.G.; Ramos, S.; Pulido, M.I.; Bravo, L.; Goya, L. Cocoa flavonoids up-regulate antioxidant enzyme activity via the erk1/2 pathway to protect against oxidative stress-induced apoptosis in hepg2 cells. *J. Nutr. Biochem.* **2010**, *21*, 196–205. [CrossRef]

39. Hirota, A.; Kawachi, Y.; Yamamoto, M.; Koga, T.; Hamada, K.; Otsuka, F. Acceleration of uvb-induced photoageing in nrf2 gene-deficient mice. *Exp. Dermatol.* **2011**, *20*, 664–668. [CrossRef]

40. Tao, S.; Park, S.L.; Rojo de la Vega, M.; Zhang, D.D.; Wondrak, G.T. Systemic administration of the apocarotenoid bixin protects skin against solar uv-induced damage through activation of nrf2. *Free Radic. Biol. Med.* **2015**, *89*, 690–700. [CrossRef]

41. Tao, S.; Justiniano, R.; Zhang, D.D.; Wondrak, G.T. The nrf2-inducers tanshinone i and dihydrotanshinone protect human skin cells and reconstructed human skin against solar simulated uv. *Redox Biol.* **2013**, *1*, 532–541. [CrossRef] [PubMed]

42. Ma, S.; Lv, L.; Lu, Q.; Li, Y.; Zhang, F.; Lin, M.; Gao, D.; Liu, K.; Tian, X.; Yao, J. Gallic acid attenuates dimethylnitrosamine-induced acute liver injury in mice through nrf2-mediated induction of heme oxygenase-1 and glutathione-s-transferase α 3. *Med. Chem.* **2014**, *4*, 663–669. [CrossRef]

43. Chen, H.-H.; Wang, T.-C.; Lee, Y.-C.; Shen, P.-T.; Chang, J.-Y.; Yeh, T.-K.; Huang, C.-H.; Chang, H.-H.; Cheng, S.-Y.; Lin, C.-Y. Novel nrf2/are activator, trans-coniferylaldehyde, induces a ho-1-mediated defense mechanism through a dual p38α/mapkapk-2 and pk-n3 signaling pathway. *Chem. Res. Toxicol.* **2015**, *28*, 1681–1692. [CrossRef] [PubMed]

44. Yeh, C.T.; Yen, G.C. Involvement of p38 mapk and nrf2 in phenolic acid-induced p-form phenol sulfotransferase expression in human hepatoma hepg2 cells. *Carcinogenesis* **2006**, *27*, 1008–1017. [CrossRef] [PubMed]

45. Sun, Z.; Park, S.Y.; Hwang, E.; Park, B.; Seo, S.A.; Cho, J.G.; Zhang, M.; Yi, T.H. Dietary foeniculum vulgare mill extract attenuated uvb irradiation-induced skin photoaging by activating of nrf2 and inhibiting mapk pathways. *Phytomedicine* **2016**, *23*, 1273–1284. [CrossRef] [PubMed]

46. Kim, M.; Park, Y.G.; Lee, H.J.; Lim, S.J.; Nho, C.W. Youngiasides a and c isolated from youngia denticulatum inhibit uvb-induced mmp expression and promote type i procollagen production via repression of mapk/ap-1/nf-kappab and activation of ampk/nrf2 in hacat cells and human dermal fibroblasts. *J. Agric. Food Chem.* **2015**, *63*, 5428–5438. [CrossRef]

47. Hwang, E.; Park, S.Y.; Lee, H.J.; Lee, T.Y.; Sun, Z.W.; Yi, T.H. Gallic acid regulates skin photoaging in uvb-exposed fibroblast and hairless mice. *Phytother. Res.* **2014**, *28*, 1778–1788. [CrossRef]

48. Choi, H.S.; Park, E.D.; Park, Y.; Han, S.H.; Hong, K.B.; Suh, H.J. Topical application of spent coffee ground extracts protects skin from ultraviolet b-induced photoaging in hairless mice. *Photochem. Photobiol. Sci.* **2016**, *15*, 779–790. [CrossRef]

49. Clifford, M.N.; van der Hooft, J.J.; Crozier, A. Human studies on the absorption, distribution, metabolism, and excretion of tea polyphenols. *Am. J. Clin. Nutr.* **2013**, *98*, 1619s–1630s. [CrossRef]

50. Hodgson, J.M.; Morton, L.W.; Puddey, I.B.; Beilin, L.J.; Croft, K.D. Gallic acid metabolites are markers of black tea intake in humans. *J. Agric. Food Chem.* **2000**, *48*, 2276–2280. [CrossRef]

51. Shahrzad, S.; Aoyagi, K.; Winter, A.; Koyama, A.; Bitsch, I. Pharmacokinetics of gallic acid and its relative bioavailability from tea in healthy humans. *J. Nutr.* **2001**, *131*, 1207–1210. [CrossRef] [PubMed]

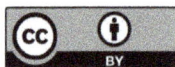

nutrients

MDPI

Article

Daily Green Tea Infusions in Hypercalciuric Renal Stone Patients: No Evidence for Increased Stone Risk Factors or Oxalate-Dependent Stones

Julie Rode [1,*], Dominique Bazin [2], Arnaud Dessombz [3], Yahia Benzerara [1],
Emmanuel Letavernier [1,4,5], Nahid Tabibzadeh [1,5], Andras Hoznek [6], Mohamed Tligui [7],
Olivier Traxer [4,7], Michel Daudon [1,4,5] and Jean-Philippe Haymann [1,4,5]

[1] Sorbonne Université, Service d'Explorations Fonctionnelles Multidisciplinaires, AP-HP, Hôpital Tenon,
   75020 Paris, France; laurent.benzerara@aphp.fr (Y.B.); emmanuel.letavernier@aphp.fr (E.L.);
   nahid.tabibzadeh@inserm.fr (N.T.); michel.daudon@aphp.fr (M.D.);
   jean-philippe.haymann@aphp.fr (J.-P.H.)
[2] Laboratoire de Chimie Physique, Université Paris-Sud, Bat 349, 91405 Orsay, France;
   dominique.bazin@u-psud.fr
[3] Centre National de la Recherche Scientifique (CNRS), Département de Physique, 91405 Orsay, France;
   arnaud.dessombz@gmail.com
[4] Sorbonne Université, GRC n°20, Groupe de Recherche Clinique sur la Lithiase Urinaire, Hôpital Tenon,
   F-75020 Paris, France; olivier.traxer@aphp.fr
[5] Institut National de la Santé et de la Recherche Médicale (INSERM), UMR-S 1155 Paris, France
[6] Service d'Urologie, Hôpital Henri Mondor, Assistance Publique-Hôpitaux de Paris, 94000 Créteil, France;
   andras.hoznek@aphp.fr
[7] Sorbonne Université, Service d'Urologie, AP HP, Hôpital Tenon, 75020 Paris, France;
   mohamed.tligui@aphp.fr
* Correspondence: rode.julie@orange.fr; Tel.: +33-156-016-774; Fax: +33-156-017-003

Received: 11 December 2018; Accepted: 22 January 2019; Published: 24 January 2019

Abstract: Green tea is widely used as a "healthy" beverage due to its high level of antioxidant polyphenol compounds. However tea is also known to contain significant amount of oxalate. The objective was to determine, in a cross-sectional observational study among a population of 273 hypercalciuric stone-formers referred to our center for metabolic evaluation, whether daily green tea drinkers ($n = 41$) experienced increased stone risk factors (especially for oxalate) compared to non-drinkers. Stone risk factors and stone composition were analyzed according to green tea status and sex. In 24-h urine collection, the comparison between green tea drinkers and non-drinkers showed no difference for stone risk factors such as urine oxalate, calcium, urate, citrate, and pH. In females, the prevalence of calcium oxalate dihydrate (COD) and calcium phosphate stones, assessed by infrared analysis (IRS) was similar between green tea drinkers and non-drinkers, whereas prevalence of calcium oxalate monohydrate (COM) stones was strikingly decreased in green tea drinkers (0% vs. 42%, $p = 0.04$), with data in accordance with a decreased oxalate supersaturation index. In males, stone composition and supersaturation indexes were similar between the two groups. Our data show no evidence for increased stone risk factors or oxalate-dependent stones in daily green tea drinkers.

Keywords: green tea; oxalate; renal stone; calcium oxalate monohydrate; hypercalciuria

---

1. Introduction

The high prevalence of urolithiasis (reaching up to 8–10% of the general population) is mainly related to environmental factors, especially the Western diet [1]. Calcium stones are encountered in

80% of cases and often contain a mixture of calcium oxalates and calcium phosphates. Among calcium oxalate crystals, the calcium oxalate monohydrate crystalline form (COM) is oxalate-dependent, whereas the calcium oxalate dihydrate crystalline form (COD) is calcium-dependent [1]. Hence, high urinary calcium and oxalate concentrations are critical factors leading to stone formation. Tea contains oxalates in varying amounts depending on the type and duration of the infusion. The amount of oxalate measured for black tea varies from 2.7 to 4.8 mg/240 mL (one cup) of tea infused for 1–5 min [2], whereas the amount of oxalate in green tea ranges from 2.08 to 34.94 mg/250 mL of tea [3]. However, the amount of oxalate in green tea depends on its origin, quality, preparation, and time of harvest, thus probably explaining why some studies report a higher oxalate concentration in black tea compared to green tea [4]. However, tea extracts, particularly green tea, are considered to have many beneficial clinical effects for centuries. Tea infusions contain polyphenol compounds, among which catechins have been of major interest due to their antioxidant properties [5]. Indeed, among the different varieties of teas, green teas as compared to black teas contain the highest concentration of catechins [6]. Other food and drinks (in particular wine and dark chocolate) may also represent a substantial dietary source of catechins, but to a lesser extent [7,8]. Catechins are mainly found under four different hydro soluble forms in green tea: epigallocatechin-3-O-gallate (EGCg), epicatechin-3-O-gallate (ECG), epigallocatechin (EGC), and epicatechin (EC) [9,10]. EGC and its metabolites are the main compounds found in the urine following the ingestion in humans and animals with concentrations up to 100 µmoles/L in humans [11–20]. As a matter of fact, several authors recommend green tea or large amounts of catechin intake in order to prevent crystallization of calcium oxalate crystals in animal models [21–23]. Conversely, tea is also known to contain high amounts of oxalate, and could have diuretic effects increasing natriuresis but potentially also calciuria, and thus its consumption is regarded by other authors as a genuine risk factor for renal stone formation [21,24,25]. The aim of this work was to study the influence of regular daily green tea intake on stone risk factors, stone morphology, and composition and to assess a potential increased risk for oxalate-dependent stones.

2. Material and Methods

2.1. Population

The data of 420 hypercalciuric renal stone formers referred to our department between 2009 and 2011 for a routine metabolic evaluation (including an oral calcium load test) were retrospectively analyzed. A careful clinical examination (including a survey related to diet and fluid intake, and noteworthy daily green tea intake) was performed. All patients gave their informed written consent for inclusion before they participated in the study. This observational cross sectional study was conducted in accordance with the Declaration of Helsinki and French legislation.

In total, 273 patients (flow chart Figure 1) were included after the exclusion of patients with a diagnosis of primary hyperparathyroidism, sarcoidosis, bowel resection, on-going steroid, bisphosphonate, antiviral, diuretic, and/or vitamin D treatments, vegetarian diet, consumption of "exotic" infusions or food supplements (in tablets or powder), and/or intermittent green tea intake or daily black tea intake. The green tea group (n = 41) was defined as patients drinking at least one cup (250–300 mL) of green tea daily, and non-drinkers as patients drinking no green tea at all (n = 232). Renal stone composition was available for 98 out of 273 patients (36%). A comparison between the two groups was performed according to sex (Figure 1).

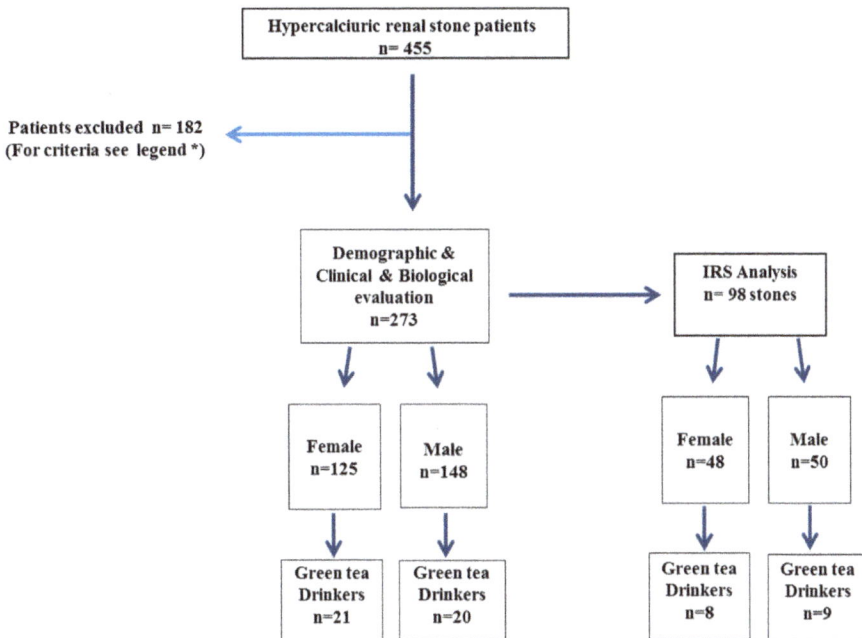

Figure 1. Flow chart. Primary hyperparathyroidism or sarcoidosis ($n = 28$); bowel resection ($n = 2$), steroid, bisphosphonate, and antiretroviral treatment ($n = 23$); vegetarian diet or "exotic" infusions ($n = 25$); food supplements ($n = 22$); intermittent green tea intake ($n = 6$); daily black tea intake ($n = 36$); diuretics, vitamin D treatment ($n = 39$); pregnancy ($n = 1$). IRS: infrared analysis.

A morpho-constitutional analysis was performed for each stones as described previously [26]. In short, the standardized protocol comprises two steps. First, a morphologic examination by means of a stereomicroscope (magnification $\times$ 10–40) of the surface and section of the calculus, with the identification of the nucleus (or core) and description of the inner organization, was carried out. The main points to be recorded in each stone were size, form, color, aspect (smooth, rough, or spiky) of the surface, presence of a papillary imprint (umbilication), presence of Randall's plaque, aspect of the section (well organized with concentric layers and/or radiating organization, or poorly organized and loose structure), and location and aspect of the nucleus. Thereafter, an analysis was performed by infrared spectroscopy (IRS) of a sample of each part of the calculus and in particular the global proportion of components in a powdered sample of the whole stone.

All of the urine collections were performed at least 3 months after lithotripsy or surgery. A 24-h urine collection under a regular diet was performed at baseline to measure the following parameters: diuresis volume, calcium, magnesium, phosphate, sodium, potassium, creatinine, urea, oxalate, uric acid, citrate, ammonium, and deoxypyridinoline excretion. A fasting blood sample was analyzed for total and ionized calcium, phosphate, magnesium, creatinine, uric acid, bicarbonates, parathyroid hormone (PTH), 25(OH)-D3, and 1,25(OH)-D3 vitamins. Bone remodeling biomarkers (serum bone alkaline phosphatase (BALP)) were also performed at that time.

Serum and urinary creatinine levels were measured by enzymatic method on a Konelab 20 analyzer from Thermo Fisher Scientific (Vantaa, Finland). Uric acid levels were measured with the Konelab analyzer (Thermo Fisher Scientific, Vantaa, Finland). Total CO_2 in blood, ionized calcium, sodium, and potassium levels were measured with an ABL 815 from Radiometer (Bronshoj, Denmark). Calcium and magnesium serum and urinary levels were measured with the PerkinElmer 3300 atomic absorption spectrometer (Courtabeuf, France). In addition, 25(OH)-D3 and 1,25(OH)-D3 were measured by radioimmunoassay kits from Immunodiagnostics Systems Ltd. (Paris, France). Parathyroid hormone was measured by the ELSA-PTH kit from Cisbio International (Codolet, France). Urinary NH4 was measured with the RANDOX Laboratories kit (Crumlin, UK). Urinary deoxypyridoline was measured by the RIA method from Immunodiagnostics Systems Ltd. (Paris, France). BALP level was measured with Ostase bone alkaline phosphatase enzyme immunoassay obtained from Immunodiagnostics Systems Ltd. (Paris, France). Citrate and oxalate measurements were performed by ionic chromatography (Metrohm, Courtabeuf, France). Ionic strength and supersaturation indexes for calcium oxalate, urate, and brushite were calculated using molar concentrations [24,25].

2.2. Statistical Analyses

Statistical analyses were performed by two different operators using StatView (SAS Institute, Inc., Cary, NC, USA) and *R* software (The *R* Foundation, Lincoln, NE, USA). Quantitative data were expressed as the mean and SD unless otherwise indicated and as a percentage for categorical variables. Because of sex differences for many biologic parameters, analyses were performed separately in women and men. Comparisons were performed using the *t*-test or a nonparametric Wilcoxon and Mann–Whitney test, whenever required. Comparisons of qualitative parameters were performed using a chi-squared test or Fisher's exact test when necessary. $p < 0.05$ was considered statistically significant.

3. Results

3.1. Demographic and Clinical Data

Among our population, 13.5% of males and 17% of females were regular green tea drinkers (i.e., drinking at least one cup a day) ($p = 0.61$). Median age in hypercalciuric renal stone patients was 47 years old (ranging from 18 to 82 years). Cardiovascular risk factors were not infrequent findings in this population: overweight status was present in 54.4% of our population, dyslipidemia was encountered in 24.4% of cases, ongoing smoking or tobacco exposure in 24% and 41% of cases, respectively, 5.7% had type 2 diabetes, and 24% had high blood pressure. However, no difference was detected between green tea drinkers and non-drinkers (Table 1).

Table 1. Demographic and clinical data.

Population	Female (n = 125)			Male (n = 148)		
	Non-Drinkers (n = 102)	Green Tea (n = 21)	p	Non-Drinkers (n = 122)	Green Tea (n = 20)	p
Age (years)	46 (34–59)	42 (33–53)	NS	48 (38–58)	44 (37–57)	NS
BMI (kg/m^2)	24.9 (21.4–29.4)	23.5 (21.2–25.6)	NS	25.7 (23.2–29.0)	25.8 (24.5–29.6)	NS
MAP (mmHg)	83.3 (76.7–92.5)	81.7 (76.7–93.4)	NS	90.0 (80.0–96.7)	86.7 (82.5–93.3)	NS
Hypertension	37%	33%	NS	47%	50%	NS
Dyslipidemia	22%	9%	NS	26%	15%	NS
Diabetes	4%	9%	NS	8%	0%	NS
Age first stone (years)	27.0 (19.0–41.0)	30.0 (18.7–41.2)	NS	29.5 (21.0–41.5)	27.5 (22.5–39.5)	NS
SWL (% of patients)	37.3%	33.3%	NS	47.5%	50.0%	NS
URS (% of patients)	45.1%	47.6%	NS	51.6%	40.0%	NS

BMI: body mass index. MAP: mean arterial pressure. NS: not significant. SWL: Shock waves lithotripsy. URS: flexible ureteroscopy.

3.2. Diet, Metabolic, and Urinary Stone Risk Factors

Comparison between male and female groups showed similar urine output (1.9 vs. 1.8 L/day, $p = 0.22$), urinary calcium (6.4 vs. 6.7 mmol/day, $p < 0.45$), oxalate (0.33 vs. 0.33 mmol/day, $p = 0.63$), urate (3.8 vs. 3.6 mmol/day, $p < 0.31$), urea (404 vs. 400 mmol/day, $p < 0.86$), and sodium (134 vs. 140 mmol/day, $p < 0.44$). Surprisingly, a higher fluid intake (declarative survey) in female green tea drinkers compared to non-drinkers was not confirmed by a higher daily urine output (Table 2). Nevertheless, as shown Table 2, the analysis according to sex showed no difference for stone risk factors between green tea drinkers and non-drinkers such as oxalate, calcium, urate, and citrate with even a trend for a lesser oxaluria in the green tea female population (0.32 vs. 0.27, $p = 0.09$). Moreover, 24-h urine supersaturation indexes were similar between green tea drinkers and non-drinkers noteworthy for the calcium oxalate relative supersaturation index (CaOx RSS) and the calcium oxalate (CaOx) product (Table 3). However, a significant higher Ca/Ox ratio is noticed in female green tea drinkers, suggesting a relatively lower risk for oxalate-dependent stones (though the other Ca Ox indexes appear similar).

Table 2. Food intake evaluation, biological data, and metabolic risk factors.

Population	Female ($n = 125$)			Male ($n = 148$)		
	Non-Drinkers ($n = 102$)	Green Tea ($n = 21$)	p	Non-Drinkers ($n = 122$)	Green Tea ($n = 20$)	p
Fluid intake ≥ 2 L/day (%)	11.2%	50.0%	<0.0001	30.3%	22.2%	0.47
Blood						
Sodium (mmol/L)	139 (138–140)	139 (138–140)	0.84	139 (138–140)	140 (138–140)	0.35
Potassium (mmol/L)	4.0 (3.8–4.3)	4.1 (3.8–4.3)	0.37	4.0 (3.9–4.3)	4.1 (3.9–4.3)	0.39
Fasting glucose (mmol/L)	5.5 (5.1–6.3)	5.1 (5.06–5.5)	0.06	5.4 (5.0–5.9)	5.8 (5.5–6.4)	0.008
tCO$_2$ (mmol/L)	27.5 (26.0–29.0)	27.9 (25.1–29.7)	0.70	27.6 (26.3–29.7)	27.6 (25.3–29.6)	0.78
Creatinine clearance (mL/min)	126 (95–145)	109 (84–138)	0.16	121 (97–153)	118 (101–157)	0.94
Ionized calcium (mmol/L)	1.18 (1.15–1.21)	1.19 (1.16–1.21)	0.43	1.18 (1.15–1.21)	1.17 (1.14–1.21)	0.82
PTH (pg/mL)	35 (26–49)	31 (25–40)	0.31	35 (27–49)	40 (33–55)	0.11
25 OH vitamin D (pg/mL)	24 (17–34)	25 (19–37)	0.52	25 (16–37)	24 (20–30)	0.95
1-25 (OH)$_2$ vitamin D (ng/mL)	66 (55–85)	79 (54–90)	0.5	66 (52–84)	58 (57–87)	0.48
BALP (UI/L)	13.5 (10.3–17.0)	12.3 (10.3–15.1)	0.36	13.5 (10.0–17.0)	10.6 (9.5–13.0)	0.06
Deoxypyridin (mmol/mmol creat)	5.7 (4.5–8.1)	6.6 (4.1–9.7)	0.7	5.4 (4.2–7.5)	5.2 (3.9–6.4)	0.29
Urine						
Diuresis (mL/day)	1880 (1460–2582)	1908 (1757–2368)	0.89	1865 (1433–2337)	1836 (1231–2301)	0.62
Calcium (mmol/day)	6.2 (4.6–8.1)	7.0 (5.5–10.0)	0.08	5.7 (4.0–8.5)	6.3 (4.5–8.1)	0.95
Oxalate (mmol/day)	0.32 (0.24–0.42)	0.27 (0.32–0.34)	0.09	0.30 (0.19–0.41)	0.29 (0.21–0.43)	0.77
Urate (mmol/day)	3.5 (2.6–4.7)	3.2 (2.7–3.7)	0.33	3.5 (2.9–4.5)	3.8 (3.0–4.7)	0.51
Citrate (mmol/day)	2.4 (1.1–3.4)	2.0 (1.7–3.4)	0.98	2.5 (1.5–3.5)	2.2 (0.4–2.7)	0.22
Fasting pH	6.33 (5.68–6.66)	6.2 (6.0–6.6)	0.83	6.18 (5.62–6.61)	5.74 (5.32–6.32)	0.06
Sodium (mmol/day)	113 (84–157)	121 (84–149)	0.25	127 (95–173)	126 (90–146)	0.4
Ammonium (mmol/day)	35 (26–45)	30 (26–45)	0.28	35 (25–48)	44 (31–54)	0.39
Magnesium (mmol/day)	4.1 (3.2–5.0)	5.0 (3.3–7.0)	0.08	4.4 (3.2–5.9)	4.2 (2.7–4.9)	0.48

BALP: bone alkaline phosphatase. tCO$_2$: plasma bicarbonate. PTH: parathyroid hormone.

Table 3. Twenty-four hour urine supersaturation indexes.

Population	Female			Male		
	Non-Drinkers	Green Tea	p-Value	Non-Drinkers	Green Tea	p Value
AP CaOx index	0.74 (0.39–1.30)	0.71 (0.28–1.31)	0.42	0.67 (0.37–1.10)	0.76 (0.41–1.28)	0.73
Br RSS	1.3 (0.3–2.5)	1.0 (0.1–1.7)	0.27	0.9 (0.3–1.9)	0.6 (0.2–1.3)	0.39
UA RSS	0.54 (0.25–1.81)	0.75 (0.19–1.48)	0.95	1.08 (0.41–2.26)	1.99 (0.33–3.96)	0.47
CaOx RSS	5.6 (3.7–8.6)	3.7 (2.0–8.3)	0.16	5.3(3.2–7.7)	6.0 (3.7–8.7)	0.64
Ca.Ox	0.53 (0.26–1.03)	0.59 (0.23–1.15)	0.67	0.47 (0.25–0.89)	0.57 (0.30–0.91)	0.57
Ratio Ca/Ox	19 (12.5–30)	26 (20.5–40.5)	0.01	19 (12–34)	18.5 (12–28.5)	0.65
Ionic Strength	0.08 (0.06–0.12)	0.09 (0.07–0.12)	0.72	0.09 (0.05–0.12)	0.07 (0.075–0.105)	0.43

RSS: relative super saturation; AP CaOx index: Tiselius index; Br RSS: brushite relative super saturation; CaOx RSS: calcium oxalate relative super saturation; Ca.Ox: calcium oxalate product. Ca/Ox: calcium/oxalate ratio. UA RSS: uric acid relative super saturation.

As shown Table 2, other biological data were similar between drinkers and non-drinkers in the male and female population in terms of noteworthy renal function, calcium phosphate homeostasis, and bone remodeling biomarkers.

Among the 98 renal stones available, 48 samples were collected from female and 50 from male patients. Within male or female groups, comparison of the major stone component identified by IRS analysis revealed no significant difference between drinkers and non-drinkers. Of note, no COM stones were detected in the female drinkers group compared to female non-drinkers (0% vs. 42%, $p = 0.04$) whereas in male drinkers, the prevalence of COM was similar between groups (33% vs. 44%, $p =$ NS) (Table 4).

Table 4. IRS analysis of stones collected from drinkers and non-drinkers.

Population	Female			Male		
	Non-Drinkers (*n* = 40)	Green Tea (*n* = 8)	*p* Value	Non-Drinkers (*n* = 41)	Green Tea (*n* = 9)	*p* Value
Major COM component (%)	42	0	0.036	33	44	0.99
Major COD component (%)	26	50	0.23	41	55	0.72
Carbapatite major component (%)	16	12.5	0.99	7	0	0.99
Type Ia or Ib (%)	23	0	0.32	18	11	0.99
Type IIa or IIb (%)	50	62	0.7	64	78	0.69
Type IVa (%)	10	12	0.99	8	0	0.99

Type Ia, Ib morphology refers to COM subtype crystalline forms. Type IIa and IIb refer to COD subtype crystalline forms (Type IIb also includes the presence of COM crystalline form). Type IVa refers to carbapatite subtype crystalline forms.

4. Discussion

The aim of the present study was to acknowledge whether drinking green tea on a daily basis would exert any influence on stone risk factors and/or calcium stone structure or composition. In the first part of our work, based upon a cross sectional observational study, we found no difference between green tea drinkers and non-drinkers for stone risk factors in particular oxalate excretion in 24-h urine collections but also urine pH, calcium, urate, and citrate. These results were further confirmed by supersaturation indexes. These data have a clinical relevance as renal stone patients are commonly advocated against regular tea drinking based upon the oxalate content reported in tea leaves [3,4]. According to the view that green tea intake would increase stone activity, one study reported an increased urinary calcium excretion in an experimental setting [21]. Conversely, in two other animal studies, the administration of catechins or green tea prevented crystallization, especially monohydrate CaOx crystal deposits within tubular lumen [22,23]. However a recent study in a very large prospective Chinese cohort reports that green tea intake was associated with a lower risk of incident kidney stones [27]. Our results are in accordance with these findings and suggest that drinking daily green tea (assessed by a detailed survey) would not be detrimental in both sexes. As a matter of fact, drinking daily green tea was reported to have also other pharmacological effects such as weight loss, cardiovascular protection, and bone mineralization [28,29]. Though this study is not designed to assess these issues, our data show no difference for body mass index, cardiovascular risk factors, bone remodeling biomarkers, or calcium and phosphate blood levels between drinkers and non-drinkers.

The second part of our work was to study a potential calcium stones composition difference between green tea drinkers and non-drinkers. Of note, among 98 stones available from this idiopathic hypercalciuric population, 34% contained COM as a major component. However, the major component of COM was similar between regular green tea drinkers and non-drinkers in the whole population ($p = 0.26$). Accordingly, similar CaOx supersaturation indexes are detected, thus ruling out green tea as a potential additional stone risk factor for COM stones. Surprisingly, in female green tea drinkers, no COM stone was detected at all (Table 4), thus suggesting either a pharmacological effect illustrated by the increased Ca/Ox ratio (Table 3) and/or a potential role of green tea catechins (or antioxidants) directing CaOx crystallization from COM to COD as previously shown in vitro [30]. Alternatively, catechins could exert a potential inhibition of COD to COM conversion. This exciting speculation however requires to be specifically addressed in further studies.

Indeed, a high prevalence of COD in the female green tea group is very unusual as COM and calcium phosphate stones are the usual major compounds reported in the female renal stone population [26,31]. Conversely, in male stone-formers, COD and COM are the two main compounds encountered in both groups, with a similar prevalence between the two groups. Thus according to stone composition drinking daily green tea has no demonstrated over risk for oxalate-dependent stones in our studied population.

Our study suffers some limitations as it is an observational study with a declarative diet survey and thus did not take into account the total amount of catechins intake in the diet. Indeed, the amount of catechins in green tea beverage depends upon green tea leaves, temperature, and the duration of infusion [3]. Moreover, substantial amount of catechins are found in a significant number of food including wine, which consumption is usually underestimated, and thus represent a bias in our study. However, despite the lack of dietary questionnaire (except for calcium intake and water), sodium and protein intake appeared similar between the two groups as assessed by 24-h urine sodium and urea. Last, similar oxaluria values in 24-h urine collection support the view that regular green tea intake is not a risk factor for oxalate-dependent stones (assessed also by stone composition). The 50% prevalence of COD stones in female green tea drinkers is related to idiopathic hypercalciuria; however, this finding may also raise the issue as to whether green tea would be an additional risk factor for an increased prevalence of calcium-dependent stones (illustrated by an increased Ca/Ox ratio in the female green tea group). Further studies are required to assess whether in non-hypercalciuric renal stone patients and/or in the general population green tea would prevent COM stone occurrence or recurrence. This specific issue is however beyond the goal of the present study.

5. Conclusions

Our data show no evidence for increased oxalate-dependent stones in daily green tea drinkers, with no increased oxaluria or calciuria in 24-h urine collection and, to our surprise, no reported COM stones in our female green tea drinkers group. A clinical trial testing the hypothesis that high catechin intakes may prevent COM stone recurrence would be most welcome.

Author Contributions: All coauthors have contributed to the work presented here. J.R., M.D. and J.-P.H. contributed to the writing and data collection, A.D., Y.B., D.B. and N.T. to data collection, E.L., A.H., M.T. and O.T. to the review.

Funding: This work was supported by UPMC, UMRS-1155, and the Association Française d'Urologie. J.R. was supported by a fellowship from the Association Française d'Urologie.

Conflicts of Interest: The authors declare no conflicts of interest.

Abbreviations

BMI	body mass index
COM	calcium oxalate monohydrate
COD	calcium oxalate dihydrate
CaOx	Calcium oxalate
EGC	epigallocatechin
IRS analysis	infrared spectroscopy analysis
MAP	mean arterial pressure
NS	not significant
SWL	shock wave lithotripsy
URS	flexible ureteroscopy
RSS	relative super saturation

References

1. Daudon, M.; Knebelmann, B. Epidemiology of urolithiasis. *Rev. Prat.* **2011**, *61*, 372–378.
2. Mahdavi, R.; Lotfi Yagin, N.; Liebman, M.; Nikniaz, Z. Effect of different brewing times on soluble oxalate content of loose-packed black teas and tea bags. *Urolithiasis* **2013**, *41*, 15–19. [CrossRef]
3. Hönow, R.; Gu, K.L.R.; Hesse, A.; Siener, R. Oxalate content of green tea of different origin, quality, preparation and time of harvest. *Urol. Res.* **2010**, *38*, 377–381. [CrossRef]
4. Charrier, M.J.; Savage, G.P.; Vanhanen, L. Oxalate content and calcium binding capacity of tea and herbal teas. *Asia Pac. J. Clin. Nutr.* **2002**, *11*, 298–301. [CrossRef]

5. Lotito, S.B.; Frei, B. Consumption of flavonoid-rich foods and increased plasma antioxidant capacity in humans: Cause, consequence, or epiphenomenon? *Free Radic. Biol. Med.* **2006**, *41*, 1727–1746. [CrossRef]
6. Jin, Y.; Jin, C.H.; Row, K.H. Separation of catechin compounds from different teas. *Biotechnol. J.* **2006**, *1*, 209–213. [CrossRef]
7. Neveu, V.; Perez-Jiménez, J.; Vos, F.; Crespy, V.; Du Chaffaut, L.; Mennen, L.; Knox, C.; Eisner, R.; Cruz, J.; Wishart, D.; et al. Phenol-Explorer: An online comprehensive database on polyphenol contents in foods. *Database (Oxford)* **2010**. [CrossRef]
8. Perez-Jiménez, J.; Neveu, V.; Vos, F.; Scalbert, A. Systematic analysis of the content of 502 polyphenols in 452 foods and beverages: An application of the phenol-explorer database. *J. Agric. Food Chem.* **2010**, *58*, 4959–4969. [CrossRef]
9. Lambert, J.D.; Sang, S.; Yang, C.S. Biotransformation of green tea polyphenols and the biological activities of those metabolites. *Mol. Pharm.* **2007**, *4*, 819–825. [CrossRef]
10. Sang, S.; Lambert, J.D.; Ho, C.T.; Yang, C.S. The chemistry and biotransformation of tea constituents. *Pharmacol. Res.* **2011**, *64*, 87–99. [CrossRef]
11. Warden, B.A.; Smith, L.S.; Beecher, G.R.; Balentine, D.A.; Clevidence, B.A. Catechins are bioavailable in men and women drinking black tea throughout the day. *J. Nutr.* **2001**, *131*, 1731–1737. [CrossRef] [PubMed]
12. Yang, C.S.; Chen, L.; Lee, M.J.; Balentine, D.; Kuo, M.C.; Schantz, S.P. Blood and urine levels of tea catechins after ingestion of different amounts of green tea by human volunteers. *Cancer Epidemiol. Biomark. Prev.* **1998**, *7*, 351–354.
13. Lee, M.J.; Maliakal, P.; Chen, L.; Meng, X.; Bondoc, F.Y.; Prabhu, S.; Lambert, G.; Mohr, S.; Yang, C.S. Pharmacokinetics of tea catechins after ingestion of green tea and (−)-epigallocatechin-3-gallate by humans: Formation of different metabolites and individual variability. *Cancer Epidemiol. Biomark. Prev.* **2002**, *11*, 1025–1032.
14. Lee, M.J.; Wang, Z.Y.; Li, H.; Chen, L.; Sun, Y.; Gobbo, S.; Balentine, D.A.; Yang, C.S. Analysis of plasma and urinary tea polyphenols in human subjects. *Cancer Epidemiol. Biomark. Prev.* **1995**, *4*, 393–399.
15. Henning, S.M.; Niu, Y.; Lee, N.H.; Thames, G.D.; Minutti, R.R.; Wang, H.; Go, V.L.W.; Heber, D. Bioavailability and antioxidant activity of tea flavanols after consumption of green tea, black tea, or a green tea extract supplement. *Am. J. Clin. Nutr.* **2004**, *80*, 1558–1564. [CrossRef] [PubMed]
16. Chow, H.H.; Cai, Y.; Alberts, D.S.; Hakim, I.; Dorr, R.; Shahi, F.; Crowell, J.A.; Yang, C.S.; Hara, Y. Phase I pharmacokinetic study of tea polyphenols following single-dose administration of epigallocatechin gallate and polyphenon E. *Cancer Epidemiol. Biomark. Prev.* **2001**, *10*, 53–58.
17. Chow, H.H.; Hakim, I.A.; Vining, D.R.; Crowell, J.A.; Ranger-Moore, J.; Chew, W.M.; Celaya, C.A.; Rodney, S.R.; Hara, Y.; Alberts, D.S. Effects of dosing condition on the oral bioavailability of green tea catechins after single-dose administration of polyphenon E in healthy individuals. *Clin. Cancer Res.* **2005**, *11*, 4627–4633. [CrossRef] [PubMed]
18. Van Amelsvoort, J.M.; Van Hof, K.H.; Mathot, J.N.J.J.; Mulder, T.P.J.; Wiersma, A.; Tijburg, L.B.M. Plasma concentrations of individual tea catechins after a single oral dose in humans. *Xenobiotica* **2001**, *31*, 891–901. [CrossRef] [PubMed]
19. Li, C.; Meng, X.; Winnik, B.; Lee, M.J.; Lu, H.; Sheng, S.; Buckley, B.; Yang, C.S. Analysis of urinary metabolites of tea catechins by liquid chromatography/electrospray ionization mass spectrometry. *Chem. Res. Toxicol.* **2001**, *14*, 702–707. [CrossRef]
20. Baba, S.; Osakabe, N.; Natsume, M.; Muto, Y.; Takizawa, T.; Terao, J. In vivo comparison of the bioavailability of (+)-catechin, (−)-epicatechin and their mixture in orally administered rats. *J. Nutr.* **2001**, *131*, 2885–2891. [CrossRef]
21. Itoh, Y.; Yasui, T.; Okada, A.; Tozawa, K.; Hayashi, Y.; Kohri, K. Preventive effects of green tea on renal stone formation and the role of oxidative stress in nephrolithiasis. *J. Urol.* **2005**, *173*, 271–275. [CrossRef] [PubMed]
22. Grases, F.; Prieto, R.M.; Gomila, I.; Sanchis, P.; Costa-Bauzá, A. Phytotherapy and renal stones: The role of antioxidants. A pilot study in Wistar rats. *Urol. Res.* **2009**, *37*, 35–40. [CrossRef] [PubMed]
23. Jeong, B.C.; Kim, B.S.; Kim, J.I.; Kim, H.H. Effects of green tea on urinary stone formation: An in vivo and in vitro study. *J. Endourol.* **2006**, *20*, 356–361. [CrossRef] [PubMed]
24. Werness, P.G.; Brown, C.M.; Smith, L.H.; Finlayson, B. EQUIL2: A BASIC computer program for the calculation of urinary saturation. *J. Urol.* **1985**, *134*, 1242–1244. [CrossRef]

25. Tiselius, H.G. Aspects on estimation of the risk of calcium oxalate crystallization in urine. *Urol. Int.* **1991**, *47*, 255–259. [CrossRef] [PubMed]
26. Daudon, M.; Bader, C.A.; Jungers, P. Urinary calculi: Review of classification methods and correlations with etiology. *Scanning Microsc.* **1993**, *7*, 1081–1104. [PubMed]
27. Shu, X.; Cai, H.; Xiang, Y.B.; Li, H.; Lipworth, L.; Miller, N.L.; Zheng, W.; Shu, X.-O.; Hsi, R. Green tea intake and risk of incident kidney stones: Prospective cohort studies in middle-aged and elderly Chinese individuals. *Int. J. Urol.* **2018**. [CrossRef]
28. Shen, C.L.; Chyu, M.C.; Cao, J.J.; Yeh, J.K. Green tea polyphenols improve bone microarchitecture in high-fat-diet-induced obese female rats through suppressing bone formation and erosion. *J. Med. Food.* **2013**, *16*, 421–427. [CrossRef]
29. Shen, C.L.; Chyu, M.C.; Wang, J.S. Tea and bone health: Steps forward in translational nutrition. *Am. J. Clin. Nutr.* **2013**, *98*, 1694S–1699S. [CrossRef]
30. Chen, Z.; Wang, C.; Zhou, H.; Sang, L.; Li, X. Modulation of calcium oxalate crystallization by commonly consumed green tea. *CrystEngComm* **2010**, *12*, 845–852. [CrossRef]
31. Daudon, M.; Doré, J.C.; Jungers, P.; Lacour, B. Changes in stone composition according to age and gender of patients: A multivariate epidemiological approach. *Urol. Res.* **2004**, *32*, 241–247. [CrossRef] [PubMed]